RECENT PROGRESS IN ANTIFUNGAL CHEMOTHERAPY

RECENT PROGRESS IN ANTIFUNGAL CHEMOTHERAPY

Edited by

Hideyo Yamaguchi

Teikyo University School of Medicine
Tokyo, Japan

George S. Kobayashi

Washington University School of Medicine
and
Barnes Hospital
St. Louis, Missouri

Hisashi Takahashi

Teikyo University
Tokyo, Japan

Marcel Dekker, Inc. **New York • Basel • Hong Kong**

Library of Congress Cataloging-in-Publication Data

Recent progress in antifungal chemotherapy / edited by Hideyo Yamaguchi, George S. Kobayashi, and Hisashi Takahashi.
p. cm.
Proceedings of the First International Conference on Antifungal Chemotherapy held in Oiso, Japan, Sept, 24-26, 1990.
Includes bibliographical references and indexes.
ISBN 0-8247-8529-0
1. Antifungal agents--Congresses. 2. Mycoses--Chemotherapy--Congresses. I. Yamaguchi, Hideyo. II. Kobayashi, George S. III. Takahashi, Hisashi.
IV. International Conference on Antifungal Chemotherapy (1st: 1990: Oiso-machi, Japan)
[DNLM: Antifungal Agents--therapeutic use--congresses.
2. Mycoses--drug therapy--congresses. QV 252 R295 1990]
RM410.R43 1991
616.9'69061--dc20
DNLM/DLC
for Library of Congress 91-34283
CIP

This book is printed on acid-free paper.

MARCEL DEKKER, INC.
270 Madison Avenue, New York, New York 10016

Current printing (last digit):
10 9 8 7 6 5 4 3 2 1

PRINTED IN THE UNITED STATES OF AMERICA

Preface

During the last few decades, the incidence of fungal infections has increased remarkably. In particular, life-threatening systemic infections caused by *Candida* spp., *Aspergillus fumigatus, Cryptococcus neoformans* and other opportunistic or pathogenic fungi are now becoming a major threat to many hospitalized patients, especially those compromised by severe underlying diseases such as leukemia, acquired immunodeficiency syndrome (AIDS) and bone marrow transplants, and who are often further compromised by intensive antineoplasmic chemotherapy or the administration of immunosuppressive drugs and/or broad-spectrum antibacterial antibiotics. Moreover, severe endemic fungal infections - coccidioidomycosis, histoplasmosis and chromomycosis - create increasing problems for clinicians working with certain populations of patients in the more rapidly growing regions of the world.

In addition to these deep-seated fungal infections, there is a larger population in the world who suffer from superficial forms of fungal diseases (*e.g.*, dermatomycoses and oral candidiasis). Although these mycoses are not life-threatening *per se*, they are prone to recur and often take months or years to treat. There can therefore be no doubt that the development of new active substances as well as newer strategies for antifungal chemotherapy represents a challenging objective.

It was against this background that the First International Conference on Antifungal Chemotherapy (ICAFC '90) was held in Oiso, Japan. This conference was a multi-disciplinary forum for review and evaluation of the rapidly progressing and expanding knowledge in the field of antifungal chemotherapy. Included were sections of clinical, preclinical and investigational aspects of varying classes of old and new antifungal drugs for systemic and/or topical use, along with the current development of drug delivery systems applicable to this scientific field and of immunomodulatory agents as adjunctive therapy. Some papers presented were rather comprehensive dealing with historical perspectives and future prospects of antifungal drugs of major chemical classes and/or with certain important biological activities. Others were dedicated to specific antifungal drugs (or drug classes) and drug formulations or usages, as well as promising biological response modifiers or cytokines for antifungal therapy. These papers were presented by scientists representing the forefront of this vital and contemporary field of research, *i.e.*, antifungal chemotherapy, in the world.

This volume of the Proceedings of ICAFC '90 provides the reader with the material covered by the invited speakers and, in briefer form, the work presented in poster sessions. It represents where we are in this field today - our current knowledge and much that we still want to know. For those of us intimately involved with the progress of this scientific area, the future needs and awaits the help that we, as scientists and doctors, can offer to those suffering from fungal diseases.

As Chairman or members of the Organizing Committee and the Editors of this volume, we would like to thank the publisher, Marcel Dekker, Inc., and extend special thanks to Jane Clarkin, the Secretary of these Proceedings, who has helped nurture and guide this production to a successful conclusion. We would also like to express our gratitude to sponsors and co-sponsors for their help in organizing the conference and to the many companies and Teikyo University for their generous financial support.

Hideyo Yamaguchi
George S. Kobayashi
Hisashi Takahashi

Contents

PART IX: APPENDIX: POSTER PRESENTATIONS

1

Recent Trends in HIV Infection in Japan

Soroku Yamagata, M.D., Ph.D.

Executive Director
Japanese Foundation for AIDS Prevention
Nakano-Kudan-Minami Building 4F
3-4-14, Kudan-Minami, Chiyoda-ku, Tokyo 102, Japan

The subject of my talk (which I must say in advance will be non-scientific) will be the recent trend of HIV (human immunodeficiency virus) infection in Japan. I wish to tell you of measures carried out by the government through its Ministry of Health and Welfare in coping with the AIDS problem since the disease was discovered in Japan, and also something of the campaign carried out by the Japanese Foundation for AIDS Prevention.

Following the first reported death of an AIDS patient in Japan in July 1983, the next recognized case was a homosexual male in March 1985, followed in January 1987 by a report that an unmarried female in the city of Kobe was the first of her sex in this country. Thus, the AIDS 'whirlwind' began in this country.

The Japanese government immediately held a cabinet meeting of the ministers concerned and drew up an outline of overall measures to be taken on the AIDS problem:

..Dissemination of correct knowledge and information on AIDS

..Identification and understanding of the sources of infection

..Improvement in the system of consultation and guidance to those worried about the disease in order to prevent secondary infections

..Since it is an international problem, cooperate internationally through joint research and other means

..Consider the legislative measures to be taken to clarify the social rules, since the human rights of the individual are involved

The following system of AIDS prevention was established on February 17, 1989: (1) The state and local authorities were asked to take responsibility for the dissemination of correct facts on AIDS, and at the same time the public and physicians were expected to take the responsibility of assuring they have accurate knowledge; (2) To learn the extent of the infection and by what route it is increasing, this law requires that the state, with the cooperation of 2,000 medical institutions throughout the country ask all physicians to voluntarily report when a diagnosis is made of an HIV-infected person (surveillance). The purpose of this is to determine the epidemiological situation by infection source on the extent of the infection; (3) The physician is to report to the prefectural governor items such as sex, age, infection source and clinical symptoms of the infected individual, but the name, place of residence and other personal facts are not required; (4) Although it is thought that most HIV-infected persons will obey the physician's instructions, for those who do not or if there is danger of others becoming infected, the physician is to report this and, in this case, the name of the infected individual to the prefectural governor; (5) The law also states that physicians and public officials who, for no justifiable reason, disclose the fact that someone suffers from this disease which they have learned during the course of their work shall be punished.

Table 1 shows the number of AIDS patients in Japan as of June 1990. The total number is 285, 21 of those foreigners. By risk groups the number of incidences due to medical use of blood products is highest with 72% of the total. Next is the male homosexual group

TABLE 1

NUMBER OF AIDS PATIENTS IN JAPAN

	Male	Female	Total
Heterosexual contact	14 (4)*	7 (2)	21 (6)
Male homosexual	39 (12)		39 (12)
Medical use of blood products**			207 (0)
Others/unknown	15+ (3)	3	18 (3)
Total	(19)	(2)	285 (21)

* Figures in parentheses denote cases among foreigners
** Report as of the end of June 1990 by the Research Committee on Prevention of Developing Illnesses and Therapy for HIV Infected Patients. Since enforcement of the AIDS Control Law on Feb. 17, 1990, cases presumed to be caused by the medical use of blood have been excluded.
\+ Includes male bisexual cases

at 14%; the heterosexual contact group accounts for 7% and 'other/unknown' for 6%.

HIV-infected persons in Japan as of June 1990 totalled 1,406 (Table 2). The highest risk group for this condition too is medical users of blood products: 1,209 or 86%. Second is the male homosexual group, and third is the heterosexual contact group, both accounting

TABLE 2

NUMBER OF HIV-INFECTED PERSONS IN JAPAN

	Male	Female	Total
Heterosexual contact	42	37	79
Male homosexual	86		86
Medical use of blood products*			1,209
Others/unknown	13	18	32**
Total			1,406

* Report as of end of June 1990 by the Research Committee on Prevention of Developing Illnesses and Therapy for HIV-Infected Patients. As in Table 1, since enforcement of the AIDS Control Law on Feb. 17, 1989, cases presumed to be caused by the medical use of blood products have been excluded.
**One case of unknown sex is included.

for 6%. We are now carefully watching the gradual increase in the heterosexual contact group.

The Ministry of Health and Welfare has been providing various benefits to patients infected by HIV through the use of blood products, in accordance with the Relief System for Sufferers from Adverse Drug Reactions, and also for families of AIDS patients who died due to treatment of hemophilia with blood products. Briefly, the benefits are: a medical care allowance, special allowances to those age 18 or over and to those under 18, consolation compensation (to family members) and funds for funeral expenses.

Although there are researchers surveying the situation of the gay community in Japan, we do not presently know its actual state. I believe personally that this community here is not as strongly organized as in some other countries, although recently the AIDS campaign carried out by the Tokyo Metropolitan Government has had the cooperation of certain groups of the gay community in Tokyo.

Our Japanese Foundation for AIDS Prevention puts its greatest emphasis on disseminating facts about the disease, thus hopefully countering some of the incorrect and fearful rumors which apparently abound elsewhere. First, the government and our Foundation sponsor a World AIDS Day memorial symposium in Tokyo once a year, where key lectures are given by specialists in this disease and followed by panel discussions. Last year in 1989, the theme was "AIDS and Youth" and panelists from various areas participated.

Then, in rural areas where the number of AIDS cases and HIV-infected persons is small, general symposia on HIV/AIDS are held targeting the health and medical personnel and those engaged in education. Mobilizers are usually the prefectural government, the Board of Education and the medical association.

In densely populated cities where there is a comparatively large number of patients and infected persons. symposia are offered on AIDS treatment, practical aspects of counselling and what type of AIDS education should be offered young people. In these areas the targets and mobilization are handled similarly to the rural areas.

Japan has 47 prefectures and 850 health centers, and the medical institutions in various parts of the country are cooperating with these health centers and local governments. Initial consultation on the disease generally takes place by telephone and then a system is established with the individual to conduct screening and confirmation tests and whatever else proves to be necessary.

The Ministry of Health and Welfare commissioned our Foundation with trust money to carry out and expand these counselling activities utilizing the result of the meetings of the Research Committee on Prevention of Developing Illness and Therapy for HIV-Infected Patients. There are 750 medical doctors in this research group representing 15 institutions who are cooperating in the 9 areas in Japan. Counselling is done by telephone and personal interview by a staff composed mainly of medical doctors and nurses. Recently there has been an increase in the number of institutions with clinical psychologists and social workers also. Research and training courses are held in each area, and our Foundatior has begun holding training courses for AIDS counsellors.

We have undertaken various public relations activities in regard to the preparation of posters to be shown to the general public, although our experience in this area is limited.

Photo 1 shows the first poster we designed and printed at the time of the 1988 AIDS campaign. In discussing the photo with the person who was to create it, I strongly emphasized the following two points: Sex was to be expressed "beautifully", and careful consideration was to be given to the selection of the models. Also, as the first step in making Japanese aware of the condom, the letter 'O' of "Love is forever" was designed to look like a condom. The Japanese slogan translates: Protect your loved one from exposure to HIV.

Many comments regarding this poster made by the Japanese public had to do with (1) association with the AIDS campaign was not clear, and (2) that unless there were instructions, one could not understand how the condom could be used to prevent AIDS. A sarcastic newspaper reporter commented that he had a feeling of repulsion at the imperious nature of the slogan. He said since it stated

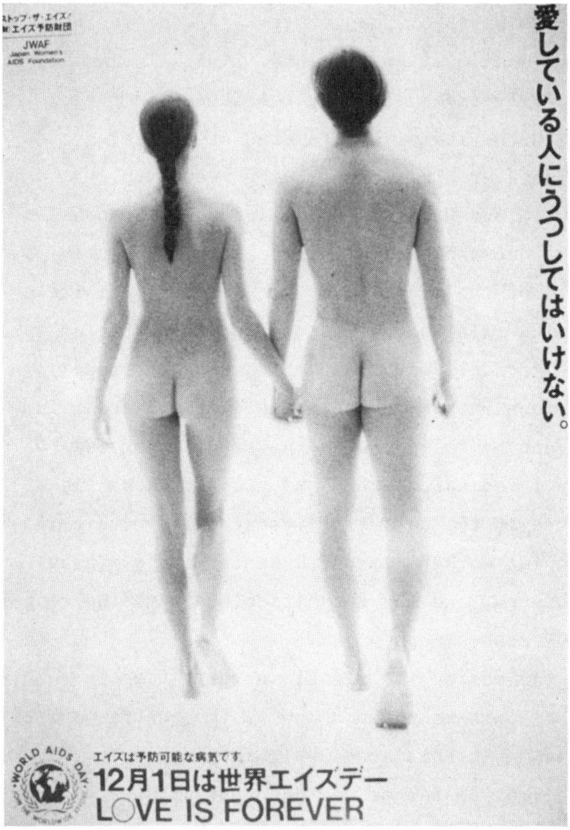

Photo 1 The caption in Japanese reads "Protect your loved one from exposure to HIV. AIDS is a disease that can be prevented!"

"Protect <u>your</u> loved one from exposure to HIV," then this could mean that it is okay for one you do not love to be exposed to this virus.

Foreigners wondered why non-Japanese models were used when the poster was in Japanese and intended for use in Japan. I agreed and redressed the individual responsible. He replied that of the many candidates the style of these two models was conspicuously good, that the mother of the male model was Japanese and so he selected them without discussing it with me or obtaining my approval.

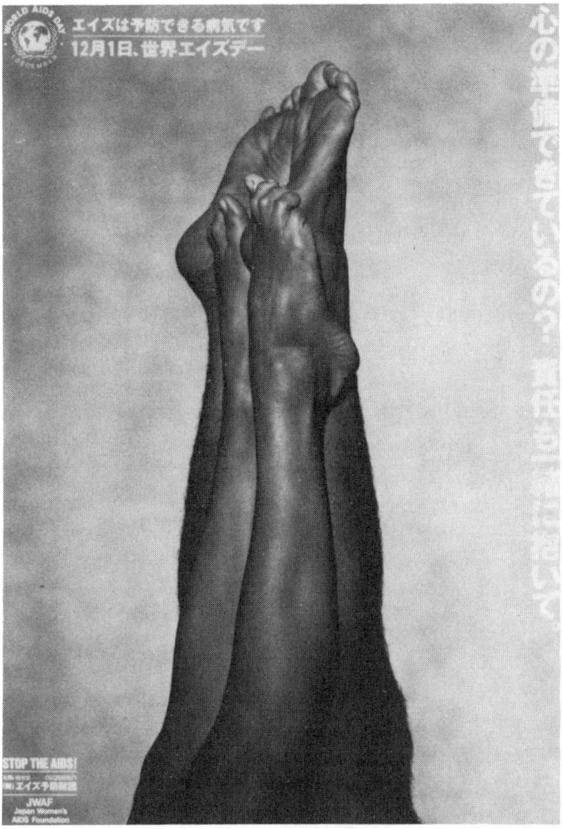

Photo 2 The caption in Japanese reads "Are you prepared to take the risk? You will take the responsibility for the risk to your partner! AIDS is a disease that can be prevented!"

From these experiences I clearly realized the many difficulties involved in the design and printing of posters of this nature.

Photo 2 is the second poster released at the time of the 1989 AIDS campaign and was based on the idea of synchronized swimming. The idea was good but the photograph itself not of good quality. The meaning of the slogan in Japanese is shown beside it. We received many favorable comments on this poster. However, as WHO's slogan for 1989 was "AIDS and Youth," our poster was considered by the principals of high schools and other schools as too explicit. Therefore, we quickly had to prepare another one.

In Photo 3 two teenagers are openly discussing AIDS. Standing at right is the mother of one of them and at left the teacher, both watching apprehensively. The Japanese wording: "They say they know about AIDS, but do they <u>really</u> know?" was readily accepted by schools and was well received nationwide.

Recently I had the opportunity to visit a friend at the University of Hawaii. When I saw this poster (Photo 4) on the wall of her

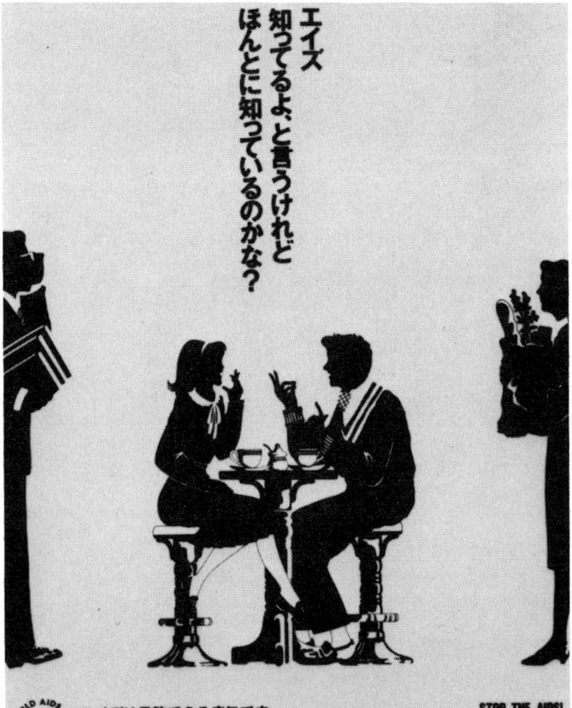
エイズ
知ってるよ、と言うけれど
ほんとに知っているのかな?
WORLD AIDS DAY
DECEMBER
エイズは予防できる病気です
12月1日、世界エイズデー
STOP THE AIDS!
(財)エイズ予防財団

Photo 3 The caption in Japanese reads "They say that they know about AIDS—but do they <u>really</u> know? AIDS is a disease that can be prevented!"

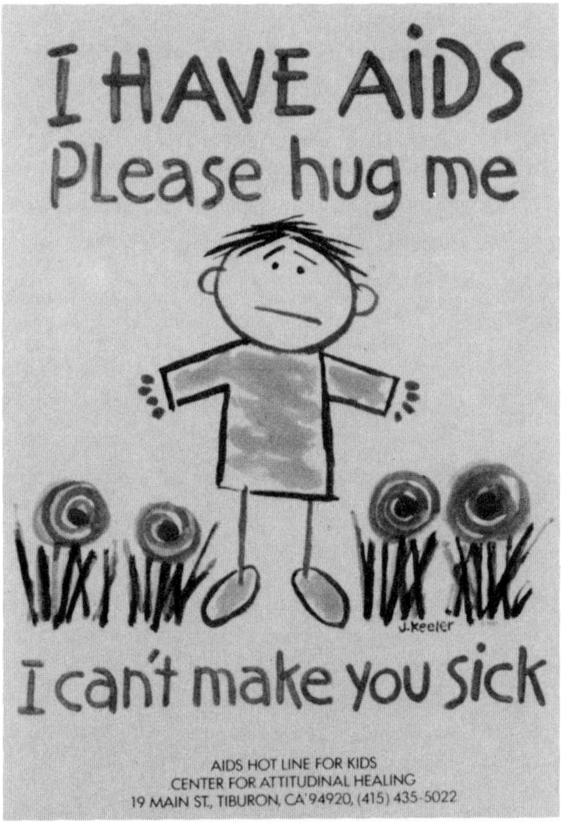
I HAVE AIDS
Please hug me
J.Keeler
I can't make you sick
AIDS HOT LINE FOR KIDS
CENTER FOR ATTITUDINAL HEALING
19 MAIN ST., TIBURON, CA 94920, (415) 435-5022

Photo 4

room, I was quite impressed. WHO's 1990 slogan is "AIDS and Women"; using my friend's poster as a basis, I am now preparing one for this year's World AIDS Day in Japan which will be strongly appealing and, I hope, easily accepted by everyone.

As I said, the posters our Foundation prepared were recognized as being vague in expression, perhaps because of their content which was directed at the emotional as opposed to the intellectual level of the Japanese public; we should have expressed the message in a more straightforward manner.

Our Foundation hopes to narrow down those whom we perceive to be the "target group" in society, i.e., those who are most at risk from HIV, and to address them directly with an awareness campaign which is pertinent both to their special needs and to the general needs of the Japanese public. To achieve this, we hope to conduct concentrated publicity through more diverse media than have previously been utilized, and to set up a system of survey and research to determine the effectiveness of this activity as well as of our AIDS information program in general.

I wish to take this opportunity to request of you, my colleagues, the following: Since it will hereafter be essential that publicity activity be conducted in harmony among various countries, I hope to see concrete measures taken for the exchange of information concerning what is being done in the target communities within each country, and to seek international cooperation regarding information campaigns and other such publicity that will have the impact we need to arrest and eventually stamp out this deadly disease of AIDS.

Thank you.

2

Fungal Cell Envelope and Mode of Action of Antimycotic Drugs

Vassil St. Georgiev

Orion Research & Technologies Corporation
P.O. Box 463, Tampa, Florida 33601-0463

Over the past 25 years, the incidence of invasive fungal infections in man has risen dramatically [1]. Patients who become severely immunocompromised because of underlying diseases such as leukemia or, more recently, acquired immune deficiency syndrome, or patients who undergo cancer chemotherapy or organ transplantation, are particularly susceptible to opportunistic fungal infections. Although Candida species continue to be the major pathogenic fungi in these patients, cryptococcosis, aspergillosis, and coccidioidomycosis, among others, have become increasingly important [2].

Antifungal drugs currently being used in clinic include polyene antibiotics, azole derivatives and 5-fluorocytosine. With the exception of the latter, all other drugs possess mechanisms of action aimed at disrupting the integrity of the fungal cell membrane by either interfering with the biosynthesis of membrane sterols or inhibiting sterol functions [3].

The fungal cell envelope consists of cell wall and cell membrane. The cell wall which is essential for the survival of the fungus is not present in mammalian cells. It determines the cell shape and confers rigidity and strength to the cell. In addition, it serves as permeability barrier for large molecules because of its limited porosity. The cell wall represents a multilayer structure composed largely of carbohydrates (glucan, chitin and mannoproteins). According to Zlotnik et al. [4], the mannoproteins form a surface layer which penetrates the wall to some depth and shields the glucans from attack by Z-glucanase. Some mannan-containing exoenzymes may be concentrated in the periplasmic space next to the plasmalema [5,6]. Fungal mannoproteins consist of branched mannose polymers attached to the protein through an N-acetylglucosamine - N-acetylglucosamine group. All linkages are alpha, with the exception of those between the two N-acetylglucosamine residues and between the mannose and N-acetylglucosamine, which are beta [7].

Structurally, glucans represent mixtures of branched beta-1,3- and beta-1,6-linked glucose polymers [8]. Glucans are synthesized on the cytoplasmic surface of the plasma membrane, then extruded and deposited on the outer surface of the cell wall as microfibrils which subsequently aggregate to form crystalline structures [3,8]. It has also been suggested that a predominantly beta-(1,6)glucan layer is deposited near the cell surface where it may serve as a barrier protecting the beta-(1,3)glucan. Such deposition was suggested because of the need to remove the beta-(1,6)glucan from intact cells prior to solubilization of beta-(1,3)glucan [8]. Stimulation of glucan biosynthesis by nucleotides that may be involved in the regulation of glucan synthetase in vivo, was investigated in detail by Shematek and Cabib [9], and some structural requirements for an activator of this enzyme and hypothetical sites of interaction with it, have emerged [10]. Guanosine triphosphate (GTP) was found to be the most potent activator of glucan synthetase having an $S_{0.5}$ (concentration for half-maximal stimulation) value of 0.2 μM. By comparison, the corresponding $S_{0.5}$ value for ATP is approximately 100-fold higher [9]. In addition to nucleoside triphosphates, there are other effective stimulants of glucan synthetase - although at higher concentrations, guanosine diphosphate, some inorganic pyrophosphates and higher polyphosphates, have stimulated the enzyme [10]. An array of structural requirements for stimulating enzyme activity have been determined [10]. For example, conversion of the terminal phosphate group of nucleoside triphosphates to methyl ester, or attaching it to another nucleoside molecule reduced the potency by competitively inhibiting the stimulatory effect. Other findings suggested that either glucan synthetase itself or a regulatory subunit of the enzyme may possess, in addition to an activation site that interacts with the terminal phosphate group, also a binding site for the nucleoside residue of the stimulatory molecule [8,10]. Other structural analogues of ATP and GTP which have imino or methylene groups in place of the α,β- or β,γ-oxygen have also demonstrated enzyme-activating properties with $S_{0.5}$ values similar to those of the parent nucleosides. Compounds having a sulfur atom attached to the terminal phosphate group were also found to be active [10]. When used in the same experiment, adenosine-β,γ-imino-triphosphate and guanosine-β,γ-imino-triphosphate did not show any additive effect suggesting interaction with the same domain on the enzyme [10].

A tentative structure of yeast cell wall is depicted in Figure 1.

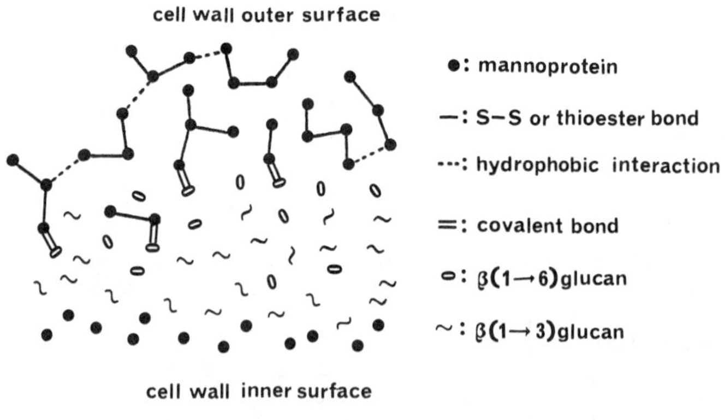

Figure 1. Tentative structure of yeast cell wall (From Refs. 4 and 8).

Chitin, the third major polysaccharide of the fungal cell wall consists predominantly of unbranched chains of β-(1→4)-2-acetamido-2-deoxy-D-glucose, also known as N-acetyl-D-glucosamine (GlcNAc) [8]. Similarly to glucan, chitin is synthesized at the cytoplasmic surface of the plasma membrane and then extruded and deposited on the outer surface [3]. More than 90% of chitin in a normal yeast wall is found in the region of the bud scars in the form of an annulus with an external thinner rim and a thin central plate [8]. The remainder of chitin is dispersed over the whole cell wall [11,12]. Experiments by Duran et al. [13] have provided evidence that chitin synthetase, the enzyme catalyzing the formation of the polysaccharide, is also exclusively located in the plasma membrane.

The second major structural component of the fungal envelope is the cell membrane. It represents a barrier between the cytoplasm and the environment and regulating the transport of molecules in and out of the cell [3]. One important feature of the cell membrane is to serve as a matrix for the membrane-bound enzymes such as glucan- and chitin synthetases. Structurally, the cell membrane is a lipid bilayer with phosphatidyl choline, phosphatidyl ethanolamine and ergosterol (or in certain cases, zymosterol) being its major lipids. Kaneko et al. [14] have studied the lipid composition of 30 different species of yeasts and found that the greater part of them contained 7-15% total lipids and 3-6% total phospholipids per dry cell weight. Qualitatively, all of the yeast membranes studied had similar neutral lipid constituents (triglycerides, sterol esters, free fatty acids and free sterols) and polar lipid components (phosphatidyl choline, phosphatidyl ethanolamine, phosphatidyl serine, phosphatidyl inositol, cardiolipin and ceramide monohexoside); minor constituents were nearly absent [14]. Marriott [15] reported a significant difference in the contents of plasma membranes from the yeast and mycelial forms of C. albicans with the latter form being richer in carbohydrates; marked differences were also observed between the phospholipids, free and esterified sterols and total fatty acids from the two forms of C. albicans.

As we have mentioned earlier, the integrity of the fungal cell membrane may be compromised in two ways: (a) by inhibition of sterol biosynthesis, and (b) by interrupting the proper interaction between membrane sterols and membrane phospholipids.

Polyene antibiotics are fungal metabolites isolated from various Streptomyces sp. Macrolides by chemical nature, they possess a large lactone ring (containing between three and seven conjugated double bonds) with a sugar residue (most often mycosamine but also perosamine) attached to it by a glycosidic bond [16,17]. Certain members of the heptaene subgroup (candicidin, ascosin, hamycin) contain an aromatic amine side chain (such as p-aminoacetophenone) which is alkali-sensitive; in other heptaene antibiotics such as candimycin, the aromatic side chain is N-methylated [17]. The conjugated polyene region of the lactone ring confers both rigidity and lipophilicity to the molecule, while the hydroxyl-containing region is conformationally flexible and hydrophilic. In general, the presence of sugar residue imparts basicity on the polyene molecule. It should be noted, however, that because of the presence of an equal number of basic (hexosamine or aromatic side chain) and acidic (carboxyl) groups, some of the polyene antibiotics (amphotericin B, nystatin, candicidin) are amphoteric by nature. Other polyenes (filipin, fungichromin) contain no ionizable functions at all, and are therefore, nonpolar.

The mechanism of action of polyene antibiotics is related to their ability to bind to membrane sterols resulting in the formation of transmembrane pores which disrupt the structural integrity of the cell membrane as seen by its increased permeability, the leakage of cytoplasmic contents such as potassium cations, and ultimately cell death [17-19]. It is important to understand that the polyenes may interact with both fungal (ergosterol) and mammalian (cholesterol) sterols; however, at least in the case of clinically useful antibiotics (amphotericin B, nystatin) the affinity towards the fungal ergosterol is higher [20,21]. It has been reported that both amphotericin B and nystatin did not affect the lipid biosynthesis in vivo at concentrations as high as 0.1 μM [3].

A partial model explaining the formation of amphotericin B-cholesterol transmembrane pores has been suggested by Andreoli [18] (Figure 2). The dotted lines between the phospholipid hydrocarbon chains indicate London-van der Waals forces which stabilize, at least partially, the aliphatic residues of the phospholipids and assure their parallel alignment within the hydrophobic core of the bilayer. One fundamental functional property of membrane sterols is to interact with membrane phospholipids. By doing so, sterols are able to either increase the order and rigidity of relatively fluid phospholipid bilayers [22-24], or to increase the fluidity and permeability of tightly organized condensed phospholipid bilayers [24-26], thus regulating the dissipative permeability of the membrane and controlling the phase transition from condensed, gel-like crystalline arrays into fluid, liquid crystal structures [18]. During such transition from crystalline to "melted" fluid state [27-30], the mobility and ordering of the hydrocarbon chains in the membrane interior would be, respectively, increased and decreased [18]. In general, organized crystalline bilayer membranes are less permeable to water and solutes as compared to more fluid liquid crystal membranes [31-35]. The increased permeability of the more "fluid" bilayer membranes towards water and solutes is thought to be the result of molecular cavities or defects in the ordering of the hydrocarbon region of the membranes [36,37] caused, for example, by greater water content in the lipid lamellae [38] and shortening, branching or unsaturation of phospholipid hydrocarbon residues [31-33]. In the context of the sterol-phospholipid interaction, the polyene will act as a "counterfeit" phospholipid. The polyene molecule will position itself in such a manner that its C_{15} hydroxyl, C_{16} carboxyl and C_{19} mycosamine amino groups will be situated at the membrane-water interface, while the C_1-C_{14} and C_{20}-C_{33} regions will be parallel to each other and within the membrane interior. Because of its hydrophobic nature, the C_{20}-C_{33} heptaene chain will also align itself along the cholesterol molecule in a hydrophobic environment, whereas the hydroxyl groups of the C_1-C_{14} moiety will face the aqueous interface and align along the inner side of the pore. The overall result of such arrangement will be an increased fluidity and hydration of the pore interior approaching that of bulk water. As demonstrated by light microscopy, the formation of polyene-sterol pores will cause significant morphological changes in the fungal cell - marked granularity, loss of organelle definition and ultimately cell death [18].

Since the total lenght of the polyene-sterol complex approximates the lenght of the fatty acid and glycerol moieties of the phospholipid molecule, the complex will be sufficient to form only a "half pore" through the lipid bilayer. A conducting "full lenght" pore would need two "half pores" to join

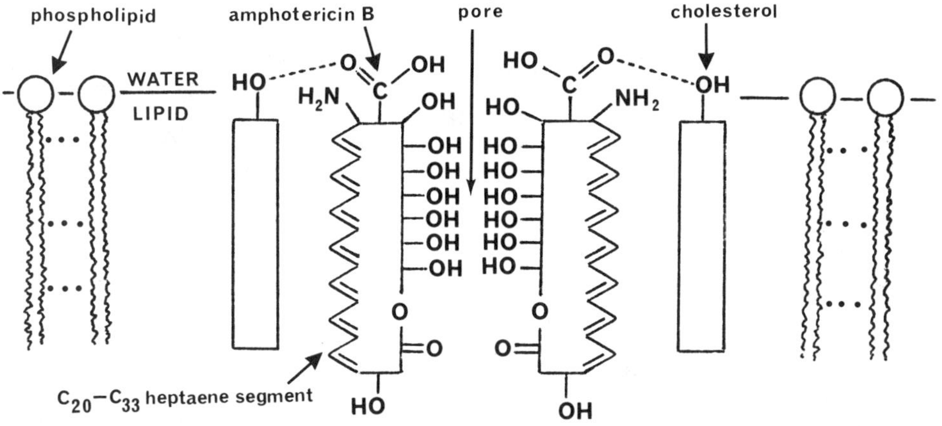

Figure 2. Partial model for amphotericin B-cholesterol pores (From Ref. 18).

together [17]. Half pores may float independently in the lipid environment; usually, a full pore would require between 5 and 10 antibiotic molecules [39, 40]. It has been found that the diameter of each pore approximates that of a glucose molecule [39-41]. Furthermore, only intact polyene molecules may participate in the construction of pore models since either hydrolysis of the lactone ring of the antibiotic or saturation of its chromophore would make pore formation theoretically impossible - experimentally, no pore formation by such modified polyene molecules has ever been demonstrated either [40].

The structure of nystatin, another clinically useful polyene antibiotic, differs from that of amphotericin B in that its conjugated double bond system is interrupted by saturation leaving two separate tetraene and diene chromophores. Such double bond arrangement should allow the bending of an otherwise rigid conformation. A structure similar to the amphotericin B-cholesterol pore model was suggested for the nystatin-sterol complex in lipid membrane bilayers [40,42,43]. Since the permeability characteristics of nystatin-sterol pores closely match that of an amphotericin B-sterol pore, it has been possible to form mixed pores when nystatin was added to one side of the lipid bilayer and amphotericin B to the other [44].

Contrary to both amphotericin B and nystatin, the pentaene antibiotic filipin possesses no ionizable groups or a sugar residue and is therefore nonpolar. Filipin contains a hydrophobic alkyl side chain adjacent to the hydrophilic hydroxylated portion of the molecule. These structural elements should make it possible for the construction of a filipin-sterol complex that may be oriented parallel to the plane of the lipid bilayer, which is a radical change from the perpendicular arrangement characteristic for the amphotericin B-cholesterol complex. Moreover, several of these parralel structures may further join together to form aggregates. One of the sides of such aggregate will become hydrophobic by the presence of the pentaene chromophore, while the opposite side will be hydrophilic due to the polyol surface [18]. Two of these planar aggregates may then combine to create a "sandwich"-like structure which would have its hydrophilic regions facing each other towards the center, whereas the hydrophobic regions will be situated on the outside surface of the "sandwich" and in a position to interact with the membrane sterols. Although such filipin-sterol complexes will bear no resemblance to amphotericin B-cholesterol pores, they still should be able to disrupt the integrity of the lipid membrane structure by effectively removing sterols from the environment thus preventing sterol-phospholipid interaction [45-47]. Similarly to amphotericin B-sterol complexing, the filipin-sterol interaction is hydrophobic by nature [46,47]. It has also been observed that lysis of lipid bilayers by filipin-sterol complexes was much faster and with no prior formation of pores [48].

Experimental evidence have revealed that the major effect taking place immediately following treatment with polyene antibiotics is the leakage of potassium cations. In order to replace their loss, a transfer of H^+ from the environment will occur [49]. The ensuing inflow of protons will cause acidification of the fungal cytoplasm - for example, the pH of the cell cytoplasm of C. albicans treated with a lethal dose of candicidin fell from 6.12 to 5.20 [49]. Such drastic change in the cytoplasmic pH value would lead, in

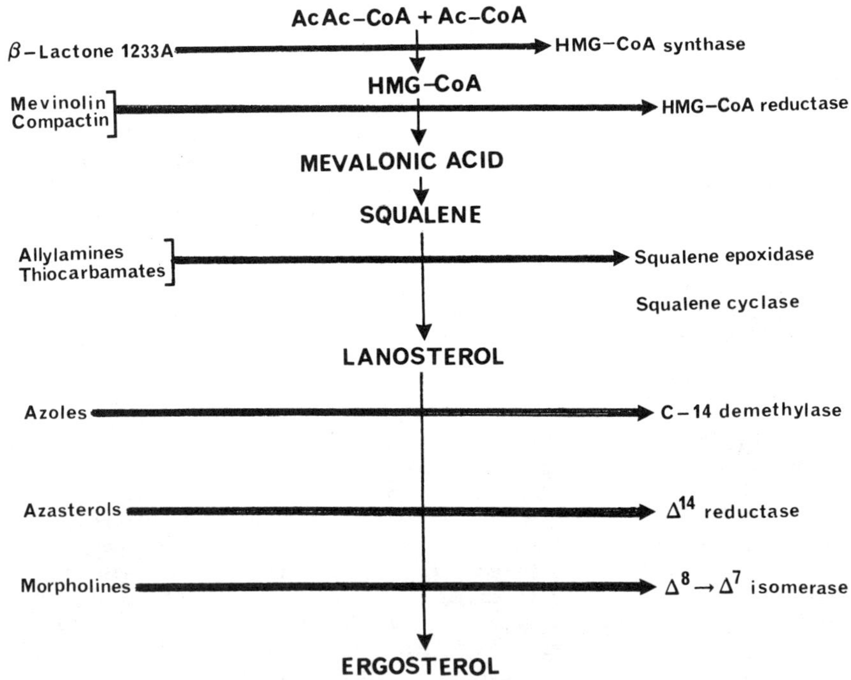

Figure 3. Biosynthesis of ergosterol showing the potential sites of its inhibition by antifungal agents (From Ref. 3).

turn, to an increase in the optical density and precipitation of cytoplasmic components [50].

The second major mode of action by which drugs exert antifungal activity is through inhibition of sterol biosynthesis. Any impairment of the biosynthesis of membrane sterols will slow down the normal fungal growth without however, causing cell lysis. Ergosterol is the major sterol component of the fungal cell membrane. Similarly to mammalian cholesterol, ergosterol plays an important role in controlling membrane fluidity and integrity (a nonspecific function), as well as specifically regulating cell growth and proliferation [51-54]. While the nonspecific function requires large ("bulk") quantities of ergosterol, its specific control of membrane-associated processes should require only minute ("sparking") amounts of the sterol [3]. In general, antifungal agents which substantially (but not completely) inhibit the ergosterol biosynthesis are likely to affect its nonspecific function thereby suppressing the fungal growth [3].

The biosynthesis of ergosterol may be divided into four distinct stages: (a) formation of mevalonic acid; (b) polymerization of mevalonic acid into squalene; (c) cyclization to lanosterol; and (d) modification of lanosterol leading to ergosterol. Enzymes that control the first stage are mitochondrial, while those of the second stage are mainly cytosolic; the enzymes involved in the third and fourth stages are microsomal [3,55]. All four stages of the ergosterol biosynthesis may serve as potential targets for antifungal drugs (Figure 3).

3-Hydroxy-3-methylglutaryl CoA synthase (HMG-CoA synthase) is the enzyme which activates the condensation of acetoacetyl-CoA (1) with acetyl-CoA (2) to generate 3-hydroxy-3-methylglutaryl CoA (HMG-CoA) (3). Subsequent reduction of the carbonyl group of HMG-CoA produces mevalonic acid (4). The reduction is catalyzed by HMG-CoA reductase and similarly to the cholesterol biosynthesis, it represents the rate-limiting step of the biosynthesis of ergosterol [56-58].

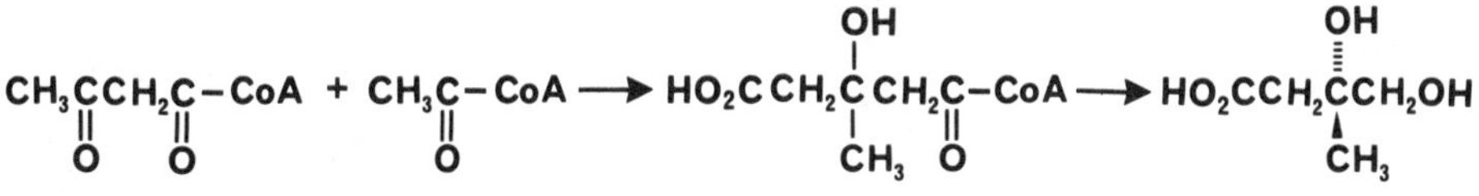

1 2 3 4

Sesquiterpenes such as mevinolin and compactin have been shown to suppress in a specific manner the activity of HMG-CoA reductase [59]. The inhibition was reversible and competitive with respect to HMG-CoA [60,61]. The latter finding comes as no surprise because of the existing structural similarity between the acid form of sesquiterpenes and HMG-CoA; experiments by Endo [62] have shown that the affinity of HMG-CoA reductase for compactin is 10,000-fold higher than its affinity for the natural substrate HMG-CoA. Structure-activity relationship studies have indicated that the lactone ring of the sesquiterpenes is critical for activity; for example, the 5'-phosphonocompactin acid showed only 1/10 of the potency of compactin [62]. So far, the enzyme-inhibiting activity of sesquiterpenes has been of little clinical value due to their poor permeability into fungal cells [3].

The lactone antibiotic 1233A was demonstrated to exert a potent and specific inhibition of HMG-CoA synthase without affecting acetoacetyl-CoA thio-

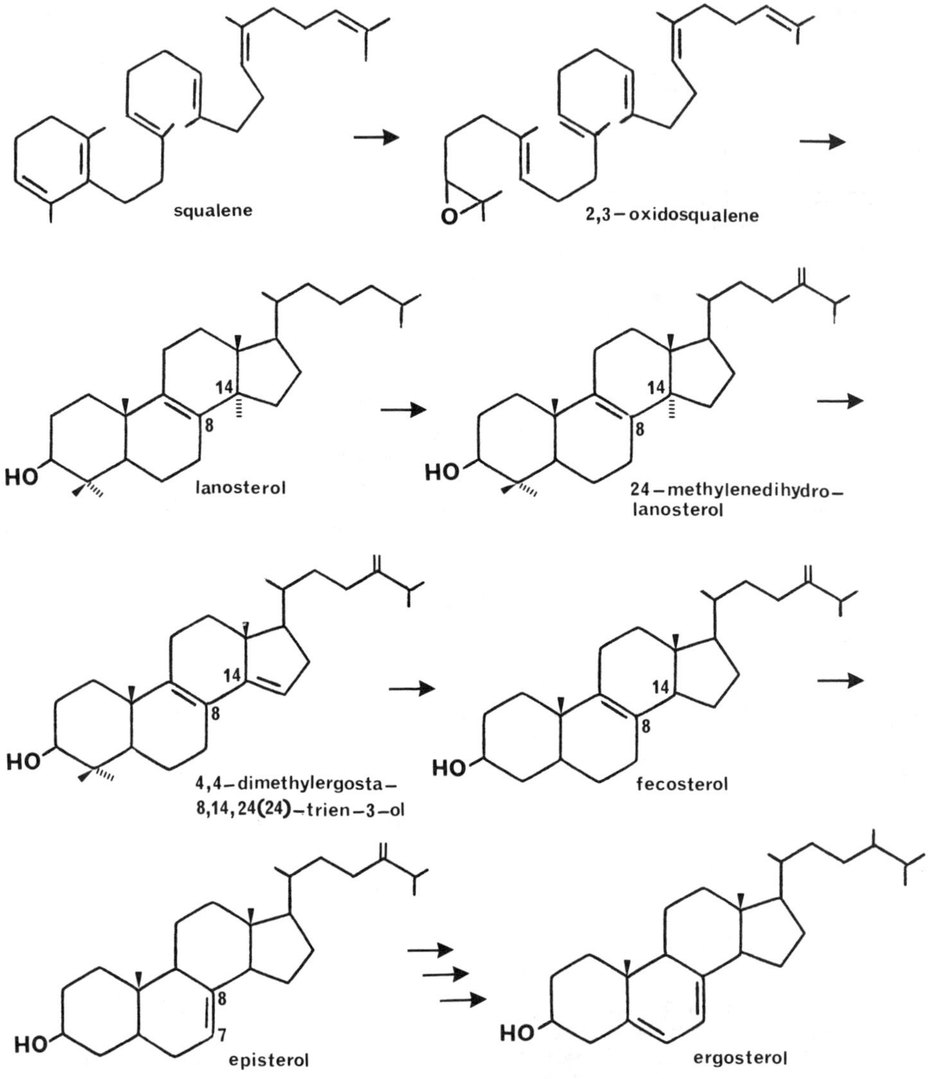

Figure 4. Biosynthetic conversion of squalene to ergosterol.

lase or HMG-CoA reductase [63]. As with the case of sesquiterpenes, the poor permeability of lactone 1233A into fungal cells significantly curtails its therapeutic effect and precludes clinical application [3].

The formation of squalene - the second stage of ergosterol biosynthesis, is carried out by tail-to-tail condensation of two farnesyl pyrophosphate molecules [64-66] with squalene synthase serving as the catalyst [67]. The oxidation of squalene to 2,3-oxidosqualene utilizes molecular oxygen with the help of squalene epoxidase. 2,3-Oxidosqualene, in turn, is cyclized to lanosterol; the enzyme involved in this conversion, squalene cyclase [67-69] showed optimal activity at low ionic strength [70]. Between the two enzymes which control the formation of lanosterol, squalene epoxidase and squalene cyclase, inhibition of squalene epoxidase is more preferable since accumulation of 2,3-oxidosqualene would be more damaging to host cells than accumulation of squalene [3,71]. A number of allylamine (terbinafine, naftifine) and thiocarbamate (tolnaftate, tolciclate) derivatives were found to elicit antifungal activity by suppressing the activity of squalene epoxidase [72-75]. The IC_{50} values (that is, the concentration at which the sterol-to-squalene ratio is decreased to 50% of control) may range from less than 1 μM for terbinafine to 100 μM for tolnaftate [3]. In addition, allylamines also reduced the unsaturated-to-saturated fatty acid ratio and caused a shift from C_{18} to C_{16} fatty acids in vivo [3].

The conversion of lanosterol to ergosterol is rather complex and may involve the synthesis of as many as 13 sterols as either end products or potential biosynthetic intermediates with lanosterol being the key precursor [76-79] (Figure 4).

Among the known in vivo enzymes participating in the sterol biosynthesis of fungi [80,81], the activities of three of them, C-14 demethylase, Δ^{14} reductase and $\Delta^8 \rightarrow \Delta^7$ isomerase have been the target of numerous antifungal agents, especially azole derivatives [2]. The azole class of antimycotics are invariably C-14 demethylase inhibitors [1,2]. The oxidative 14α-demethylation of sterols is P-450 dependent; its suppression results from the binding of nitrogen from the heterocyclic portion of the azole molecule (imidazole, 1,2,4-triazole, pyridine, pyrimidine) to the heme iron of cytochrome P-450 [82-84]. First reported for two imidazole compounds, clotrimazole [85] and ketoconazole [86,87], the inhibition of C-14 demethylation reaction was associated with profound morphological and functional damage to the fungal cell membrane (loss of permeability to potassium cations and leakage of intracellular phosphorus-containing components) [88,89]. At higher concentrations, clotrimazole and miconazole were found to be fungicidal by their action on the cell membrane; however, at lower doses both drugs were only fungistatic [90,91]. In recent years, some azole derivatives (fluconazole, itraconazole) having a 1,2,4-triazole ring in place of imidazole, have been shown to possess better pharmacokinetic profile resulting in a more potent antimycotic activity with lesser toxicity [2]. In addition to causing accumulation of methylated sterols (as demonstrated by the decrease in ergosterol-to-methylated sterols ratio), the azoles, in general, decreased the unsaturated-to-saturated fatty acid ratio and initiated a shift from C_{18} to C_{16} fatty acids in vivo [3]. Furthermore, stimulation of chitin synthase activity in vivo (likely as a result of ergosterol depletion in the plasma membrane) has also been observed [3].

A number of N-containing sterols were also found to elicit antifungal activity by suppressing the ergosterol biosynthesis. For example, the 15-azasterol antibiotic A28522B was reported to inhibit the activity of Δ^{14} reductase leading to accumulation of 8,14-diene sterol [92]. Another derivative, the 23-azasterol was able to inhibit the 24-methylene-24(28) reductase in yeast fungi [93], whereas some 25-azasterols were potent inhibitors of the 24-methylation reaction in yeasts [94]. To date, however, none of the antifungal azasterols have found any clinical application.

Among other antimycotic agents suppressing the ergosterol biosynthesis, morpholines (tridemorph, fenpropimorph) have been known primarily as agricultural fungicides active against powdery mildews [95,96]. In 1980, Kato et al. [97] provided evidence for the accumulation of fecosterol after treatment with tridemorph suggesting inhibition of $\Delta^8 \rightarrow \Delta^7$ isomerization reaction. Later, Kerkenaar et al. [98] observed that tridemorph suppressed the Δ^{14} reductase step. Such dual action by the morpholines may eventually lead to lower incidence of drug resistance by fungi [3]. Recently, amorolfine, a structural analogue of fenpropimorph was found active against several fungal pathogens in humans [99,100].

In conclusion, it may be said that although great progress has been achieved in the development of newer and more potent antifungal agents, the need for antimycotic drugs with broader spectrum of activity and lesser toxicity is still very acute [1]. Future efforts should be directed towards the development of agents having fungicidal rather than fungistatic properties. In this context, the fungal envelope will remain as potentially the most attractive site for drug action. Ways leading to disruption of cell wall integrity and the biosynthesis of cell-wall polysaccharides will remain the goal of antimycotic research and development since any antifungal agent affecting the fungal cell wall will not only be fungicidal but also more selective in its mode of action because of the lack of cell wall in mammalian cells. Such newer mechanisms of action will have a clear advantage over those of the fungistatic drugs presently used in the clinic.

REFERENCES

1. V. St. Georgiev, Ann. N.Y. Acad. Sci., 544: 1 (1988).
2. Antifungal Drugs (V. St. Georgiev, ed.), The New York Academy of Sciences, New York, pp. 431-589 (1988).
3. N. H. Georgopapadakou, Perspectives in Antiinfective Therapy (G. G. Jackson, H. D. Schlumberger, and H. J. Zeiler, eds.), Friedr. Vieweg & Sohn, Braunschweig/Wiesbaden, pp. 60-67 (1989).
4. H. Zlotnik, M. P. Fernandez, B. Bowers, and E. Cabib, J. Bacteriol., 159: 1018 (1984).
5. W. N. Arnold, Physiol. Chem. Physics, 5: 117 (1973).
6. W. N. Arnold, and R. G. Garrison, Curr. Microbiol., 5: 57 (1981).
7. C. E. Ballou, Adv. Microb. Physiol., 14: 93 (1976).
8. E. Cabib, R. Roberts, and B. Bowers, Annu. Rev. Biochem., 51: 763 (1982).
9. E. M. Shematek, and E. Cabib, J. Biol. Chem., 255: 895 (1980).
10. V. Notario, H. Kawai, and E. Cabib, J. Biol. Chem., 257: 1902 (1982).
11. M. Horisberger, and M. Volanthen, Arch. Microbiol., 115: 1 (1977).
12. J. Molano, B. Bowers, and E. Cabib, J. Cell Biol., 85: 199 (1980).
13. A. Duran, B. Bowers, and E. Cabib, Proc. Natl. Acad. Sci. USA, 72: 3952 (1975).
14. H. Kaneko, M. Hosohara, M. Tanaka, and T. Itoh, Lipids, 11: 837 (1976).
15. M. S. Marriott, J. Gen. Microbiol., 86: 115 (1975).
16. J. M. T. Hamilton-Miller, Adv. Appl. Microbiol., 17: 109 (1977).
17. S. M. Hammond, Progr. Med. Chem., 14: 105 (1977).
18. T. E. Andreoli, Kidney Internat., 4: 337 (1973).
19. S. M. Hammond, P. A. Lambert, and B. N. Kliger, J. Gen. Microbiol., 81: 325 (1974).

20. T. Teerlink, B. De Kruijff, and R. A. Demel, Biochim. Biophys. Acta, 599: 484 (1980).
21. G. Medoff, G. S. Kobayashi, C. N. Kwan, D. Schlessinger, and P. Venkov, Proc. Natl. Acad. Sci. USA, 69: 196 (1972).
22. D. Ghosh, M. A. Williams, and J. Tinoco, Biochim. Biophys. Acta, 291: 351 (1973).
23. J. M. Boggs, and J. C. Hsia, Biochim. Biophys. Acta, 290: 32 (1972).
24. D. Marsh, and I. C. P. Smith, Biochim. Biophys. Acta, 298: 133 (1973).
25. R. Bittman, and L. Blau, Biochemistry, 11: 4831 (1972).
26. J. L. Lippert, and W. L. Peticolas, Proc. Natl. Acad. Sci. USA, 68: 1572 (1971).
27. J. M. Steim, M. E. Tourtellotte, J. C. Reinert, R. N. McElhaney, and R. L. Rader, Biochemistry, 63: 104 (1969).
28. M. C. Phillips, R. M. Williams, and D. Chapman, Chem. Phys. Lipids, 3: 234 (1969).
29. D. L. Melchior, H. J. Morowitz, J. M. Sturtevant, and T. Y. Tsong, Biochim. Biophys. Acta, 219: 114 (1970).
30. G. B. Ashe, and J. M. Steim, Biochim. Biophys. Acta, 233: 810 (1971).
31. L. L. M. van Deenen, Chem. Phys. Lipids, 8: 366 (1972).
32. B. de Kruyff, W. J. de Greef, R. V. W. van Eyk, and L. L. M. van Deenen, Biochim. Biophys. Acta, 298: 479 (1973).
33. R. N. McElhaney, J. de Gier, and E. C. M. van der Neuf-Kok, Biochim. Biophys. Acta, 298: 500 (1973).
34. V. Graziani, and A. Livne, J. Membr. Biol., 7: 275 (1972).
35. A. Finkelstein, and A. Cass, Nature, 216: 717 (1967).
36. H. Träuble, J. Membr. Biol., 4: 193 (1971).
37. E. Sackman, and H. Träuble, J. Am. Chem. Soc., 94: 4482 (1972).
38. V. Luzzati, Biological Membranes: Physical Fact and Function (D. Chapman, ed.), Academic Press, New York, p. 71 (1968).
39. B. de Kruijff, W. J. Geritsen, A. Oerlemans, R. A. Demel, and L. L. M. Deenen, Biochim. Biophys. Acta, 339: 30 (1974).
40. A. Cass, A. Finkelstein , and V. Krepsi, J. Gen. Physiol., 56: 100 (1970).
41. V. W. Denis, N. W. Stead, and T. E. Andreoli, J. Gen. Microbiol., 55: 375 (1970).
42. B. de Kruijff, and R. A. Demel, Biochim. Biophys. Acta, 339: 57 (1974).
43. A. Finkelstein, and R. Holz, Membranes (G. Eisenman, ed.),Marcell Dekker, New York, vol. 2, p. 377 (1972).
44. Kh. Kasumov, E. A. Liberman, V. A. Nenashev, and I. S. Yurkov, Biofizika, 20: 62 (1975).
45. A. W. Norman, R. A. Demel, B. de Krujiff, W. S. M. Guerts van Kessel, and L. L. M. van Deenen, Biochim. Biophys. Acta, 290: 1 (1972).
46. A. W. Norman, R. A. Demel, B. de Kruijff, and L. L. M. van Deenen, J. Biol. Chem., 247: 1918 (1972).
47. B. de Kruijff, W. J. Geritsen, A. Oerlemans, P. W. M. van Dijk, R. A. Demel, and L. L. M. van Deenen, Biochim. Biophys. Acta, 339: 44 (1974).
48. H. van Zutphen, L. L. M. van Deenen, and S. C. Kinsky, Biochim. Biophys. Acta, 22: 393 (1966).
49. S. M. Hammond, P. A. Lambert, and B. N. Kliger, J. Gen. Microbiol., 81: 331 (1974).
50. S. M. Hammond, and B. N. Kliger, Microbios., 13: 15 (1975).

51. R. J. Rodriguez, F. R. Taylor, and L. W. Parks, Biophys. Res. Commun., 106: 435 (1982).
52. M. Ramgopal, and K. Bloch, Proc. Natl. Acad. Sci. USA, 80: 712 (1983).
53. W. J. Pinto, R. Lozano, B. C. Sekula, and W. R. Nes, Biochem. Biophys. Res. Commun., 112: 47 (1983).
54. R. J. Rodriguez, C. Low, C. D. K. Bottema, and L. W. Parks, Biochim. Biophys. Acta, 837: 336 (1985).
55. T. Nishino, S. Hata, S. Taketani, Y. Yabusaki, and H. Katsuki, J. Biochem., 89: 1391 (1981).
56. M. Boll, M. Lowel, J. Still, and J. Berndt, Eur. J. Biochem., 54: 435 (1975).
57. J. D. Brodie, G. Wasson, and W. Porter, J. Biol. Chem., 238: 1294 (1963).
58. R. B. Clayton, Quart. Rev. Chem. Soc., 19: 168 (1965).
59. A. Endo, M. Kuroda, and Y. Tsujita, J. Antibiot., 29: 1346 (1976).
60. A. Endo, M. Kuroda, and K. Tanzawa, FEBS Lett., 72: 323 (1976).
61. K. Tanzawa, and A. Endo, Eur. J. Biochem., 98: 195 (1979).
62. A. Endo, J. Med. Chem., 28: 401 (1985).
63. J. C. Onishi, G. K. Abbruzzo, R. A. Fromtling, G. M. Garrity, J. A. Milligan, B. A. Pelak, W. Rozdilsky, and B. Weissberger, Ann. N.Y. Acad. Sci., 544: 230 (1988).
64. L. J. Altman, R. C. Kowerski, and H. C. Rilling, J. Am. Chem. Soc., 93: 1782 (1971).
65. G. Popjak, and J. W. Cornforth, Biochem. J., 101: 553 (1966).
66. B. H. Amdur, H. C. Rilling, and K. Bloch, J. Am. Chem. Soc., 79: 2646 (1957).
67. F. Lynen, H. Eggerer, V. Henning, and I. Kessel, Angew. Chem., 70: 738 (1958).
68. I. Shechter, and K. Bloch, J. Biol. Chem., 246: 7690 (1971).
69. P. D. G. Dean, P. R. Ortiz de Montellano, K. Bloch, and E. J. Corey, J. Biol. Chem., 242: 3014 (1967).
70. E. I. Mercer, and M. W. Johnson, Phytochemistry, 8: 2329 (1969).
71. I. Shechter, F. W. Sweat, and K. Bloch, Biochim. Biophys. Acta, 220: 463 (1970).
72. F. Paltauf, G. Daum, G. Zuder, G. Hogenauer, G. Schulz, and G. Seidl, Biochim. Biophys. Acta, 712: 268 (1982).
73. N. S. Ryder, and M.-C. Dupont, Biochem. J., 230: 765 (1985).
74. T. Morita, and Y. Nozawa, J. Invest. Dermatol., 85: 434 (1985).
75. N. S. Ryder, I. Frank, and M.-C. Dupont, Antimicrob. Agents Chemother., 29: 858 (1986).
76. J. D. Weete, Phytochemistry, 12: 1845 (1973).
77. D. H. R. Barton, U. M. Kempe, and D. A. Widdowson, J. Chem. Soc., Perkin I, 1: 513 (1972).
78. D. H. R. Barton, J. E. T. Corrie, P. J. Marshall, and D. A. Widdowson, Bioorg. Chem., 2: 363 (1973).
79. D. H. R. Barton, J. E. T. Corrie, D. A. Widdowson, M. Bard, and R. A. Woods, J. Chem. Soc., Chem. Commun., 30 (1974).
80. J. B. M. Rattray, A. Schibeci, and D. K. Kidby, Bacteriol. Rev., 39: 197 (1975).
81. J. L. Gaylor, Biochemistry of Lipids (T. W. Goodwin, ed.),Biochemistry Series One, Butterworth, London, vol. 4, pp. 1-37 (1974).
82. B. C. Baldwin, Biochem. Soc. Trans., 11: 659 (1983).

83. P. Gadher, E. I. Mercer, B. C. Baldwin, and T. E. Wiggins, Pestic. Biochem. Physiol., 19: 1 (1983).
84. T. E. Wiggins, and B. C. Baldwin, Pestic. Sci., 15: 206 (1984).
85. H. Buchenauer, Pestic. Biochem. Physiol., 8: 15 (1978).
86. H. Van den Bossche, G. Willemsens, W. Cools, W. F. J. Lauwers, and L. Le Jeune, Chem.-Biol. Interact., 21: 59 (1978).
87. H. Van den Bossche, G. Willemsens, W. Cools, W. F. J. Lauwers, and L. Le Jeune, Curr. Chemother., 3: 228 (1978).
88. K. Iwata, H. Yamaguchi, and T. Hiratani, Sabouraudia, 11: 158 (1973).
89. S. De Nollin, and M. Borgers, Antimicrob. Agents Chemother., 7: 704 (1975).
90. I. J. Sud, and D. S. Feingold, Antimicrob. Agents Chemother., 20: 71 (1981).
91. I. J. Sud, and D. S. Feingold, J. Invest. Dermatol., 76: 438 (1981).
92. R. J. Rodriguez, and L. W. Parks, Antimicrob. Agents Chemother., 20: 184 (1981).
93. D. Pierce, A. M. Pierce, R. Srinivasan, A. M. Unrau, and A. C. Oehlschlager, Biochim. Biophys. Acta, 529: 429 (1978).
94. L. Avruch, S. Fischer, H. Pierce, and A. C. Oehlschlager, Can. J. Biochem., 54: 657 (1975).
95. K. H. Konig, E. H. Pommer, and W. Sanne, Angew. Chem., int. ed. Engl., 4: 336 (1965).
96. W. Himmele, and E. H. Pommer, Angew. Chem., int. ed. Engl., 19: 184 (1980).
97. T. Kato, M. Shaomi, and Y. Kawase, J. Pestic. Sci., 5: 69 (1980).
98. A. Kerkenaar, M. Uchiyama, and G. G. Versluis, Pestic. Biochem. Physiol., 16: 97 (1981).
99. A. Polak, Sabouraudia, 21: 205 (1983).
100. A. Polak, Ann. N.Y. Acad. Sci., 455: 221 (1988).

PART I

ACTION MECHANISM AND NEW CLINICAL APPLICATIONS OF ANTIFUNGAL DRUGS

3

Azole Antifungals: Mode of Action

Hugo Vanden Bossche and Patrick Marichal

Department of Comparative Biochemistry
Division of Medicinal Chemistry and Pharmacology
Janssen Research Foundation
B 2340 Beerse
Belgium

I. INTRODUCTION

In the last two decades antifungal therapy has completely changed. The broad-spectrum imidazole and triazole derivatives (the azole antifungals) improved topical treatment and oral therapy with the imidazole derivative, ketoconazole, was a major therapeutic breakthrough.

Studies of Wilkinson et al.(1) indicated that a number of N-1 substituted imidazole derivatives inhibited cytochrome P450-dependent reactions. They proved that the unhindered nitrogen (N-3 in the imidazole ring) binds to the heme iron of cytochrome P450 (P450) at the site occupied by the exchangeable sixth ligand (2). It has been proven that the azole antifungals also bind to P450s and specially to that involved in the synthesis of ergosterol, the major sterol in fungal cells (3). It is the aim of this paper to overview the effects of a number of azole antifungals on this fungal P450 and ergosterol synthesis.

II. CYTOCHROMES P450

The cytochrome P450-dependent enzymes are among the more ubiquitous enzymes in living organisms. They are present in bacteria, protozoa, yeasts and fungi, insects, fishes, plants and mammals. A large family of structurally related cytochromes, P450 monooxygenases metabolize a vast majority of exogenous (xenobiotics) and endogenous (endobiotics) compounds. Examples of endobiotics are sterols, steroids, bile acids, vitamins A and D, and products of the arachidonic acid cascade. In prokaryotes P450s are soluble proteins, the eukaryotic forms are located in the mitochondrial inner membrane, the nuclear envelope and the endoplasmic reticulum.

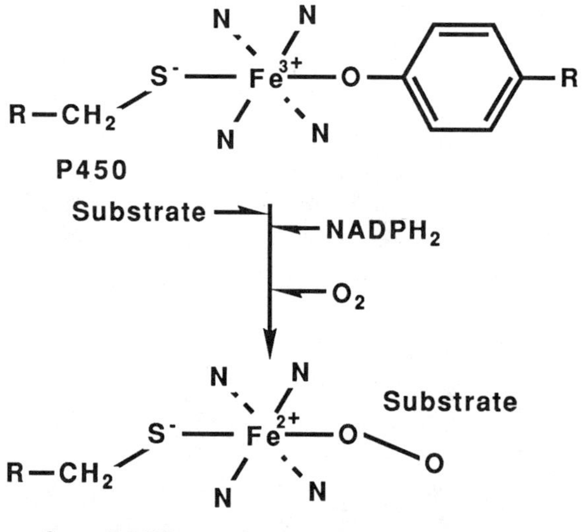

FIG. 1. Models of P450 and Oxy-P450. The 5th ligand is the sulfur of the thiol from a cysteyl residue; as 6th ligand part of the thyrosyl residue is shown. The substrate binds to the oxidized form of P450 (Fe^{3+}), after reduction molecular oxygen is bound.

The catalytic site of P450 is the heme-iron linked to the protein by a thiol residue (the fifth ligand) of cysteine (Fig. 1). The sixth ligand is a hydroxyl group from a seryl, threonyl or thyrosyl residue (4). P450 enzymes generally insert an atom of oxygen into their substrates. This reaction requires a source of reducing equivalents and molecular oxygen (Fig. 1). The reducing equivalents originate from $NADPH_2$ and the cytochrome P450 reductase. One oxygen atom of the dioxygen is activated for insertion into the substrate, the other is reduced to water.

Carbon monoxide is capable to compete with oxygen for the binding site of the reduced heme iron (Fe^{2+}). CO-binding results in inhibition of the P450-dependent reaction and in the spectrophotometer this binding results in the typical absorption spectrum maximum of 450nm. Indeed, the name of this hemoprotein describes a **P**igment which absorbs at about **450**nm when reduced and complexed with carbon monoxide.

The ability to activate oxygen for insertion into a substrate is also the key property of the P450 ($P450_{14DM}$) involved in the 14α-demethylation of lanosterol (in *Saccharomyces cerevisiae*, *Candida* (*Torulopsis*) *glabrata* and mammalian liver) or of 24-methylenedihydrolanosterol in a number of *Candida albicans* isolates and all filamentous fungi studied so far. $P450_{14DM}$ purified to homogenity from rat liver(5,6), *S. cerevisiae* (3) and *C. albicans* (7) microsomes catalyses three oxidative steps:

1. the hydroxylation of the C-32-methyl group of lanosterol to give the 14α-hydroxymethyl compound, 32-hydroxy-lanosterol;
2. the oxidation of the 14α-hydroxymethyl compound to the 14α-carboxyaldehyde, 3ß-hydroxylanost-8-en-32-aldehyde;
3. the oxidative elimination of the aldehyde [at least in liver via the formation of 14α-formyl-lanost-8-en-3ß-ol (6)] as formic acid, resulting in the formation of 4,4-dimethyl-$\Delta^{8,14,24(28)}$-ergostatrienol in fungi, and 4,4-dimethyl-$\Delta^{8,14,24}$-cholestatrienol in *S. cerevisiae* and liver.

As already mentioned above, N-1 substituted imidazole derivatives bind to the 6th coordination position of the heme iron and thus interfere with oxygen or CO-binding. Interference with CO-binding will result in a decreased absorption at 450 nm. Binding to the heme iron (Fe^{3+}) can also be visualised spectrophotometrically as an increase in absorbance at about 420nm and a decrease at about 390nm. These difference spectra have been designated type II spectra.

N-1 Substituted azole antifungals have been found to yield type II spectra and to compete with CO for binding to the heme iron in P450(s) present in *C. albicans*, *Candida glabrata*, *Aspergillus fumigatus* and/or *S. cerevisiae* microsomes (3, 8-20). Yoshida and Aoyama (21) titrated $P450_{14DM}$, purified from *S. cerevisiae* microsomes, with ketoconazole and showed the stoichiometric binding of the antifungal to this P450. Effects of some antifungal agents on CO-binding by *C. albicans* microsomal P450 are presented in Fig. 2.

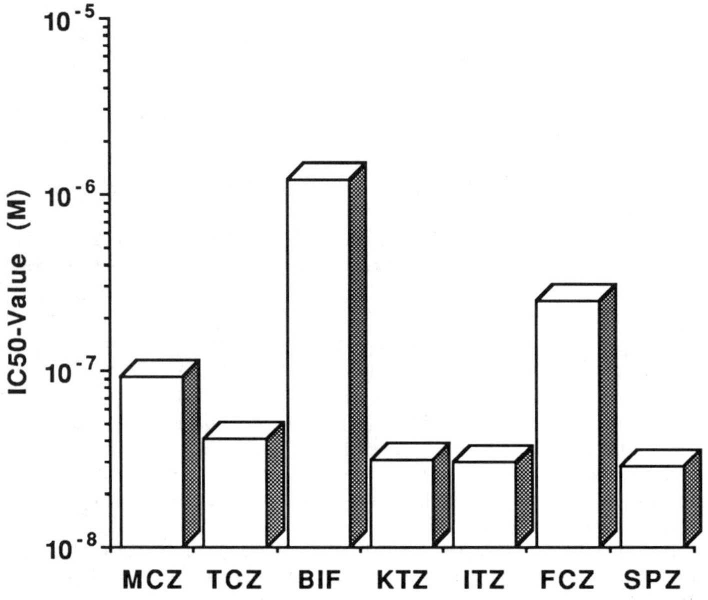

FIG. 2. Effects of azole antifungals on microsomal P450 from *C.albicans* (ATCC 28516). IC_{50}-values= concentrations needed to inhibit CO binding to the heme iron for 50% (P450 content= 0.1 nmole/ml). MCZ: miconazole, TCZ: terconazole, BIF: bifonazole, KTZ: ketoconazole, ITZ: itraconazole, FCZ: fluconazole, SPZ: saperconazole.

Differences in affinity (i.e. competition with CO for the binding place) are found between the different imidazole and triazole antifungals. Bifonazole (an imidazole derivative) and fluconazole (a triazole derivative) showed the lowest affinity. This indicates that activity is not only determined by the affinity of the unhindered nitrogen (N-3 of the imidazole ring; N-4 of the triazole ring) for the heme iron but also by the affinity of the N-1 substituent for the apoprotein moiety. The importance of this N-1 substituent was proven by titrating $P450_{14DM}$, purified from *S. cerevisiae* microsomes, with ketoconazole (21). Upon addition of hydrosulfite to the P450-ketoconazole complex, the Fe^{3+}-complex was reduced to the corresponding Fe^{2+}-complex. Addition of CO to the reduced complex showed a slow replacement of ketoconazole by CO.

Similar results were obtained by using microsomal preparations of *C. albicans* (22). Furthermore, the reactivity of the reduced azole-$P450_{14DM}$ complex was not affected by replacing the imidazole moiety in ketoconazole by a triazole ring (22).

Itraconazole forms an even more stable complex with $P450_{14DM}$ purified from *S. cerevisiae* microsomes (21) and with P450 in *C. albicans* microsomes (22).

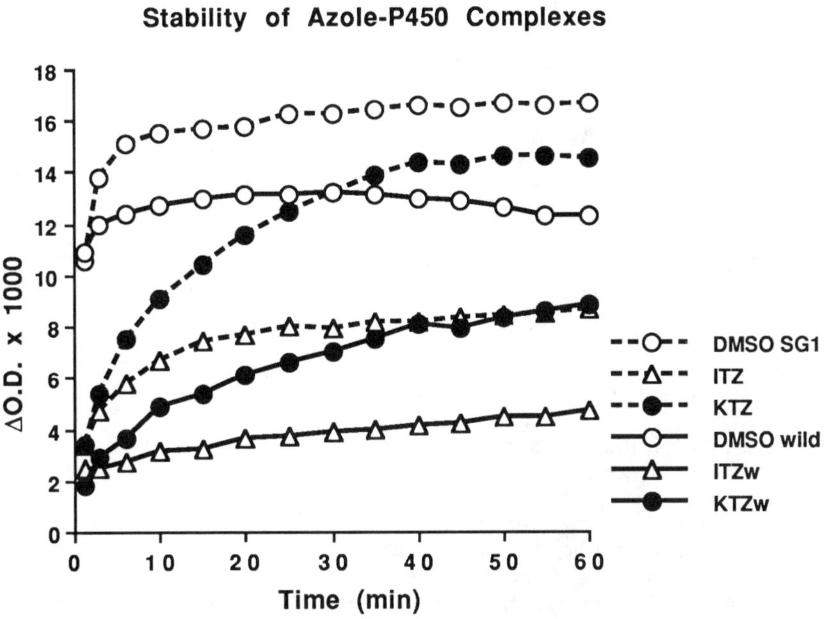

FIG. 3. Stability of the azole-P450 complexes. The microsomal suspensions (0.1 nmol P450 ml^{-1}; pH 7.4) obtained from *S. cerevisiae* SG_1 (ATCC 46786) or its parent (wild) (D587) were divided between reference and sample cuvettes and increasing concentrations (up to $5x10^{-6}$M) of itraconazole (ITZ) or ketoconazole (KTZ) were added to the sample cuvette. Equal amounts of DMSO were added to the reference cuvette and the resulting difference spectra recorded. The same amount of azole antifungal or DMSO was added to the reference and sample cuvette, respectively and the P450 was reduced with a few grains of sodium dithionite. The sample cuvette was bubbled for 30 sec with CO and tightly closed. The difference spectrum was recorded 45 sec later and at different time intervals up to 60 min after the addition of the reductant. Control spectra were obtained in the presence of DMSO. Results are taken from Ref. 16.

When the triazole ring of itraconazole was replaced by an imidazole ring, a complex with P450 from *C. albicans* microsomes as stable as that seen with itraconazole was obtained (22).

Further proof for the role both the apoprotein and the N-1 substituent of the azole antifungals play in the formation of drug-P450 complexes was obtained by comparing the affinity of ketoconazole and itraconazole for microsomal P450 of a wild (D587) and a mutant strain of *S. cerevisiae* (SG_1, ATCC 46786). It has been found that in the $P450_{14DM}$ of this mutant glycine-310 is replaced by an aspartic acid residue (23). This results in a modification of the conformation of the apoprotein so that a histidyl residue is becoming the 6th ligand. As shown in Fig. 3, this mutation not only replaces the tyrosyl residue (or a seryl or threonyl residue, see above) by a histidyl residue, but also affects the stability of the ketoconazole- and itraconazole-P450-complexes. Indeed, both itraconazole and ketoconazole are more easily replaced by CO from the SG_1 P450 than from the microsomal P450 of the parent strain.

III. ERGOSTEROL SYNTHESIS

Binding of antifungals to the heme iron and to the apoprotein moiety of $P450_{14DM}$ will result in an inhibition of the 14-demethylation of lanosterol. Indeed, Aoyama and colleagues (24) proved that the pyridyl derivative, buthiobate and the triazole derivative, triadimefon (21) bound to $P450_{14DM}$ from *S.cerevisiae* and inhibited lanosterol 14α-demethylation in a reconstituted system consisting of $P450_{14DM}$ and NADPH-P450 reductase, both purified from *S. cerevisiae* microsomes. Yoshida and Aoyama (3, 21) also proved that ketoconazole and itraconazole inhibited lanosterol 14α-demethylase activity of this reconstituted system. The inhibition was linearly dependent on the amount of ketoconazole or itraconazole and reached 100% when an equal amount of azole antifungal to $P450_{14DM}$ was added. This again proves that azole antifungals inactivate the 14α-demethylase system by forming a stoichiometric complex with $P450_{14DM}$. Yoshida and colleagues,using the reconstituted system also found that ketoconazole inhibited the 14α-demethylation of 24,25-dihydrolanosterol and of 32-hydroxy-24,25-dihydrolanosterol [i.e. the product of the hydroxylation of the C-32 methyl (14α-methyl group) of lanosterol] but the inhibitory effect on the removal of the 32-hydroxymethyl group was weaker(24). This suggests that ketoconazole preferentially inhibits the hydroxylation step and not so much the formation and oxidative elimination of the aldehyde as formic acid.

Inhibition of ergosterol synthesis has been shown in, for example, *C. albicans* (8-13, 17, 20, 25-26), *C. glabrata* (20), *Pityrosporum ovale* (27), *A. fumigatus* and *A. niger* (14, 17, 28), *Trichophyton mentagrophytes* (17), *Histoplasma capsulatum* (20), *Paracoccidioides brasiliensis* (unpublished results) and *Penicillium italicum* (9). To get an idea of the potency of some of the azole antifungals, concentrations needed to reach 50% inhibition of ergosterol synthesis by intact *C. albicans* and *C. glabrata* are listed in Table 1. As could be expected from fluconazole's low affinity for fungal P450 (Fig. 2), high concentrations are needed to inhibit ergosterol synthesis.

TABLE 1

Effects of Azole Antifungals on Ergosterol Synthesis*

Azole Antifungal	IC_{50}-Values (10^{-8}M)	
	C. albicans	*C. glabrata*
Fluconazole	>1000	45.7
Itraconazole	8.3	4.8
Ketoconazole	7.7	5.3
Saperconazole	6.3	3.3

*Cells were first grown for 16h (8h of which in an orbital shaker) at 30°C in a polypeptone:yeast extract:glucose (10:10:40 g/l) medium, then washed and resuspended in a 0.1M potassium phosphate buffer containing 56 mM glucose (pH 6.5). ^{14}C-Acetate, azole antifungal and/or DMSO were added and the cell suspensions were incubated for 2h at 30°C in an orbital shaker (300rpm). At the end of the incubation period sterols were extracted and separated by TLC. IC_{50}-values: concentrations needed to get 50% inhibition of ^{14}C-incorporation into ergosterol (17).

Inhibition of ergosterol synthesis by interaction with $P450_{14DM}$ results in an accumulation of 14-methylated sterols. For example, the sterols found in *C. albicans* grown for 24h in the presence of itraconazole and/or DMSO are shown in Fig. 4. The results presented indicate that at 3×10^{-8}M itraconazole cells lost the capacity to synthesize ergosterol. Of interest are also the high amounts of 14α-methyl-ergosta-$\Delta^{8,24(28)}$-dien-3ß,6α-diol (3,6-diol) found in treated cells. Studies of Watson et al. (29-30) suggest that at least in *S. cerevisiae*, azole-

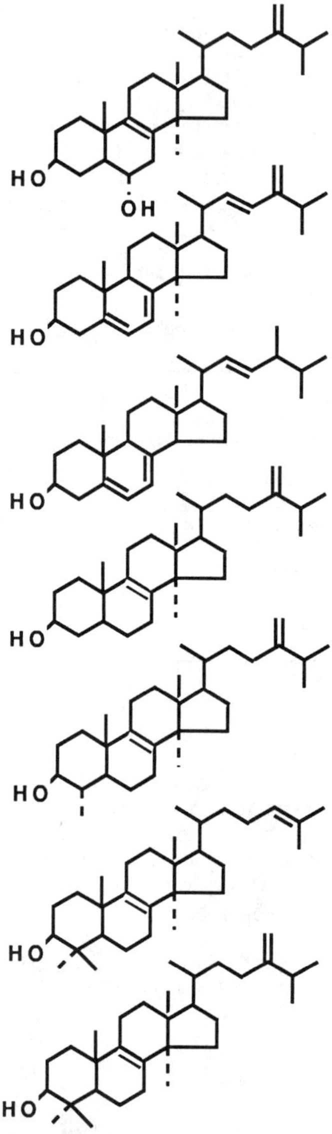

Compound	Percent of total radioactivity (0)	Percent of total radioactivity (30nM)
14α-Methyl-ergosta-$\Delta^{8,24(28)}$-dien-3ß,6α-diol	0.0	69.0
14α-Methyl-ergosta-$\Delta^{5,7,22,24(28)}$-tetraen-3ß-ol	0.0	1.3
Ergosterol	96.3	0.0
14α-Methylfecosterol	0.0	7.0
Obtusifoliol	0.0	15.8
Lanosterol		
24-Methylenedihydrolanosterol	0.0	3.8

FIG. 4. *C. albicans*

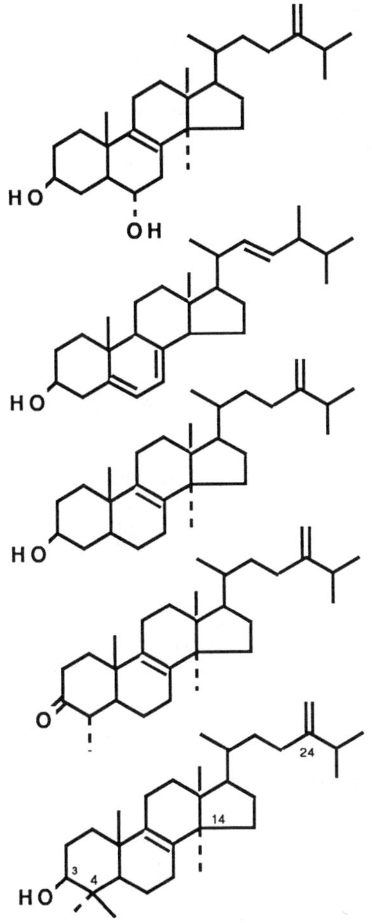

	Percent of total radioactivity	
	(0)	(30nM)
14α-Methyl-ergosta-$\Delta^{8,24(28)}$-dien-3ß,6α-diol	0.0	4.0
Ergosterol	63.0	0
14α-Methylfecosterol	37.0	0.0
Obtusifolione	0.0	44.0
24-Methylenedihydrolanosterol	0.0	52.0

FIG. 5. *H. capsulatum*

FIG. 4. Effects of itraconazole on ergosterol synthesis in *C. albicans* grown for 24h in CYG-medium supplemented with ^{14}C-acetate and itraconazole and/or DMSO. Homogenisation of the cells, saponification, extraction and separation of the sterols by HPLC was as previously described (13). ^{14}C-Acetate and drug and/or solvent were added at inoculation. 30 nM is the itraconazole concentration needed to get 100% inhibition of ergosterol synthesis; (0)= the control. Obtusifoliol and lanosterol were not separated by the HPLC method used. Taken from Ref. 48.

FIG. 5. Sterols and ketones formed by *H. capsulatum* (G217-B) after 48 h of growth in GY medium (2% glucose- 1% yeast extract- 0.03% L-cysteine) supplemented with ^{14}C-acetate and 30 nM itraconazole and/or DMSO (0). Taken from Ref. 20.

induced growth inhibition originates from inhibition of the 14α-demethylase and the consequent accumulation of this 3,6-diol. Their hypothesis is based on the inability of the 3,6-diol to support growth. This might be true for *S. cerevisiae* and for the *C. albicans* isolate used in this study. However, as shown in Fig. 5, of the sterols found in *H. capsulatum* (yeast form), incubated for 48h in the presence of $3x10^{-8}$M itraconazole, the 3,6-diol represented only 4 %. Most of the radioactivity derived from ^{14}C-acetate is found in obtusifolione and 24-methylenedihydrolanosterol. The accumulation of the 3-ketosteroid, obtusifolione, indicates that itraconazole (and also ketoconazole, 20) not only inhibits the 14α-demethylase but also the 3-ketosteroid reductase, an enzyme involved in the conversion of 24-methylenedihydrolanosterol into obtusifoliol. In this species the 3-ketosteroid might have the same destabilising effect as 3,6-diol in *S. cerevisiae*. Indeed, it has been shown that 3-ketosteroids greatly increase permeability and fragility of membranes and this might be related to their strong bilayer-destabilizing effect (31). The high amount of 14-methylfecosterol found in *H. capsulatum* under control conditions suggests that the accumulation of obtusifolione may be more important for the antifungal effects on *H. capsulatum* than that of the 14-methylsterols.

IV. CONSEQUENCES OF ERGOSTEROL BIOSYNTHESIS INHIBITION

The interaction of the more potent azoles antifungals (e.g. ketoconazole, itraconazole and saperconazole) with the $P450_{14DM}$ results in ergosterol depletion. For example, ergosterol could not be detected in *H. capsulatum* (48h) and *C. albicans* (24h) incubated in the presence of 10^{-7}M ketoconazole or itraconazole. Since the presence of ergosterol in most fungi is a prerequisite for cell proliferation (for reviews see refs. 33, 42), the observed azole-induced depletion might be the prime cause for the effect on fungal growth.

Although it is possible that 14-methylfecosterol is not affecting the growth of *H. capsulatum*, it is known that the 14-methylsterol, lanosterol, has detrimental effects on membrane properties (for reviews see 32-33). The effects of lanosterol might originate from the fact that the C-14 methyl group of lanosterol protrudes from the sterol α-face in the lipid-lipid contact region and diminishes as such the van der Waals contacts allowing greater motional freedom to fatty acyl chains and thus changing membrane fluidity (32).

Parks et al. (34) showed that structural changes in the sterols affect not only the physical but also enzymatic properties of membranes. An example is the chitin synthetase. Chitin is a major component of the primary septum in the yeast form and of the septa and primary wall of the mycelium form of *C. albicans* (35). Chiew et al.(36) showed that high concentrations of ergosterol inhibit chitin synthesis. Furthermore, mutants of *C. albicans* , with a low ergosterol content, showed increased activity of the chitin synthetase (37). These studies indicate that ergosterol biosynthesis inhibitors could disturb chitin synthesis. An itraconazole-induced increase in the ratio chitin:total carbohydrate was found in *C.albicans* (10). This enhanced chitin synthesis corresponds with the increased and irregular distribution of chitin observed in itraconazole- (10) or bifinazole-treated (39-39) *C. albicans* (yeast and mycelium forms). In budding *C. albicans*, irregular deposition of chitin will disturb the normal sequence of cell separation, resulting in chains and clusters of interconnected cells and in filamentous fungi; such a defect may be lethal, causing abnormal swelling and bursting of cells (39). Such effects have been observed with miconazole (40), bifonazole (38-39, 41), ketoconazole (10) and itraconazole (28).

Effects of azole antifungals on the activity of other membrane-bound enzymes might also be related to changes in sterol composition (for reviews see refs. 10, 19, 33, 42). For example, *C. albicans* incubated in the presence of 14α-demethylase inhibitors is not able to maintain the synthesis of unsaturated fatty acids (10, 33, 43). The unsaturated fatty acids have been partly replaced by palmitic acid. This indicates that the azole antifungals affect the microsomal Δ^9 desaturase. In *S. cerevisiae* the Δ^9 desaturase system contains NADH, NADH-cytochrome b_5 reductase, cytochrome b_5, a cyanide-sensitive factor and phospholipids. The requirement for phospholipids indicates that this enzyme, as other membrane-bound enzymes, is only active at a defined fluidity of the environment. Thus, it is possible that the azole-induced ergosterol depletion and accompanying accumulation of 14α-methylsterols alter the fluidity in such a way that the desaturase is inhibited. Effects of azole antifungals on for, example, the $Mg^+Na^+K^+$-ATPase (10), cytochrome oxidase (44), and cytochrome c peroxidase (44-45) might also originate from inhibition of ergosterol synthesis. Indeed, in contrast to mammalian cells, in yeast cells sterols are not only components of the microsomal but also of the mitochondrial membranes (10, 34). Furthermore, ergosterol and unsaturated fatty acids have an essential role in the biogenesis of organelles, particularly of mitochondria, and a great number of experiments suggest that there may be a specific dependency of the synthesis of mitochondrial enzymes on the synthesis of mitochondrial lipids (33, 46-47).

IV. CONCLUSIONS

Most of the azole antifungals show high affinity for the cytochrome P450-dependent 14α-demethylase in fungal cells. The affinity is depending on the nitrogen heterocycle, and, even more on the N-1 substituent of the azole antifungal. Binding to $P450_{14DM}$ results in an inhibition of ergosterol synthesis and accumulation of 14-methylated sterols such as 14α-methyl-ergosta-$\Delta^{8,24(28)}$-dien-3ß,6α-diol and 24-methylenedihydrolanosterol, and in *Histoplasma capsulatum* the membrane destabilizing 3-ketosteroid, obtusifolione is also accumulating. It is hypothesized that ergosterol depletion, achieved with, for example, ketoconazole and itraconazole, and the coinciding accumulation of precursors are at the origin of alterations in membrane permeability, activity of membrane-bound enzymes and morphology.

REFERENCES

1. C.F. Wilkinson, K. Hetnarski, and T.O. Yellin, Imidazole derivatives- A new class of microsomal enzyme inhibitors, Biochem. Pharmacol., 21: 3187 (1972).
2. P.R. Ortiz de Montellano and N.O. Reich, Inhibition of cytochrome P-450 enzymes, Cytochrome P-450 Structure, Mechanism and Biochemistry (P.O.Ortiz de Montellano, ed.), Plenum Press, New York, p. 273 (1986).
3. Y. Yoshida, Cytochrome P450 of fungi: primary target for azole antifungal agents, Current Topics in Medical Mycology (M.R. McGinnis, ed.)., Springer Verlag, New York, Vol 2, p. 388 (1988).
4. K. Ruckpaul and R. Bernhardt, Biochemical aspects of the monooxygenase system in the endoplasmic reticulum of mammalian liver (K. Ruckpaul, and H. Rein H, eds.) Cytochrome P-450, Akademie-Verlag, Berlin, p. 9 (1984).
5. J.M. Trzaskos, S. Kawata, and J.L. Gaylor, Microsomal enzymes of cholesterol biosynthesis. Purification of lanosterol 14α-methyl demethylase cytochrome P-450 from hepatic microsomes, J. Biol. Chem., 261: 14651 (1986).
6. J.M. Trzaskos, R.T. Fischer, R.L. Magolda, S.S. Ko, C.S. Brosz, and B. Larson, The lanosterol 14α-demethylase: metabolic and kinetic studies which define the final oxidative process, Drug Metbolizing Enzymes: Genetics, Regulation and Toxicology, Proceedings of the VIIIth International Symposium on Microsomes and Drug Oxidations (M.I. Ingelman-Sundberg, J-A Gustafson, and S. Orrenius, eds.), Karoliska Institutet, Stockholm, p. 22. (1990)

7. C.A. Hitchcock, K. Dickinson, S.B. Brown, E.G.V. Evans, and D.J. Adams, Purification and properties of cytochrome P-450-dependent 14α-sterol demethylase from *Candida albicans*, Biochem. J., 263: 573 (1989).
8. H. Vanden Bossche, G. Willemsens, W. Cools, P. Marichal, and W. Lauwers, Hypothesis on the molecular basis of the antifungal activity of *N*-substituted imidazoles and triazoles, Biochem. Soc. Trans., 11: 665 (1983).
9. H. Vanden Bossche, W. Lauwers, G. Willemsens, P. Marichal, F. Cornelissen, and W. Cools, Molecular basis for the antimycotic and antibacterial activity of *N*-substistuted imidazoles and triazoles: the inhibition of isoprenoid biosynthesis, Pestic. sci., 15: 188 (1984).
10. H. Vanden Bossche, Biochemical targets for antifungal azole derivatives: hypothesis on the mode of action, Current Topics in Medical Mycology (M.K. McGinnis ed.). Springer Verlag, New York, Vol 1, p. 313 (1985).
11. H. Vanden Bossche, D. Bellens, W. Cools, J. Gorrens, P. Marichal, H. Verhoeven, G. Willemsens, R. De Coster, D. Beerens, C. Haelterman, M-C. Coene, W. Lauwers, and L. Le Jeune, Cytochrome P-450: target for itraconazole. Drug Dev. Res., 8: 287 (1986).
12. H. Vanden Bossche, Itraconazole: a selective inhibitor of the cytochrome P-450 dependent ergosterol biosynthesis (R.A. Fromtling, ed.), Recent Trends in the Discovery, Development and Evaluation of Antifungal Agents, JR Prous Science Publishers, S.A., Barcelona, p. 207 (1987).
13. H. Vanden Bossche, P. Marichal, J. Gorrens, D. Bellens, H. Verhoeven, M-C. Coene, W. Lauwers, and P.A.J. Janssen, Interaction of azole derivatives with cytochrome P-450 isozymes in yeast, fungi, plants and mammalian cells, Pestic. Sci. 21: 289 (1987).
14. H. Vanden Bossche, P. Marichal, H. Geerts, and P.A.J. Janssen, The molecular basis for itraconazole's activity against *Aspergillus fumigatus*, Aspergillus and Aspergillosis (H. Vanden Bossche, D.W.R. Mackenzie and G. Cauwenbergh, eds.), Plenum Press, New York, p. 171 (1988).
15. P. Marichal, H. Vanden Bossche, J. Gorrens, D. Bellens, and P.A.J. Janssen, Cytochrome P-450 in *Aspergillus fumigatus*- Effects of itraconazole and ketoconazole, Cytochrome P-450: Biochemistry and Biophysics (I. Schuster, ed.), Taylor and Francis, London, p. 171 (1989).
16. H. Vanden Bossche, P. Marichal, J. Gorrens, D. Bellens, H. Moereels, and P.A.J. Janssen, Mutation in cytochrome P-450-dependent 14α-demethylase results in decreased

affinity for azole antifungals, Biochem. Soc. Trans., 18, 56 (1990).
17. H. Vanden Bossche, P. Marichal, G. Willemsens, D. Bellens, J. Gorrens, I. Roels, M-C. Coene, L. Le Jeune and P.A.J. Janssen, Saperconazole: a selective inhibitor of the cytochrome P450-dependent ergosterol synthesis in *Candida albicans*, *Aspergillus fumigatus* and *Trichophyton mentagrophytes*, Mycoses, in press.
18. J.T.B.Shaw, M.H. Tarbit and P.F. Troke, Cytochrome P-450 mediated sterol synthesis and metabolism: differences in sensitivity to fluconazole and other azoles, Recent Trends in the Discovery, Development and Evaluation of Antifungal Agents (R.A.. Fromtling, ed.), JR Prous Science Publishers, S.A., Barcelona, p. 125 (1987).
19. S.L. Kelly, S. Kenna, H.F.J.Bligh, P.F. Watson, I. Stansfield, S.W. Ellis and D.E. Kelly, Lanosterol to ergosterol-enzymology, inhibition and genetics, Biochemistry of Cell Walls and Membranes in Fungi (P.J. Kuhn , A.P.J. Trinci, M.J. Jung, M.W. Goosey L.G., and Copping, eds.), Springer Verlag,Berlin, p. 223 (1990).
20. H. Vanden Bossche, P. Marichal, J. Gorrens, D. Bellens, M-C. Coene, W. Lauwers, L. Le Jeune, H. Moereels, and P.A.J. Janssen, Mode of action of antifungals of use in immunocompromised patients. Focus on *Candida glabrata* and *Histoplasma capsulatum*, Mycoses in Aids Patients (H. Vanden Bossche, D.W.R. Mackenzie, G. Cauwenbergh, J. Van Cutsem, E. Drouhet, and B. Dupont, eds.), Plenum Press, New York, London, p. 223 (1990).
21. Y. Yoshida and Y. Aoyama, Interaction of azole fungicides with yeast cytochrome P-450 which catalyzes lanosterol 14α-demethylation, In vitro and In Vivo Evaluation of Antifungal Agents (K. Iwata, and H. Vanden Bossche, eds.) Elsevier Science Publishers, Amsterdam, p. 123 (1986).
22. H. Vanden Bossche, P. Marichal, J. Gorrens, H. Geerts, and P.A.J. Janssen, Mode of action studies basis for the search of new antifungal agents, Ann. N.Y. Acad. Sci., 544: 191 (1988).
23. N.Y. Ishida, Y. Aoyama, R. Hatanaka, Y. Oyama, S. Imajo, M. Ishiguro, T. Oshima, H. Nakazato, T. Noguchi, U.S. Maitra, V.P. Mohan, D.B. Sprinson, and Y. Yoshida, A single amino acid substitution converts cytochrome $P450_{14DM}$ to an inactive form, cytochrome $P450_{SG1}$: complete primary structures deduced from cloned DNA, Biochem. Biophys. Res. Commun., 155: 317 (1988)
24. Y. Aoyama, Y. Yoshida, Y. Sonoda,and Y. Sato, Metabolism of 32-hydroxy-24,25-dihydrolanosterol by purified cytochrome $P\text{-}450_{14DM}$ from yeast. Evidence for contribution of the cytochrome to whole process of

lanosterol 14α-demethylation, J. Biol. Chem., 262: 1239 (1987).
25. H. Vanden Bossche, G. Willemsens, W. Cools, W. Lauwers, and L. Le Jeune, Biochemical effects of miconazole on fungi. II. Inhibition of ergosterol biosynthesis in *Candida albicans*, Chem-Biol. Interact., 21: 59 (1978).
26. H. Vanden Bossche, G. Willemsens, W. Cools, F. Cornelissen, W. Lauwers, and J. Van Cutsem, In vitro and in vivo effects of the antimycotic drug ketoconazole on sterol synthesis, Antimicrob. Ag. Chemother., 17: 922 (1980).
27. P. Marichal, J. Gorrens, J. Van Cutsem, F. Van Gerven, and H. Vanden Bossche, Effects of ketoconazole and itraconazole on growth and sterol synthesis in *Pityrosporum ovale*, J. Med. Vet. Mycol., 24: 487 (1986).
28. P. Marichal, J. Gorrens, and H. Vanden Bossche, The action of itraconazole and ketoconazole on growth and sterol synthesis in *Aspergillus fumigatus* and *Aspergillus niger*, J. Med. Vet. Mycol., 23: 13 (1985).
29. P.F. Watson, M.E. Rose, and S.L. Kelly, Isolation and analysis of ketoconazole resistant mutants of *Saccharomyces cerevisiae*, J. Med. Vet. Mycol., 26: 153 (1988).
30. P.F. Watson, M.E. Rose, S.W. Ellis, H. Englannd, and S.L. Kelly Defective sterol C5-6 desaturation and azole resistance: a new hypothesis for the mode of action of azole antifungals, Biochem. Biophys. Res. Commun., 164: 1170 (1989)
31. J. Gallay, and B. Kruijff, Correlation between molecular shape and hexagonal H_{II} phase promoting ability of sterols, FEBS Lett., 143: 133 (1982).
32. K.E. Bloch, Sterol structure and membrane function, Crit. Rev. Biochem., 14: 47 (1983).
33. H. Vanden Bossche, Importance and role of sterols in fungal membranes, Biochemistry of Cell Walls and Membranes in Fungi (P.J. Kuhn , A.P.J. Trinci, M.J. Jung, M.W. Goosey L.G., and Copping, eds.), Springer Verlag,Berlin, p. 135 (1990).
34. L.W. Parks, D.K. Bottema, and R.J. Rodriguez, Physical and enzymatic function of ergosterol in fungal membranes, Isopentenoids in Plants. Biochemistry and Function (W.D. Nes, G. Fuller, and K-S. Tsai, eds.), Marcel Dekker, Inc, p. 433 (1984).
35. D.R. Soll, *Candida albicans*, Fungal Dimorphism (P.J. Szanislo, and J.L. Harris, eds.), Plemum Press, New York, London, p. 167 (1985).
36. Y.Y. Chiew, P.A. Sullivan, and M.G. Shepherd, The effects of ergosterol and alcohols on germ-tube formation and chitin synthase in *Candida albicans*, Can. J. Biochem., 60: 15 (1984).

37. M. Pesti, J.M. Campbell, J.F. Peberdy, Alteration of ergosterol content and chitin synthase activity in *Candida albicans*, Current. Microbiol., 5: 187 (1981).
38. D. Barug, R.A. Samson, and A. Kerkenaar, Microscopic studies of *Candida albicans* and *Torulopsis glabrata* after in vitro treatment with bifonazole, Arzneim.-Forsch., 33: 528 (1983).
39. D. Barug, C. de Groot, and R.A. Samson, Morphology and ultrastructure of *Candida albicans* after in vitro treatment with bifonazole, Recent Trends in the Discovery, Development and Evaluation of Antifungal Agents (R.A. Fromtling, ed.), JR Prous Science Publishers, S.A., Barcelona, p. 353, (1987)
40. S. De Nollin, and M. Borgers, Scanning electron microscopy of *Candida albicans* after in vitro treatment with miconazole, Antimicrob. Ag. Chemother., 7: 704 (1975).
41. H. Yamaguchi, Morphological aspects of azole action, Sterol biosynthesis inhibitors. Pharmaceutical and Agrochemical Aspects (D. Berg, and M. Plempel, eds.), Ellis Horwood Ltd., Chichester, England, p. 56 (1988).
42. H. Vanden Bossche, Mode of action of pyridine, pyrimidine and azole antifungals, Sterol biosynthesis inhibitors. Pharmaceutical and Agrochemical Aspects (D. Berg and M. Plempel, eds.), M Ellis Horwood Ltd., Chichester, England, p.79 (1988).
43. N.H. Georgopapadakou, B.A. Dix, S.A. Smith, J. Freudenberger, and P.T. Funke, Effect of antifungal agents on lipid biosynthesis and membrane integrity in *Candida albicans*, Antimicrob. Ag. Chem., 31: 46 (1987).
44. S. De Nollin, H. Van Belle, F. Goossens, F. Thoné, and M. Borgers, Cytochemical and biochemical studies of yeasts after in vitro exposure to miconazole, Antimicrob. Ag. Chemother., 11: 500 (1977).
45. M. Borgers, Mechanism of action of antifungal drugs with special reference to the imidazole derivatives. Rev. Infect. Dis., 2: 520 (1980).
46. D. Lloyd, The Mitochondria of Microorganisms, Academic Press, London, New York, p. 173 (1974).
47. P.Z. Margalith, Steroid Microbiology, Charles C. Thomas, Publisher, Sringfield, Illinois, p. 47 (1986).
48. H. Vanden Bossche, P. Marichal, J. Gorrens, M-C. Coene, G. Willemsens, D. Bellens, I. Roels, H. Moereels, and P.A.J. Janssen, Biochemical approaches to selective antifungal activity. Focus on azole antifungals, Mycoses, 32 (suppl. 1): 35 (1989).

4

Mechanism of Action of Allylamine Antifungal Drugs

Neil S. Ryder

Department of Dermatology
SANDOZ FORSCHUNGSINSTITUT
A-1235 Vienna, Austria

I. INTRODUCTION

The allylamines are a recently developed class of synthetic antifungal agents which inhibit the enzyme squalene epoxidase [1]. Extensive chemical derivatisation of naftifine, the prototype of the allylamines, has produced more than a thousand related compounds, many with significant antifungal activity [2,3]. Amongst these, terbinafine (Fig. 1) was selected as a potent antimycotic which is clinically effective after both topical and oral application (see article by Mieth & Villars, this volume. The biological and clinical properties of the allylamines have recently been reviewed [4]. Their distinguishing features include: primary fungicidal action against many fungi; extremely high activity against dermatophytes; more

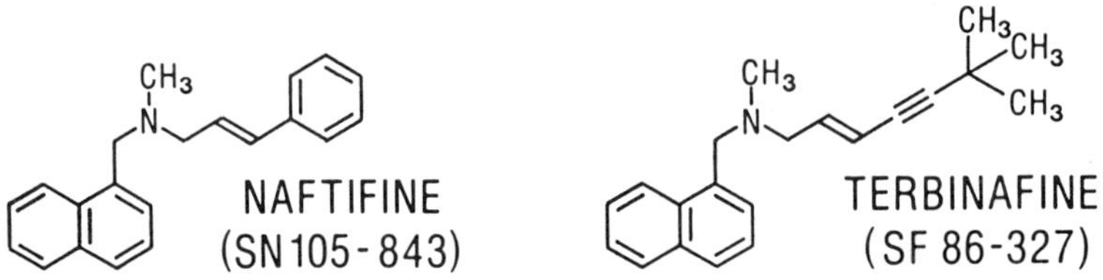

FIG. 1 Structures of naftifine and terbinafine

variable activity against yeasts; and a high degree of selectivity.- This report summarises our current understanding of the biochemical basis for these properties.

II. INHIBITION OF ERGOSTEROL BIOSYNTHESIS

Numerous experiments have demonstrated that the allylamines act as ergosterol biosynthesis inhibitors [5-7]. Ergosterol is essential for membrane integrity and growth in virtually all fungi, its importance being reflected in the fact that several other classes of antifungals also act on this pathway, including the azoles, morpholines and thiocarbamates. Fungal cells treated with naftifine or terbinafine rapidly become deficient in ergosterol and accumulate the intermediate squalene. The precursor sterols found in control cells disappear during this treatment [5], indicating that the inhibited step is prior to formation of the sterol backbone. The inhibition can be evaluated quantitatively in fungal cells by incorporation of radiolabelled acetate [5,6], or alternatively with methyl-labelled methionine which is specifically incorporated into the ergosterol side-chain [7]. While control cells incorporate acetate almost entirely into the ergosterol fraction of the nonsaponifiable lipids, those treated with an allylamine exhibit a dose-dependent inhibition of sterol biosynthesis and accumulate labelled squalene. A similar inhibition is observed using the sterol side-chain methylation technique, which also assesses the degree of residual biosynthesis occurring distal to the point of inhibition by methylation of endogenous sterol precursors [7]. The lack of inhibition of this residual activity by allylamines is evidence that only a single biosynthetic step is inhibited.

Direct inhibition of ergosterol biosynthesis by allylamines was confirmed by experiments with cell-free fractions from Candida. With labelled mevalonate as substrate, naftifine and terbinafine cause a dose-dependent inhibition of incorporation into the ergosterol fraction and accumulation of labelled squalene, qualitatively and quantitatively similar to the effect in whole cells [5,6]. Further experiments using labelled substrates entering early or late stages in the pathway [6] indicate that squalene epoxidase is the sole step inhibited by therapeutically relevant concentrations of allylamines, as confirmed by subsequent work with this enzyme.

III. MECHANISM OF FUNGAL GROWTH INHIBITION

A. COMPARISON OF DIFFERENT FUNGI

Ergosterol biosynthesis inhibition by allylamines has been observed in a range of pathogenic fungi, with qualitatively similar results. The dermatophytes are extremely sensitive to inhibition, showing ergosterol biosynthesis inhibition at terbinafine concentrations below 1 ng/ml, in agreement with their high suceptibility to allylamines. Comparing results from various different fungi (Table 1), there is a clear correlation between inhibition of fungal growth (expressed as the minimum inhibitory concentration, MIC) and of ergosterol biosynthesis. From Table 1 it is clear that ergosterol biosynthesis inhibition is not the sole factor determining susceptibility to allylamines, since the range of variation between MIC values is much greater than between sterol inhibitory concentrations. Factors which might influence susceptibility include the following:

1. Uptake into fungus. In Candida, drug concentrations required for sterol biosynthesis inhibition in whole cells are virtually identical to those in cell-free extracts, indicating that allylamines readily penetrate the Candida cell envelope. It is not known

TABLE 1

Terbinafine Concentrations (μg/ml) Inhibiting Fungal Growth (MIC) and Sterol Biosynthesis

Fungus	MIC	Sterol Biosynthesis 50 %	95 %
Trichophyton rubrum	0.003	0.0005	0.02
T.mentagrophytes	0.003	0.002	0.04
Aspergillus fumigatus	0.8	0.07	1.2
Candida parapsilosis	0.4	0.006	0.3
C. albicans	3.1	0.008	0.2
C. glabrata	100	0.04	0.9

Drug concentrations causing respectively 50 % and 95 % inhibition of sterol biosynthesis (mean of 3 experiments). Source: Ref. [10].

whether this is the case in other yeasts, or whether dermatophytes specifically accumulate allylamines.

2. **Sensitivity of target enzyme.** The importance of this factor is not clear, since it has not proved possible up to now to isolate squalene epoxidase from filamentous fungi. Enzyme sensitivity is not a decisive factor in determining susceptibility of different Candida species (Table 3).

3. **Rapidity of inhibition.** When measuring inhibition by the sterol side-chain methylation method, it was found that the degree of residual biosynthesis varied considerably between different fungi treated with terbinafine concentrations which fully blocked squalene epoxidation. This is presumably due to variation in the stocks of precursor sterols which different fungi maintain. The extent of this residual biosynthesis is inversely proportional to the susceptibility of the fungus to the drug [7, 10]. Thus in dermatophytes, which apparently have negligible reserves of precursors, terbinafine-induced blockade of ergosterol production will be almost instantaneous. This may play a role in the potent activity of allylamines.

4. **Susceptibility to lipid imbalance.** Membrane lipid composition and other physiological factors may strongly influence the effect of ergosterol deficiency and squalene accumulation on fungal growth and viability. For example, yeasts such as Saccharomyces which can grow anaerobically are able to adapt to such lipid imbalance and are indeed fairly resistant to allylamines. Such factors appear to be very important in determining fungal susceptibility to allylamines.

B. MECHANISM OF FUNGICIDAL ACTION

Naftifine, terbinafine and other allylamines show primary fungicidal action in vitro against dermatophytes, dimorphic and filamentous fungi [4]. The type of activity against yeasts is variable, being cidal against C. parapsilosis and static against C. albicans. The mechanism of fungicidal action is not obvious since many other ergosterol biosynthesis inhibitors have a fungistatic action. From the data in Table 1, fungi can be separated into two groups: (a) those in which the MIC is achieved with drug concentrations causing only partial inhibition of ergosterol biosynthesis, and (b) those in which the MIC appears to require total inhibition of ergosterol biosynthesis. Group (a) contains those fungi which are subject to cidal action. This suggests that ergosterol deficiency alone is not the cause of cell death and that squalene accumulation might be the critical factor. This is supported by studies of cell death, growth inhibition and lipid content in several fungi treated with naftifine or terbinafine [11]. In all cases, cell death is associated with a massive increase in intracellular squalene levels, as shown for Trichophyton in Fig. 2. Squalene would be expected to increase membrane fluidity, but the precise mechanism of its fungal toxicity is not understood and is still under investigation.

C. ACTIVITY AGAINST CANDIDA

Allylamines inhibit both growth and sterol biosynthesis in yeast cells of C. albicans (Table 1) and are clinically effective against this organism [4]. However, higher concentrations are required than

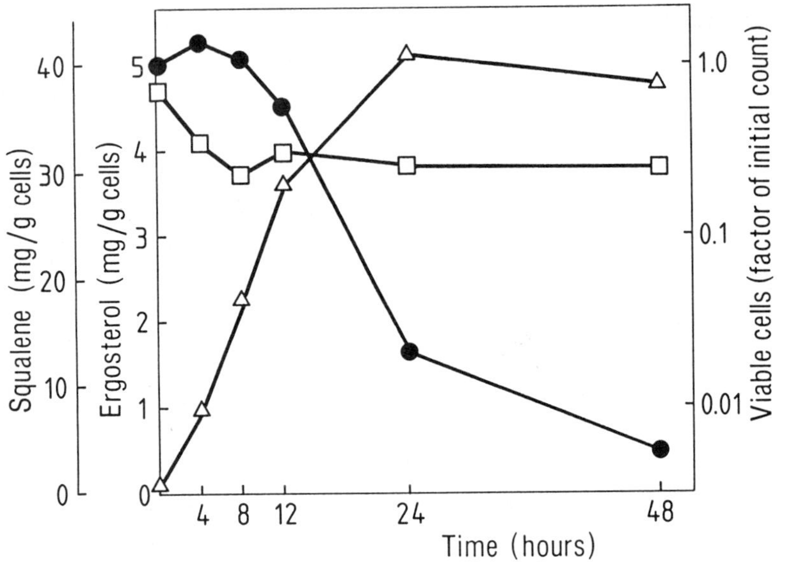

FIG. 2. Effect of terbinafine (3 ng/ml) on viable cell count (●), squalene content (△), and ergosterol content (□) in cells of T. mentagrophytes. Source: Ref. [11].

against dermatophytes, and the effect is generally fungistatic. The mycelial growth form, which is thought to be associated with pathogenicity and tissue invasion, is suppressed at drug concentrations much lower than the MIC for the yeast form [9, 12]. A system has recently been developed to provide pure mycelial form growing in a defined medium (N. S. Ryder & I. Frank, in preparation). In this system, the MIC for terbinafine is much lower in the mycelial than in the yeast form, while ergosterol biosynthesis in the two growth forms displays similar sensitivity to inhibition by terbinafine (Table 2). It appears that the mycelial growth form is more susceptible to disruption by inhibition of ergosterol biosynthesis, in agreement with the findings with other fungi (Table 1). Suppression of mycelial growth is probably fundamental to the clinical activity of the allylamines against C. albicans.

TABLE 2

Terbinafine Concentrations (μg/ml) Inhibiting Growth (MIC) and Sterol Biosynthesis in Yeast and Mycelial Forms of <u>C. albicans</u>

Growth form	MIC	Sterol Biosynthesis 50 %	Sterol Biosynthesis 95 %
Yeast	12.5	0.014	0.63
Mycelial	1.5	0.013	0.22

IV. SQUALENE EPOXIDASE INHIBITION

A. FUNGAL SQUALENE EPOXIDASE

Squalene epoxidase is a complex membrane-bound system requiring molecular oxygen, a source of reducing equivalents and phospholipids; its properties and inhibitors have recently been reviewed [13]. Naftifine and terbinafine are specific reversible inhibitors of the <u>Candida</u> epoxidase, showing non-competitive kinetics with respect to the squalene and cofactors FAD and NADH [8]. The solubilised enzyme is similarly inhibited by allylamines [9]. The potency of epoxidase inhibition by allylamines is sufficient to explain the ergosterol biosynthesis inhibition observed in <u>Candida</u> cells, and inhibitory concentrations of the drugs correlate well with their respective antifungal activities.

The mechanism of inhibition by the allylamines at the molecular level is not yet known. The inhibition is reversible and unlikely to be of the mechanism-based type. The compounds are also unlikely to be acting as analogues of squalene [13], in view of their kinetics and high degree of selectivity. Two possible models for an inhibitory mechanism have been developed [13, 14]. The allylamines might interact with an essential lipid domain of the enzyme, the activity of which is known to be modulated <u>in vitro</u> by both phospholipids and fatty acids [13]. Our current working model envisages that the

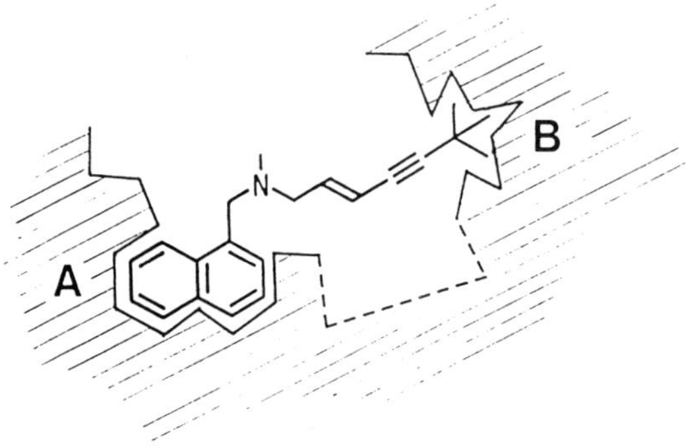

FIG. 3. Hypothetical model for inhibition of squalene epoxidase by terbinafine. The naphthalene ring interacts with squalene-binding site (A) while the side-chain binds to adjacent lipophilic site (B). Source: Ref. [14].

inhibitor might interact simultaneously with both the squalene binding site and a second lipophilic site (Fig. 3), to provide potent inhibition by the principle of entropic binding [14].

B. MAMMALIAN SQUALENE EPOXIDASE

Squalene epoxidase is also involved in the biosynthesis of cholesterol in mammals, and the fungal and mammalian enzymes have quite similar properties [13]. However, in a cell-free cholesterol biosynthesis system from rat liver [6, 15], naftifine and terbinafine showed only weak inhibitory activity at high concentrations. Later studies confirmed that orally applied terbinafine has no effect on cholesterol levels in animals or in humans. It is now known that this selectivity originates from differences at the enzymatic level. There are both qualitative and quantitative differences between the effects of terbinafine on the fungal and mammalian epoxidases [8, 9, 13]. The rat liver squalene epoxidase is orders of magnitude less sensitive than the Candida enzyme to inhibition by allylamines (Table 3). The effect of terbinafine on the rat liver epoxidase is

TABLE 3

Inhibition of Fungal and Mammalian Squalene Epoxidase

Compound	C. albicans	C.paraps.	Rat liver
Naftifine	1.1	0.34	144
Terbinafine	0.03	0.04	93
SDZ 87-469	0.01	0.02	16
Benzylamine 880-349	0.045	-	-

Concentrations (μM) for 50 % inhibition. Source: Refs [11, 23].

reversible, competitive with respect to squalene, and antagonised competitively by soluble cytoplasmic factors present in liver [9]. The nature of the difference between fungal and mammalian epoxidases responsible for this selectivity is not yet clear, but might involve differences in orientation of the two binding sites in the hypothetical model described above.

A further important point is that squalene epoxidase is not an enzyme of the cytochrome P-450 superfamily [13], so that allylamines, unlike azoles, have no intrinsic tendency to inhibit this very important class of enzymes [16].

C. STRUCTURAL REQUIREMENTS FOR EPOXIDASE INHIBITION

All the antifungally active allylamines which have been tested, of various structural types, have been found to inhibit squalene epoxidase, indicating that epoxidase inhibition is a prerequisite for activity of the allylamines. However, as discussed above, many other factors play a role in determining antifungal activity even *in vitro*. Some effective epoxidase inhibitors have only poor antifungal activity, probably on account of instability or lack of uptake into fungal cells. The carbon analogue of terbinafine is an example of this; despite good inhibition of the epoxidase, it is not readily taken up by fungi and has little antifungal activity [3]. This

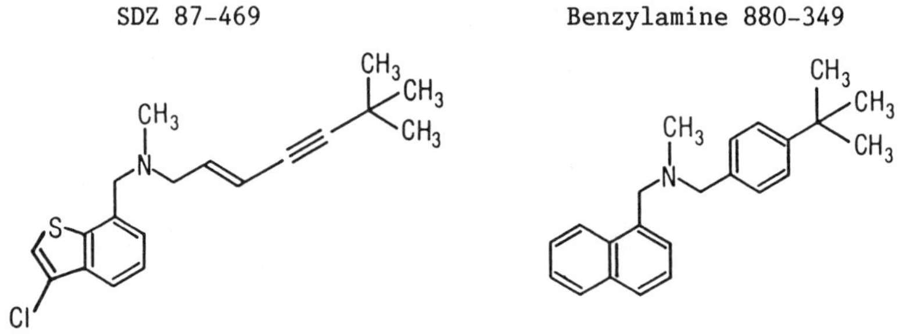

FIG. 4. Structures of SDZ 87-469 and the benzylamine 880-349.

compound is of interest in demonstrating that the nitrogen of the side-chain is not required for epoxidase inhibition. The allylamines were originally so named for the existence of this function in their side-chain, but it is now clear that neither the nitrogen nor the double bond are strictly necessary for epoxidase inhibition [3]. The benzylamine derivative 880-349 (Fig. 4) shows a further possible structural type of epoxidase inhibitor (Table 3). Some modification of the ring system is also permitted, as shown by the 3-chloro-7-benzo[b]thienyl derivative SDZ 87-469 (Fig. 4) which is a highly potent inhibitor (Table 3). The structure-activity relationships of the allylamines are consistent with the 2-site model of epoxidase inhibition, in particular the requirement for a minimum length of side-chain, which would provide the bridge between the two binding regions of the inhibitor.

V. REFERENCES

1. G. Petranyi, N. S. Ryder, A. Stütz, Allylamine derivatives: new class of synthetic antifungal agents inhibiting fungal squalene epoxidase, Science, 224: 1239 (1984).

2. A. Stütz, Synthesis and structure-activity correlations within allylamine antimycotics, Ann. N. Y. Acad. Sci., 544: 46 (1988).

3. P. Nussbaumer, N. S. Ryder, A. Stütz, Allylamine antimycotics: recent trends in structure-activity relationships and syntheses, Pestic. Sci. (in press).

4. N. S. Ryder, H. Mieth, Allylamine antifungal drugs, Curr. Top. Med. Mycol., 4: (in press).

5. N. S. Ryder, G. Seidl, P. F. Troke, Effect of the antimycotic drug naftifine on growth of and sterol biosynthesis in Candida albicans, Antimicrob. Agents Chemother., 25: 483 (1984).

6. N. S. Ryder, Specific inhibition of fungal sterol biosynthesis by SF 86-327, a new allylamine antimycotic agent, Antimicrob. Agents Chemother., 27: 252 (1985).

7. N. S. Ryder, Effect of allylamine antimycotic agents on fungal sterol biosynthesis measured by sterol side-chain methylation, J. Gen. Microbiol., 131: 1595 (1985).

8. N. S. Ryder, M.-C. Dupont, Inhibition of squalene epoxidase by allylamine antimycotic compounds: a comparative study of the fungal and mammalian enzymes, Biochem. J., 230: 765 (1985).

9. N. S. Ryder, Squalene epoxidase as the target of antifungal allylamines, Pestic. Sci., 21: 281 (1987).

10. N. S. Ryder, Mechanism of action of the allylamine antimycotics, Recent Trends in the Discovery, Development and Evaluation of Antifungal Agents (R. A. Fromtling, ed.) J. R. Prous Science Publishers, Barcelona, p. 451 (1987).

11. N. S. Ryder, G. Seidl, G. Petranyi, A. Stütz, Mechanism of the fungicidal action of SF 86-327, a new allylamine antimycotic agent, Recent Advances in Chemotherapy (J. Ishigami, ed.), University of Tokyo Press, Tokyo, p. 2558 (1985).

12. M. Schaude, H. Ackerbauer, H. Mieth, Inhibitory effect of antifungal agents on germ tube formation in Candida albicans, Mykosen, 30: 281 (1987).

13. N. S. Ryder, Squalene epoxidase: enzymology and inhibition, Biochemistry of Cell Walls and Membranes in Fungi, (P. J. Kuhn, A. P. J. Trinci, M. J. Jung, M. W. Goosey, L. G. Copping, eds.), Springer-Verlag, Berlin, p. 189 (1990).

14. N. S. Ryder, Inhibition of squalene epoxidase and sterol side-chain methylation by allylamines, Biochem. Soc. Trans., 18: 45 (1990).

15. N. S. Ryder, Mechanism of action and biochemical selectivity of allylamine antimycotic agents, Ann. N. Y. Acad. Sci., 544: 208 (1988).

16. I. Schuster, The interaction of representative members from two classes of antimycotics - the azoles and the allylamines - with cytochromes P-450 in steroidogenic tissues and liver, Xenobiotica, 15: 529 (1985).

5

Biochemical Aspects of Squalene Epoxidase Inhibition by a Thiocarbamate Derivative, Naphthiomate-T

Y.Nozawa and T.Morita

Department of Biochemistry
Gifu University School of Medicine
Gifu 500, Japan

I. INTRODUCTION

The clinical importance of fungal infections has greatly stimulated the interest in the study of the mechanism of action of the antifungal agents. Indeed, during the last decade numerous works have been done for imidazole derivatives focusing on the biochemical aspects of their abilities to inhibit the ergosterol biosynthesis (1-5). It is now widely accepted that the imidazole derivatives interfere with the sterol interconversion at the step of microsomal p-450-dependent lanosterol 14C-demethylase. It has been shown that ergosterol biosynthesis inhibition of azole derivatives originates from binding of azole moiety to the iron atom in the protoporphyrin moiety in cytochrome p-450 (6, 7), Thus such interaction results in a depletion of ergosterol coinciding with an accumulation of lanosterol and other 14C-methylsterols. The decreased availability of ergosterol together with the accumulation of 14C-methylsterols greatly disturbs the permeability of plasma membranes and the activity of membrane bound enzymes (1). On the other hand, a thiocarbamate antifungal agent, naphthiomate-T (Fig. 1) which was invented by Noguchi (8), has for many years been used clinically for topical treatment of skin infections (9), but there has been relatively limited information on the mechanism of its action. Although several modes of action have been proposed for the antifungal activity of naphthiomate-T such as inhibitions of RNA, DNA synthesis (10) and cell wall formation (11), none of them was sufficient to explain its antifungal activity. Recently, this drug was found to block ergosterol biosynthesis in several fungi, including *T. mentagrophytes* and *C. albicans*, by acting at the point of squalene epoxidase (12-16).

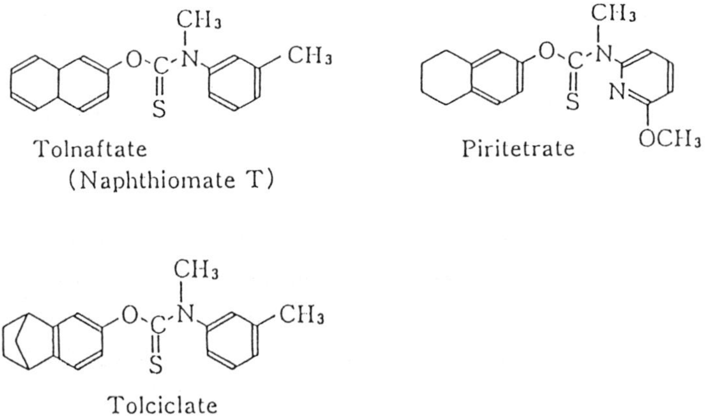

FIG. 1. Chemical structures of thiocarbamate antifungals

II. INHIBITORY EFFECT OF THIOCARBAMATES ON ERGOSTEROL BIOSYNTHESIS

A. Effect of naphthiomate-T on fungal ergosterol biosynthesis in whole cells

In order to examine the effects of naphthiomate-T on ergosterol biosynthesis, the incorporation of radioactivity into sterols and their intermediates was examined for fungal cells labeled with [^{14}C] acetate for 2 hr. Table 1 shows the distribution of radioactivity in unsaponifiable fractions analysed by gas-liquid chromatography. It was shown that naphthiomate-T caused a marked accumulation of radioactivity in squalene and a reduced radioactivity in sterol fractions in T. mentagrophytes and C. albicans (12). In T. mentagrophytes, a great increase of radioactivity was observed in squalene (83.5%) with a considerable decrease of radioactivity in ergosterol and 4,14-dimethylzymosterol as compared to the untreated control. Similar but smaller effects were observed in C. albicans ; 44.1% in squalene and 23.3% in ergosterol. These results indicate evidence that inhibition of ergosterol biosynthesis by naphthiomate-T is due to interference with squalene epoxidase activity, by interaction with either the enzyme or its soluble activator (17). It is to be noted that ergosterol biosynthesis in fungi cannot be discussed in terms of a single pathway. Instead, it appears that most fungi produce ergosterol by several alternative routes (18). Fig. 2 displays the typical but simplified pathways of ergosterol biosynthesis in fungi under normal growth conditions and when exposed to antifungal agents. As shown in Fig. 2, in contrast to the imidazole antifungal agent, miconazole which inhibits ergosterol formation at the step of sterol interconversion (e.g., 14C-demethylation)(1), naphthiomate-T blocks the utilization of squalene by blockage of squalene epoxidation.

A previous report of MIC indicated that naphthiomate-T exhibited a greater antifungal activity against dermatophytes than C. albicans (19). Thus, the superior efficacy of naphthiomate-T to T. mentagrophytes was reflected in its higher potency in the inhibition of sterol biosynthesis.

TABLE 1. Effects of naphthiomate-T and miconazole on (^{14}C)-acetate incorporation into fungal sterols

	Squalene	Lano-sterol	24-MDL	4,14-DMZ	Ergo-sterol	Others
Trichophyton mentagrophytes				(%)		
Control	2.8	1.8	9.1	30.7	38.1	17.5
Naphthiomate-T (100 ng/ml)	83.5	0.2	1.0	0.5	1.5	12.7
Miconazole (10 ng/ml)	trace	9.6	74.8	0.9	3.5	12.7
Candida albicans						
Control	0.8	4.4	13.3	16.9	50.0	14.7
Naphthiomate-T (100 ng/ml)	44.1	1.2	2.7	9.6	23.3	19.1
Miconazole (10 ng/ml)	5.9	50.5	15.8	7.5	6.9	13.2

MDL ; methylenedihydrolanosterol, DMZ ; dimethylzymosterol (From Ref. 12)

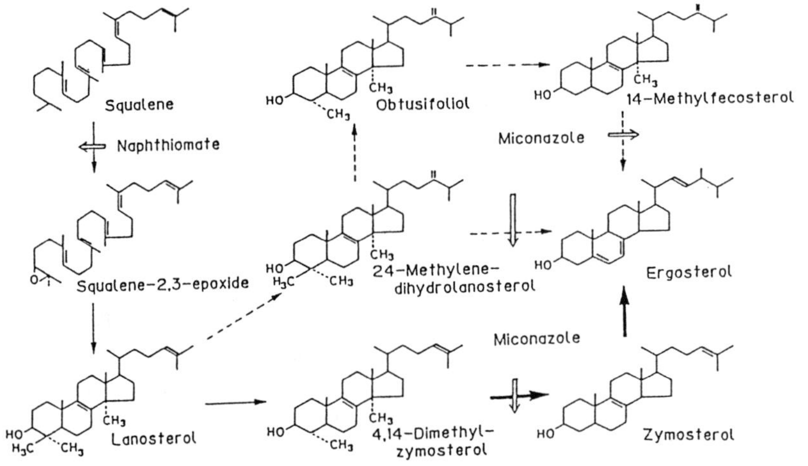

FIG. 2. Metabolic pathways of ergosterol biosynthesis and sites of action of naphthiomate-T and miconazole in the fungal cell (From Ref. 12)

B. Effect of naphthiomate-T on ergosterol biosynthesis in cell-free system of T. mentagrophytes

The cell-free system was employed to define the exact primary site of action of naphthiomate-T in the ergosterol biosynthesis of T. mentagrophytes. Not much data has been obtained with the cell-free system of dermatophytes, because some of the enzymes involved in the later steps of ergosterol biosynthesis are labile (20) and effective disruption of fungal cells is difficult. In the present experiment, therefore, we have prepared the cell-free fraction by disrupting cells in a high power-ultrasonic disintegrator followed by centrifugation at 10,000 xg for 20 min. Thus, the freshly prepared cell-free fraction (S_{10} fraction, 30 mg protein/ml) was used for examination of ergosterol biosynthesis. Ergosterol biosynthesis was examined by a modification of the method previously described by Kato and Kawase (21). After 3 hr incubation with $[^{14}C]$ mevalonate at 30°C, unsaponifiable components were extracted with petroleum ether and incorporation of $[^{14}C]$ radioactivity into sterols and their precursors was analyzed by thin layer chromatography (Silica gel 60 F_{254}). As shown in Fig. 3, there was a dose-dependent reduction in the radioactivity in the sterol fractions (4,4',14-trimethyl, 4,14-dimethyl and 4-desmethylsterols) and a concomitant increase in the squalene fraction. Thus, naphthiomate-T showed the inhibitory effect on squalene epoxidation in the cell-free system of T. mentagrophytes. The squalene epoxidation is one of essential early reactions for biosynthesis of cholesterol in mammalians as well as ergosterol in fungi. Therefore, the effect of naphthiomate-T on cholesterol biosynthesis was also investigated in the S_{10} fraction (15 mg protein/ml) isolated from rat liver. No significant change in the cholesterol metabolism was observed even at the concentration of the drug up to 5 x 10^{-4}M indicating the different sensitivity toward mammalian squalene epoxidase and fungal one (data not shown). This selective sensitivity is advantageous for therapeutic application.

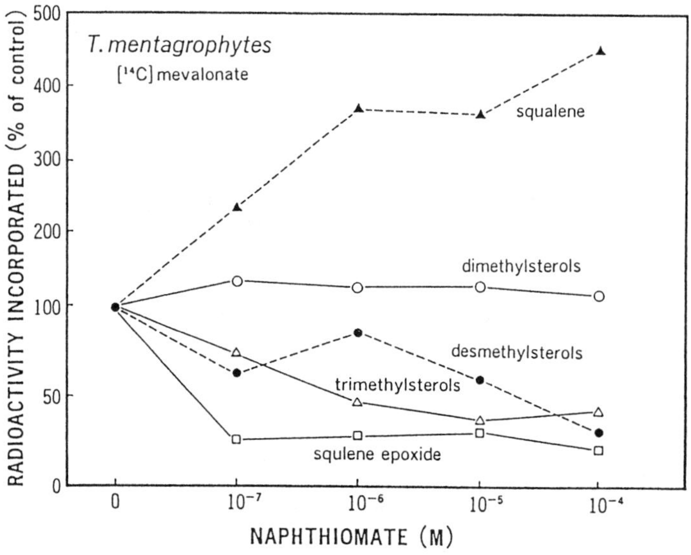

FIG. 3. Effect of naphthiomate-T on ergosterol biosynthesis in cell-free system of T. memtagophytes

C. Effect of naphthiomate-T on microsomal squalene epoxidase

All available experimental evidence mentioned above strongly indicates that the squalene epoxidation is the primary site of action of naphthiomate-T. Squalene epoxidase was well characterized for microsomes of C. albicans (17) and rat liver (22), and it is known that the enzyme requires molecular oxygen, FAD, and NADPH (for fungal microsomes) or NADH (for liver microsomes). Ryder et al. (17) have demonstrated that the squalene epoxidase from rat liver differs from the fungal enzyme in having a strong requirement for a specific factor in the cytoplasmic soluble fraction. In order to reinforce the evidence for the inhibition of squalene epoxidase by naphthiomate-T, the squalene epoxidase activity was examined in the microsomal fractions from C. albicans and rat liver. As shown in Fig. 4

naphthiomate-T exerted a dose-dependent inhibition of squalene epoxidase from C. albicans cells and the fifty percent inhibition was achieved at concentration of 5 x 10^{-6}M (23). It was also shown that the inhibiting potency of naphthiomate-T was not affected by the presence of cytoplasmic soluble fraction (23). In contrast to squalene epoxidase in C. albicans microsomes, naphthiomate-T was found to be less sensitive to the rat liver microsomal enzyme. Elucidation of such difference in the drug sensitivity has to await the comparison of molecular structures of squalene epoxidases from mammalian and fungal microsomes.

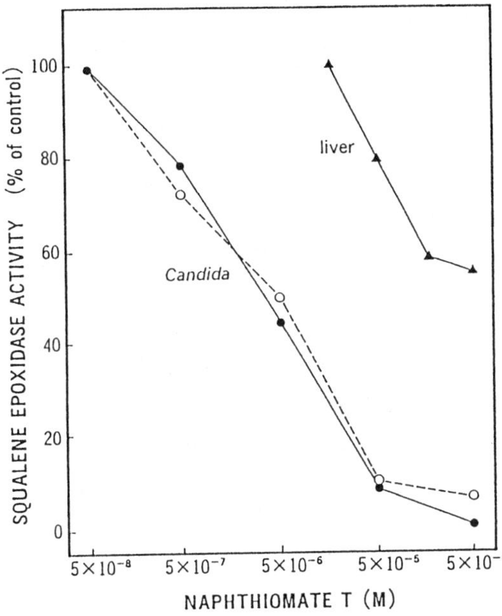

FIG. 4. Effect of naphthiomate-T on squalene epoxidase in miconazole fractions of C. albicans and rat liver (From Ref. 23)
C. albicans microsomes : in the presence (—●—) or absence (--O--) of soluble fraction.

III. EFFECT OF NAPHTHIOMATE-T ON MEMBRANE PHYSICAL STATES

It is widely accepted that sterol is an essential component to serve as an efficient bioregulator of membrane fluidity, and also that the physical state of membrane lipids is closely associated with membrane functions. It was thus postulated that the naphthiomate-T-induced alterations in membrane lipid composition may affect membrane fluidity. There was no significant change in the proportional composition of phospholipids of plasma membranes isolated from C. albicans treated with naphthiomate-T (18). However, the fatty acyl chain composition of the plasma membrane phospholipid fraction was altered by exposure to the antifungal drug. The main saturated fatty acid, palmitic acid (C16:0) was increased whereas oleic acid (C18:1) was decreased (18). Such alterations lead to the lower unsaturation index (U.I.). Two possibilities were suggested to explain this finding; inhibition of chain elongation of palmitic to stearic acid and inhibition of unsaturation of stearic to oleic acid via desaturase. The latter mechanism seems more likely but further investigations should be required to define the precise mechanism.

Then, we have measured the order parameters of plasma membranes by electron spin resonance (ESR) using 5-SAL probe. Small but significant decreases were observed in the parameter value in naphthiomate-T-treated C. albicans, indicating the enhanced membrane fluidity. Furthermore, we have examined effects of ergosterol, lanosterol and squalene which were changed in the content on the membrane fluidity (Fig. 5). Ergosterol and lanosterol showed progressive decreases in the fluidity as a function of concentration, with the latter sterol being less effective. In contrast, squalene did not exert any compacting effect on membranes. Therefore, accumulation of squalene may cause some damage in the membrane functions. Janos et al. (24) indicated that increased squalene enhanced the membrane permeability leading to disintegration of cellular organization. In our experiments, the activities of chitin synthetase and β-1,3 glucan synthetase in isolated plasma membranes were not affected in C. albicans exposed to naphthiomate-T. However, further work should be performed to disclose the effects of membrane disorganization due to accumulation of squalene and reduced ergosterol availability.

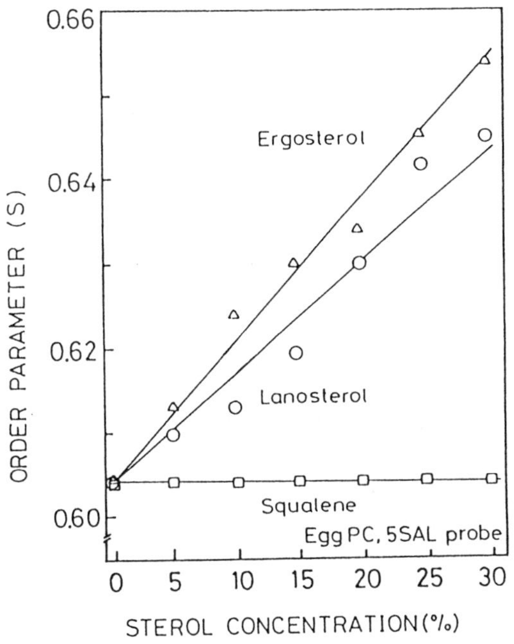

FIG. 5. Order parameters of egg PC liposomes containing ergosterol, lanosterol and squalene (From Ref. 13)

IV. EPILOGUE

A thiocarbamate antifungal agent, naphthiomate-T exerts a selective and potent inhibition on squalene epoxidase of microsomes (endoplasmic reticulum) in C. albicans and T. mentagrophytes. Compared to rat liver microsomes, the fungal microsomes show a preferential sensitivity toward the antifungal agent. This marked difference in the sensitivity provides a great benefit for the therapeutic applicaion. However, to understand the mechanism underlying such distinct selectivity, further studies at the molecular level including cDNA cloning should be performed for squalene epoxidase from mammalian and fungal microsomes.

REFERENCES

1) H.Vanden Bossche, G.Willemsens, W.Cools, W.F.J.Lauwers, and L.Le Jeune, Biochemical effects of miconazole on fungi, II. Inhibition of ergosterol biosynthesis in Candida albicans, Chem.Biol. Interact., 21:59 (1978).
2) H. Vanden Bossche, G. Willemsens, P.Marichal, W.Cools, and W.Lauwers, The molecular basis for the antifungal activities of N-substituted azole derivatives: Focus on R51211, Mode of Action of Antifungal Agents (M.R. McGiniss, ed.), Springer-Verlag, New York, p.321 (1984).
3) H.Vanden Bossche, Itraconazole, a selective inhibitor of the cytochrome p-450 dependent ergosterol biosynthesis, Recent Trend in the Discovery, Development and Evaluation of Antifungal Agents (R.A. Fromtling, ed.), Prous Scientific Publ, p.207 (1987).
4) H. Yamaguchi, Advances in research of mechanism of imidazole-antimycotic action, Filamentous Microorganisms. Biochemical Aspects (T.Arai, ed.) Japan Scientific Societies Press, Tokyo, p.355 (1985).
5) H.Vanden Bossche, Biochemical target for antifungal azole derivatives: hypothesis on the mode of action, Current Topics in Medical Mycology (M.R.Mcginnis, ed.), Springer-Verlag, New York, p.313 (1985).
6) Y. Yoshida, and Y.Aoyama, Yeast cytochrome p-450 catalyzing lanosterol 14C-demethylation, I. Purification and spectral properties, J.Biol.Chem., 259:1655 (1984).
7) Y. Aoyama, Y. Yoshida, and R. Sato, Yeast cytochrome p-450 catalyzing lanosterol 14C demethylase, II. Lanosterol metabolism by purified P-450 and by intact microsomes, J.Biol.Chem., 259: 1661 (1984).
8) T.Noguchi, A.Kaji, Y.Igarashi, A.Shigematsu, and K.Taniguchi, 1963. Antitrichophyton activities of naphthiomates, Antimicrob.Agents Chemother., p.259 (1962).
9) G.Hildick-Smith, Antifungal agent, Adv.Biol.Skin, 12:303 (1981).

10) T.Nishino, Y.Okano, Y.Isogawa, T.Koshi, and T.Tanino, Antimycotic studies on tolciclate, Chemother. (Tokyo), 29:1304 (1981).

11) T.Hiratani, H.Yamaguchi, E.Uchida, Y.Osumi, S.Watanabe, K. Okuzumi, H.Yamani, N.Tanaka, Y.Yamamoto, and K.Iwata, Mechanism of action of antifungal agents-Biochemical study, Jpn.J.Med.Mycol., 24:194 (1983).

12) T.Morita, and Y.Nozawa, Effects of antifungalagents on ergosterol biosynthesis in Candida albicans and Trichophyton mentagrophytes: Differential inhibitory sites of naphthiomate and miconazole, J.Invest.Dermatol., 85:434 (1985).

13) Y.Nozawa, and T.Morita, Molecular mechanisms of antifungal agents associated with membrane ergosterol: Dysfunction of membrane ergosterol and inhibition of ergosterol biosynthesis, In Vitro and In Vivo Evaluation of Antifungal Agents (K.Iwata, and H.Van den Bossche, ed,), Elsevier Science Publishers, B.V., p.111 (1986).

14) T.Morita, K.Iwata, and Y.Nozawa, Inhibitory effect of a new mycotic agent, piritetrate on ergosterol biosynthesis in pathogenic fungi, J.Med.Vet.Mycol., 27:17 (1989).

15) K.J.Barrett-Bee, A.C.Lane, and R.W.Turner, The mode of action of tolnaftate, J.Med.Vet.Mycol., 24:155 (1986).

16) N.S.Ryder, F.Ingerborg, and M.C.Dupont, Ergosterol biosynthesis inhibition by the thiocarbamate antifungal agents, tolnaftate and tolciclate, Antimicrob.Agents Chemother., 29:858 (1986).

17) N.S.Ryder, M.C.Dupont, Properties of a particulate squalene epoxidase for Candida albicans, Biochim.Biophys.Acta, 794:466 (1984).

18) J.D.Weete, Pathway of ergosterol biosynthesis, Lipid Biochemistry of Fungi and Other Organisms (J.D.Weete, ed.), Plenum Press, New York, p.282 (1980).

19) A.Capek, A.Simek, L.Bruna, V.Janata, and Z.Budesinsky, Antimicrobial agents, Fol. Microbiol., 17:396 (1972).

20) N.S.Ryder, Mode of action of allylamines, Sterol Biosynthesis Inhibitor (D.Berg, and M.Plempel, ed.) Ellis Horwood, p.151 (1988).

21) T.Kato, and Y.Kawase, Selective inhibition of the demethylation at C-14 in ergosterol biosynthesis by fungicide, Denmert (S-1358), Agr.Biol.Chem., 40:2379 (1976).

22) T.Ono, S.Ozawa, F.Hasegawa, and Y.Imai, Involvment of NADPH-cytochrome C reductase in rat liver squalene epoxidase system, Biochim.Biophys.Acta, 486:401 (1977).

23) T.Morita, and Y. Nozawa, The nature of squalene epoxidase inhibition by thiocarbamate derivative, naphthiomate-T, Jpn. J.Med.Mycol., 27:239 (1986).

24) K.L.Janos, Z.P.William, and K.Moris, Lipid interactions in membranes of extremely halophilic bacteria. II. Modification of the bilayer structure by squalene, Biochemistry, 13:4914 (1974).

6

Amphotericin B: Studies Focused on Improving Its Therapeutic Efficacy

J. Brajtburg[1], I. Gruda[2], and G.S. Kobayashi[1]

[1]*Department of Medicine*
Washington University School of Medicine
St. Louis, Missouri, USA 63110

[2]*University of Quebec, Trois Rivieres, Canada*

I. INTRODUCTION

At the present time amphotericin B (AmB), a heptaene macrolide, is the most effective antifungal agent used in the treatment of systemic fungal infections. However, toxicity to host cells and problems associated with its solubility and delivery limit its clinical usefulness. The cellular effects of AmB are complex and depend on the conditions used to evaluate its activity. With reasonable approximation it can be proposed that these effects occur in three dose dependent stages: (i) stimulatory - observed at the lowest concentrations of AmB and seen as adjuvant and immunological effects; (ii) permeabilization - occur at

[1]This study was supported in part by grants from the National Institutes of Health, USA, AI 25903, T32 AI 07015 and N01-AI72640 and the Engineering Council of Canada.

intermediate concentrations and can be monitored as a decrease in the retention of potassium by cells; and (iii) lysis or lethality - occurs at higher concentrations and are measured as lytic (erythrocytes) or killing (yeast cells) effects (for review see ref. 1).

The binding of AmB to sterols incorporated in cell membranes followed by disorganization of the membrane that result in increased permeability to ions and small molecules is considered the basic mechanism of its action. However, available data indicate that cell lysis or death could not be attributed solely to changes in membrane permeability. Since AmB can autooxidize and give rise to active forms of oxygen, we postulated that an oxidation dependent damage is an additional mechanism involved in the lytic or lethal effects of AmB on cells.

The diversity of AmB effects potentially leads to various novel approaches that can be exploited to improve its therapeutic efficacy: (i) facilitate entry of other antifungal drugs into cells by utilizing its permeabilizing activity; (ii) increase its lytic or lethal activity by modulating the involvement of oxidative dependent damage; and (iii) potentiate its selective toxicity to fungal cells.

Here we present our recent research on:

1. synergistic antifungal interaction of AmB and quinolones
2. effects of pro-oxidant and scavengers on AmB induced cell lysis or death
3. effects of detergents on AmB binding to sterols and toxicity to cells and animals

II. SYNERGISTIC ANTIFUNGAL INTERACTION OF AmB AND QUINOLONES

In the treatment of cryptococcal meningitis, the combination of AmB with 5-fluorocytosine is based on permeabilization of fungal cells by AmB with resultant increased uptake of 5-fluorocytosine. Potentiating uptake of second agent by using AmB to increase fungal cell membrane permeability has also been shown with other drugs (2). We are currently investigating the antifungal action of AmB and quinolones. Nalidixic acid, the first quinolone to be used clinically, has been found to have weak antifungal activity, whereas its analogues, ciprofloxacin and norfloxacin, do not demonstrate this property. We attributed the insensitive of yeast cells to quinolones to the lack of uptake and predicted that treatment of fungal cells with AmB would render them permeable to quinolones.

It has been reported that high concentrations of norfloxacin enhanced the inhibition of <u>Candida albicans</u> by AmB, however, in a recent study with AmB and either norfloxacin or ciproflaxacin no specific interaction or even antagonism was observed (3). Since quinolones act by inhibiting DNA gyrase, an enzyme from the family of topoisomerases responsible for maintaining bacterial and eukaryotic chromosomes in a spatial state necessary for DNA replication, and since fungi have a long generation time, we hypothesized that cell growth would have to be monitored over several days in order to demonstrate the combined effects of AmB and quinolones on fungi. Therefore, in our assays we used small initial inocula of fungal cells, added both the drugs to be assayed and then monitored growth over a period of several days by changes in optical density. When the difference between the control and drug-treated cultures were the most pronounced, samples were plated on Sabouraud agar and cell viability was determined by colony counts. Using these procedures, we assayed 5 quinolones alone and in combination with AmB against <u>C. albicans</u>, <u>Cryptococcus neoformans</u>, and <u>Saccharomyces cerevisiae</u> (Table I).

TABLE I. Chemical and physical properties of quinolones tested (4)

QUINOLONE	HYDROPHOBICITY*	MOL. WT.	IONIC TYPE
ENOXACIN	0.007	320.3	AMPHOTERIC
NORFLOXACIN	0.01	319.3	AMPHOTERIC
CIPROFLOXACIN	0.02	331.3	AMPHOTERIC
OFLOXACIN	0.33	360.4	AMPHOTERIC
NALIDIXIC ACID	3.92	232.2	ACIDIC

*Given in octanol: water partitioning coefficient

The greatest effects on growth were seen after 3 days exposure for <u>C. albicans</u> and <u>S. cerevisiae</u> and 7 days for <u>C. neoformans</u>. Figure 1 illustrates a representative example from our pool of data.

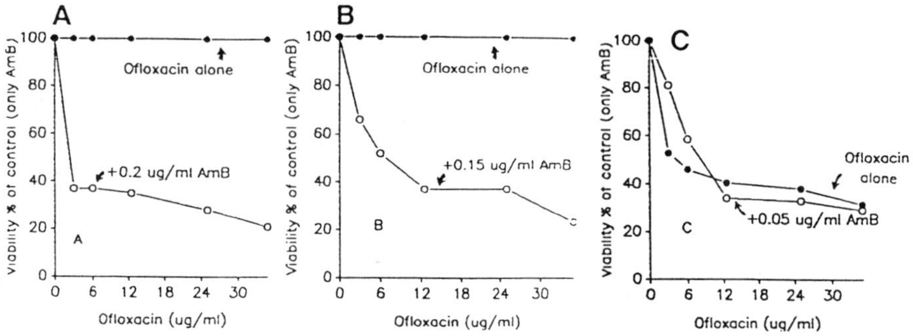

FIGURE 1. Effects of ofloxacin used alone and in combination with AmB on viability of S. cerevisiae (A), C. albicans (B), and C. neoformans (C).

Ofloxacin had no effect on either C. albicans or S. cerevisiae when used alone but when combined with AmB a synergistic effect was observed (Figure 1A and 1B). On the other hand, ofloxacin alone was toxic for C. neoformans and addition of AmB did not did not enhance this effect (Figure 1C).

Nalidixic acid, the only acidic compound assayed, was toxic to S. cerevisiae and C. neoformans but not C. albicans when used alone. As a result the combination of nalidixic acid and AmB caused a pronounced synergistic interaction using C. albicans but not with the other two organisms. When used as single agents the four amphoteric quinolones had no effect on S. cerevisiae and C. albicans when used alone but had a pronounced synergistic interaction in the presence of AmB. On the other hand, the amphoteric quinolones were toxic to C. neoformans when used alone, as a result the addition of AmB did not cause a significant increase in toxicity. The molecular size of the quinolones, which varied from 319 for norfloxacin to 360 for ofloxacin, did not appear to influence the antifungal activity of these agents either alone or when used in combination with AmB. Furthermore, there was no correlation between the hydrophobicity of the amphoteric quinolones and their synergistic antifungal combination with AmB.

III. EFFECTS OF PRO-OXIDANTS AND SCAVENGERS OF ACTIVE FORMS OF OXYGEN ON AmB-INDUCED CELL LYSIS OR DEATH

Evidence for the role of active oxygen species in the lytic or lethal action of AmB was obtained from experiments which showed that AmB injury to cells could be modulated by extracellular scavengers, or prooxidants (5,6). In these experiments, hemolysis of erythrocytes and lysis of protoplasts caused by AmB could be inhibited by extracellular catalase and potentiated in the presence of ascorbic acid but catalase and ascorbic acid had no effect on K^+ leakage from cells. These observations indicate that changes in membrane permeability are not linked to oxidative cell damage (for references see review 1).

We further showed that ascorbic acid enhanced the lethal but not the permeabilizing effects of AmB on C. albicans and C. neoformans (7). Two other ene-diol acids, D-erythorbic and dihydroxyfumaric, also enhanced the antifungal effects of AmB. We proposed that ascorbic acid and the ene-diol acids, acting as pro-oxidants, augmented the AmB-induced oxidative dependent killing of fungal cells. This assumption was recently supported by our finding that potentiation of C. albicans cell sensitivity to AmB lethality by ascorbic acid correlated with the effects of ascorbic acid on decrease in cellular catalase levels.

If AmB-induced cell damage is linked to the generation of reactive forms of oxygen, the ability to decompose them should affect cell resistance to damage. In support of this notion, erythrocytes from AKR mice with higher levels of catalase activity were less sensitive to lysis by AmB than erythrocytes from C57Bl/6 mice which had lower levels of catalase activity. These in vitro results correlated very well with in vivo characterization. AKR mice with the higher intracellular catalase levels were more resistant to the toxic effects of AmB than the C57Bl/6 mice (8). Hl-60 cultured cells, whose levels of glutathione were lowered by incubation with the 1-(2-chloroethyl)-3-cyclohexyl-1-nitrosourea (CCNU), were more sensitive to AmB-induced lysis than control HL-60 cells (9).

What is the mechanism of the AmB-induced oxidative events? The literature indicates two processes by which Amb could affect cells through oxidative dependent events. The first, unrelated to the permeabilizing effects, is by autooxidation of AmB and the formation of free radicals. The second mode of action is a result of increased membrane permeability. In isolated perfused rat kidneys it has been shown that lethal cell injury induced by AmB depends on transport activity, which is associated with a rise in oxygen demand. The cell injury that follows AmB induced permeability is probably associated with both modes of action.

The observed dependency of lytic and lethal action of AmB on cell resistance to oxidative damage suggests two types of strategy that can be considered. First, the host can be protected from the oxidative dependent damage. McDonnell et al (10) showed that in vivo administration of AmB produced an increase in the ratio of oxidized to non-oxidized glutathione in the lung and plasma of animals and also in isolated perfused lungs. The increase in this ratio in tissues taken from perfused lung was attenuated by addition of catalase or 1-phenyl-3-pyrazolidone (Phenidone), a scavenger of oxygen radicals.

Alternatively, the possibility exists of increasing sensitivity of fungal cells to AmB by decreasing their resistance to oxidative dependent damages.

IV. EFFECTS OF DETERGENTS ON AmB BINDING TO STEROLS AND TOXICITY TO CELLS AND MICE

AmB is insoluble in aqueous solution and a vehicle (carrier) has to be used to form a dispersion. The commercial preparation of AmB, Fungizone, is a combination of AmB, deoxycholate, and buffer. Since the clinical utility of AmB is limited by its toxicity to host cells, an important question is how to decrease its toxicity to host cells without impairing its action on fungal cells. One strategy is to use vehicles other than deoxycholate. Novel formulations that have been proposed include AmB complexed to phospholipid vesicles (11) or to lipids of open structures (12). The important characteristic of AmB complexed to lipids is its diminished toxicity to the host without impaired antifungal activity. Because of this decreased toxicity, AmB can be given in higher, more effective doses.

To understand the role of the detergent, deoxycholate, in Fungizone, we compared the cellular effects by AmB used as either Fungizone or added as a dispersion in dimethylsulfoxide. Figure 2 shows that AmB as Fungizone was less potent in inducing hemolysis of erythrocytes than AmB added as a dispersion in dimethylsulfoxide. This difference indicates that the presence of deoxycholate decreased the lytic potency of AmB. The two preparations of AmB did not differ in toxicity toward fungal cells.

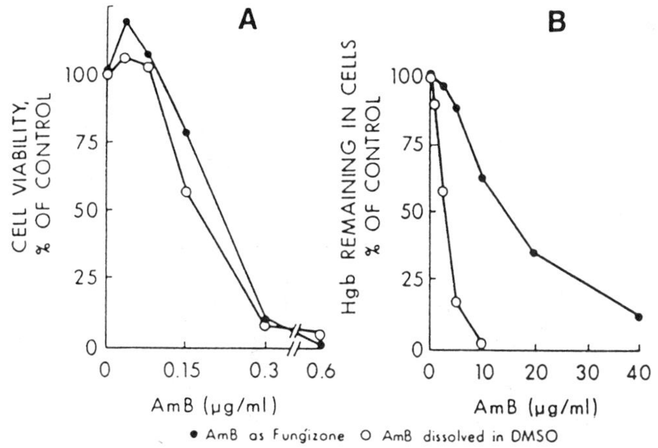

FIGURE 2. Toxic effect of AmB with or without the detergent deoxychlate on fungal cells (A) and erythrocytes (B).

Thus the selectivity in the inhibitory action of this detergent is similar to that of lipids.

To understand how a detergent may increase the selective toxicity of AmB to fungal and mammalian cells, we must first understand the basis of this selectivity. The proposed explanation is based on the so-called "sterol hypothesis": AmB damages cells by binding to sterols incorporated into their membranes; AmB binds more avidly to ergosterol (the fungal sterol) then cholesterol (the mammalian sterol) and for this reason it is more toxic to fungal than mammalian cells. The question is, how does AmB binds more to ergosterol than cholesterol and how can this preferential binding be potentiated? Figure 3, drawn according to studies by Herve et al (13) and Cybulska et al (14), illustrates two kinds of binding of AmB to sterols. Part A of this figure shows how AmB and sterols, with the participation of water, forms a "cage" by hydrogen bonding. The functional groups involved in the hydrogen bonds are the hydroxyl groups of the

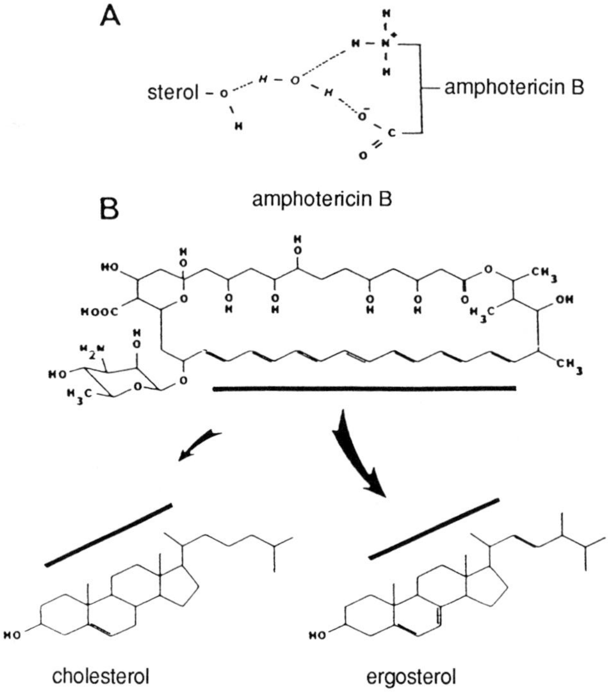

FIGURE 3. Schematic representation of hydrogen bond formation (A) and nonspecific interactions between AmB and sterols (B). Taken from reference 1.

sterols and the carboxyl and amino groups of the AmB molecule. Both ergosterol and cholesterol are 3-beta hydroxy sterols and it can be assumed that their reactions involving hydrogen bonding with AmB are equivalent.

The second type of interaction, shown in part B of this figure, is governed by hydrophobic forces and involves the rigid side chain of seven conjugated double bonds of AmB and the entire sterol molecule. Conformational analysis of ergosterol and cholesterol show that the overall shape of ergosterol conformers is flat. The flat shape of the ergosterol molecule may facilitate intermolecular contact with the polyene macrolide (15). In contrast a flat shape is only one of the possible conformations of cholesterol because the cholesterol side chain without the double bond at C-22 is more flexible. Thus hydrophobic bonding determines selectivity in the AmB sterol interaction.

It could be assumed that under some conditions that are not favorable for the formation of hydrophobic bonding, AmB may still interact with ergosterol but not with cholesterol. AmB in water forms aggregates and it was shown that the interaction of AmB with sterol depends on its state of aggregation (16). One could expect that the detergent induced changes in aggregation state of AmB may selectively inhibit its binding to ergosterol and cholesterol and toxicity to mammalian and fungal cells. To explore this possibility we investigated the effects of several mild detergents composed of sucrose esters on the activity ofAmB.

Four monoesters of sucrose, listed in Figure 4, were investigated. The effects of these esters on deaggregation and

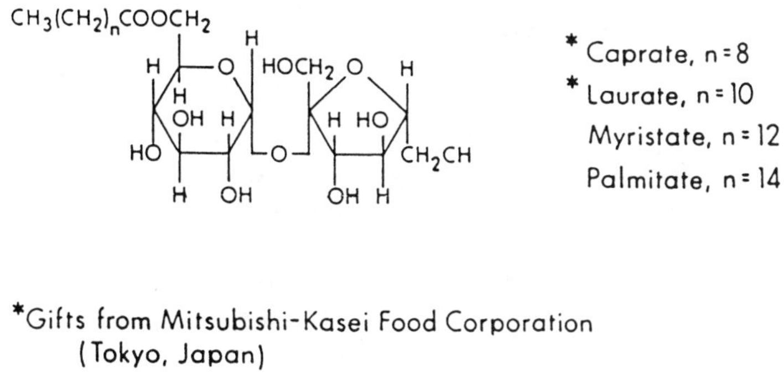

FIGURE 4. Chemical structure of sucrose esters tested.

binding of AmB to sterols were estimated from changes in the AmB spectrum in the ultra-violet-visible region. In the absorption spectrum of AmB four peaks characteristic of the heptaene chromophore can be distinguished. The peak at 408 nm is attributed to the monomeric form of AmB. The peak at 348 nm is attributed to the aggregate form of AmB or, when measured in the presence of sterol, to AmB complexed to sterol. The ratio (R) of the peaks decrease in the presence of sterol and increase in the presence of esters. Thus sterols and sucrose esters affect the spectrum of AmB in contrasting ways. The absorbance ratio of AmB in the presence of both sterols and sucrose ester demonstrated which effect prevailed, either deaggregation or binding to sterol. Progressive increases in ester concentrations, in the absence of sterol, induced an initial decrease in peak ratios followed by an increase. This increase indicated that more AmB was in a monomeric state. In the presence of cholesterol, the increase in R was the same as in its absence. However, in the presence of ergosterol, the ester-induced increase in R were smaller. The proposed interpretation is that in the wide range of ester concentrations, the change in physical state of AmB from mostly aggregated to mostly deaggregated interfered with its binding to cholesterol but not ergosterol. At very high concentrations of ester, when AmB was completely deaggregated, AmB did not bind to any sterol.

In cellular experiments we compared the effects of these esters on AmB toxicity to mouse erythrocytes, cultured mouse fibroblast cells and C. albicans cells. Toxicity was measured as a decrease in retention of K^+, hemolysis of erythrocytes or loss of viability by C. albicans cells. In all these assays, the potency of the esters in inhibiting the toxicity of AmB was about 600-fold greater when mammalian cells were assayed than when fungal cells were used as target. The order of inhibitory potency was: palmitate > myristate > laurate > caprate. At concentrations greater than inhibitory, the esters were toxic to mammalian cells. Toxicity studies with the esters in uninfected mice revealed the same order of potency in inhibiting the acute toxicity of AmB.

These observations suggest that a relationship exists between the potency of the detergent to induce changes in the physical state of AmB and its ability to inhibit AmB toxicities to cells and animal. Each of the esters assayed inhibited AmB binding to cholesterol more than to ergosterol and toxicity to mammalian cells more than to fungal cells. The implication is that esters may selectively inhibit cellular toxicity of other polyenes which bind preferentially to ergosterol, for example, nystatin, but not of filipin whose structure does not impose preferential binding to ergosterol.

V. IMPLICATIONS FOR FUTURE STUDIES

We have discussed some of the activities of AmB at the molecular and cellular levels and proposed three directions for future in vivo studies. Investigations at the molecular and cellular level, in parallel with in vivo studies, may clarify the bases of the observed effects of AmB and enlarge our perspective. The assumed increased uptake of quinolones by AmB treated cells, compared to non treated cells should be documented by direct measurement of intracellular levels of quinolones. A detailed analysis of oxidative events involved in AmB effects in vitro may help to design experiments aimed at modulation of AmB activities in vivo. The finding that detergents other than deoxycholate can be used to increase the selective toxicity of AmB towards fungal cells and decrease its animal toxicity suggests that efforts should be expended towards discovery of non-toxic detergents with increased potency to deaggregate AmB. The correlation of detergent effects at the molecular, cellular and whole animal levels suggests that initial evaluation of prospective dispersing agents may be done by spectrophotometrically measuring their effects on aggregation state of AmB and selectivity of its binding to ergosterol and cholesterol.

VI. REFERENCES

1. J. Brajtburg, W.G. Powderly, G.S. Kobayashi, and G. Medoff, Amphotericin B: Current understanding of mechanisms of action. Antimicrob. Agents Chemother. 34:183-188, (1990).

2. G. Medoff, G.S. Kobayashi, C.N. Kwan, D. Schlessinger, and P. Venkov, Potentiation of rifampin and 5-fluorocytosine as antifungal antibiotics by amphotericin B. Proc. Nat. Acad. Sci. (USA) 69:196-199 (1972).

3. M.A. Petrou and T.R. Rogers, In-vitro activity of antifungal agents in combination with four quinolones. Drugs Exptl. Clin. Res. 14:9-18 (1988).

4. K. Hirai, H. Aoyama, T. Irikura, S. Iyobe, and S. Mitsuhashi, Difference in susceptibility to quinolones of outer membrane mutants of Salmonella typhimurium and Escherichia coli. Antimicrob. Agents Chemother. 29:535-538, 1986.

5. J. Brajtburg, S. Elberg, D. Schwarz, A. Vertut-Croquin, D. Schlessinger, G.S. Kobayashi, and G. Medoff, Involvement of oxidative damage in erythrocyte lysis induced by amphotericin B. Antimicrob. Agents Chemother. 27:172-176 (1984).

6. M.L. Sokol-Anderson, J. Brajtburg, and G. Medoff, Amphotericin B-induced oxidative damage and killing of Candida albicans. J. Infect. Dis. 154:76-83 (1986).

7. J. Brajtburg, S. Elberg, G.S. Kobayashi, and G. Medoff, Effects of ascorbic acid on the action of amphotericin B on Candida albicans cells. J. Antimicrob. Chemother. 24:333-337 (1989).

8. J. Brajtburg, S. Elberg, G.S. Kobayashi, and G. Medoff, Toxicity and induction of resistance to Listeria monocytogenes infection by amphotericin B in inbred strains of mice. Infect. Immun. 54:303-307 (1986).

9. J. Brajtburg, S. Elberg, K. Schechtman, and G. Medoff, Lysis of human promyelocytic HL-60 cells by amphotericin B in combination with 2-chlorethyl-1-nitrosoureas: Role of the carbamoylating activity of nitrosoureas. Cancer Res. 50:3274-3278 (1990).

10. T.J. McDonnell, S. Chang, J.Y. Wescott, and N.F. Voelkl, Role of oxidants, eicosanoids and neutrophils in amphotericin B lung injury in rats. J. Appl. Physiol. 65:2195-2206 (1988).

11. G. Lopez-Berestein, Treatment of systemic fungal infections with liposomal-amphotericin B. In: Liposomes in Therapy of Infectious Disease and Cancer. Eds. G. Lopez-Berestein and I.J. Fidler. Alan R. Liss Inc., New York. PP. 317-327 (1989).

12. A.S. Janoff, L.T. Boni, M.C. Popescu, S.R. Minchey, P.R. Cullis, T.D. Madden, T. Taraschi, S.M. Gruner, E. Shyamsunder, M.W. Tate, R. Mendelsohn, and D. Bonner, Unusual lipid structures selectively reduce the toxicity of amphotericin B. Proc. Nat. Acad. Sci. (USA) 85:6122-6126 (1988).

13. M. Herve, J.C. Debouzy, E. Borowski, B. Cybulska, and C.M. Gary-Bobo, The role of the carboxyl and amino groups of polyene macrolides in their interactions with sterols and their selective toxicity. A ^{31}P-NMR study,. Biochim. Biophys. Acta 980:261-272 (1989).

14. B. Cybulska, M. Herve, B. Borowski, and C.M. Gary-Bobo, Effect of the polar head structure of polyene macrolide antifungal antibiotics on the mode of permeabilization of ergosterol- and cholesterol-containing lipid vesicles studies by ^{31}P-NMR. Molec. Pharmacol. 29:293-298 (1986).

15. M. Baginski, A. Tempczyk, and E. Borowski, Comparative conformational analysis of cholesterol and ergosterol by molecular mechanistics. Eur. Biophys. J. 17:159-166 (1989).

16. I. Gruda, and N. Dussault, Effect of the aggregation state of amphotericin B on its interaction with ergosterol. Biochem. Cell Biol. 66:177-183 (1988).

7

5-Fluorocytosine and Its Combination with Other Antifungal Agents

PD Dr. Annemarie Polak

Pharmaceutical Research, F. Hoffmann-La Roche Ltd, CH-4002 Basel, Switzerland

The antifungal spectrum of flucytosine (5-FC) relevant to human chemotherapy is limited to species of *Candida, Cryptococcus, Aspergillus* and *Dematiaceae. Candida* and *Cryptococcus* are highly sensitive with MICs ranging from 0.1-2 μg/ml, whereas aspergilli and dematiaceae are only moderately sensitive, their MICs being 1-25 μg/ml. A fungicidal effect is seen in yeasts and dematiaceae after prolonged contact (1).

The basic biochemical mechanism of 5-FC which leads to cessation of growth in fungal cells is the intracellular formation of 5-FDUMP, a known inhibitor of thymidylate synthetase, and incorporation of 5-FUTP into RNA. The critical enzyme, which determines the antimicrobial spectrum of 5-FC, is uracil deaminase, and only fungi which possess this enzyme are sensitive. Mammalian cells lack deaminase activity, giving 5-FC a low toxicity in humans. Only bacteria of the intestinal tract are able to convert 5-FC into

5-FU.The metabolic pathway of 5-FC in fungal is prone to various spontaneous mutations. The incidence of primary resistance and especially the selection of secondary resistance during monotherapy with 5-FC is a significant problem. In *Cryptococcus neoformans*, for example, only 1.8 % of strains tested were found to be naturally resistant, but during monotherapy resistant populations are easily selected. Most therapeutic failures could be explained by the selection of resistant strains. In *Candida albicans* the incidence of primary resistance isolates is dependent on the serotype. 30 % of type B strains are 5-FC-resistant, but only 7 % of type A (1).

A strong synergy exists between 5-FC and amphotericin B (Amph B) both in vitro (2) and in animal experiments (3). Furthermore, the appearance of mutants resistant to 5-FC was drastically reduced in this combination (2,4). A strong synergistic action between 5-FC and triazoles has also been observed in various animal models. 5-FC + itraconazole (ITRA) and 5-FC + fluconazole (FLU) exert the same degree of synergy as 5-FC + Amph B in candidosis, and 5-FC + ITRA is synergistic in *Aspergillus* infections. However, a strong antagonism was observed between ketoconazole (KETO) and Amph B in both (5,6). In actual clinical practice the detrimental influence of prophylaxis with KETO on the susceptibility of aspergilli to Amph B has been observed in two cases where aspergillosis appeared despite prophylactic treatment with KETO. This antagonism of Amph B is less pronounced with triazoles but is still present and strongly dependent on the dose (6). In recent animal experiments the triple combination of 5-FC + Amph B + triazole was tested. This triple combination was beneficial in cryptococcosis,while a slight antagonism was seen in *Candida* and *Aspergillus* infections (7).

It can be concluded from the data obtained in animal experiments that 5-FC can be combined with Amph B or triazoles in all opportunistic fungal infections, but that combination of azoles and triazoles with Amph B should be avoided. Only in the case of cryptococcosis did a double combination of Amph B + KETO or triazole and a triple combination of 5-FC + Amph B + triazole act synergistically.

Only one antifungal combination, that of 5-FC with Amph B, has actually been tested in controlled clinical trials. The superiority of the combination over monotherapy with Amph B was proven in cryptococcal meningitis by two thorough randomized prospective clinical trials (8,9). A faster sterilization of the cerebrospinal fluid was seen, a more rapid clinical response and an overall higher cure rate. During the second study (9) a high incidence of side effects (44 %) was observed, including azotemia, leukopenia and thrombocytopenia. The incidence of these toxic effects of 5-FC correlated significantly with concentrations over 100 µg/ml over a long period of time. This can be largely avoided if 5-FC levels are monitored during therapy. Since 5-FC is wholly excreted by the kidney, even a minor impairment of renal function by Amph B leads to elevated levels. Salt loading is effective in decreasing the nephrotoxicity of Amph B and should be employed if 5-FC is given in tablet form. A 5-FC infusion contains 9 grammes of sodium chloride so that patients treated with this already have a salt supplement (7,10).

Based on experience over the years this combination is in fact also recommended as the treatment of choice for other opportunistic fungal infections, particularly those due to *Candida*.

Cryptococcosis is a frequent opportunistic infection in AIDS-patients. Here, the cause of infection is different and requires a different approach. Most patients respond to initial therapy with 5-FC + Amph B, but the relapse rate is high unless some form of maintenance therapy is subsequently given. Whether a combination as the initial therapy brings advantages over monotherapy with Amph B or with FLU in AIDS-patients has been the subject of much discussion. The attitude towards this question is different in Europe to that common in the United States. In Germany, for instance, the initial treatment is still 5-FC + Amph B, but in the US a FLU monotherapy seems to be preferred (11,12). In Italy success has been achieved by both ITRA and FLU monotherapy, but combination therapy with 5-FC + ITRA was found to clear the cerebrospinal fluid more rapidly than monotherapy (13). There are also reports of successful treatment of cryptococcosis in AIDS by a combination of FLU + Amph B (14). The beneficial effect of the triple combination of 5-FC + FLU

+Amph B was also demonstrated in a clinical situation. Cryptococcosis in AIDS was treated with this combination in daily doses of 200 mg 5-FC, 400 mg FLU and 0.3 mg/kg Amph B. The initial response to this combination is highly satisfactory, and after the clearing of cryptococcosis from all body sites and the disappearance of symptoms a maintenance therapy with 200 mg FLU daily is started (15).

In the case of candidosis response of therapy is strongly dependent on both the localization of infection and the underlying disease. The following are just a few examples where combination therapy was more successful than monotherapy.

Candida fungaemia may resolve spontaneously on removal of a catheter if this is the source of infection, but it may cause endophthalmitis in neutropenic patients. In immunosuppressed patients a fungicidal therapy is clearly needed, and the only possibility at present is a combination therapy of 5-FC + Amph B or 5-FC + triazole. Monotherapy with a triazole is never sufficient.

Systemic *Candida* infections have become a significant problem in neonatal intensive care units. At present treatment is often 5-FC +Amph B, but it may be replaced by FLU-monotherapy in fungaemia or by 5-FC + FLU in more critical situations such as meningitis (16).

Antifungal chemotherapy for *Candida* sepsis in patients with neoplastic disease is usually unsuccessful if the underlying disease is not controlled. The best treatment successes for *Candida* infection in leukaemic and cancer patients have been achieved with the combination of 5-FC + Amph B (17,18), but in future 5-FC + FLU or 5-FC+ ITRA may be also successful in these settings.

Candida peritonitis can lead to complications and interruption of dialysis treatment. Monotherapy does not achieve a cure without removal of the catheter according to most authors (19). However, combination therapy with 5-FC + Amph B, 5-FC + KETO and 5-FC + FLU have all given high cure rates (> 93 %) without removal of the catheter (19,20).

The *Candida* syndrome peculiar to heroin addicts (21) responds well to monotherapy with KETO or newer triazoles if the infection is restricted to the skin. A combination therapy is, however, needed as soon as other localizations are involved. In the case of concomitant endophthalmitis combination therapy eradicates the fungus sufficiently quickly that the sight can be saved whereas with monotherapy the illness is cured but the eyesight lost.

Osteoarthritis only responds to combination therapy, although surgical removal of the infected bone is sometimes necessary to achieve 100 % cure. The choice of combination partner for 5-FC is not important, it may be Amph B, FLU or ITRA. Combinations of triazoles with Amph B should be avoided (7).

Aspergillosis responds poorly to all antifungal chemotherapy and recovery from granulocytopenia is critical for survival. Therapy with Amph B alone or in combination with 5-FC gives only 50-60 % cure rates (7). Burch et al. (22) recently reported a 90 % survival in granulocytopenic leukaemic patients treated with 5-FC + Amph B, but he used an unusually high dose of Amph B, 1.5 mg/kg in the combination which may explain the very high success rate. Walsh and Pizzo (23) have also recommended the combination of 5-FC + Amph B for aspergillosis, especially at the beginning of the therapy. ITRA monotherapy has also shown promising results in some cases (13) and may lead to high cure rates in combination with 5-FC.

Combination therapy with 5-FC and the triazoles ITRA and FLU may show synergy in some clinical cases of chromomycosis and phaeohyphomycosis. 5-FC + ITRA proved to be the therapy of choice in chromomycosis cases caused by *Fonsecaea pedrosoi* (24,25). When the disease is caused by *Cladosporium carinoii*, ITRA monotherapy leads to high cure rates. In phaeohyphomycosis a strong neurotropism of the causative dematiaceous fungi is observed. In this localization a combination of 5-FC + FLU may be needed to eradicate the fungus from the brain since both drugs cross the blood-cerebrospinal fluid barrier. Up to now no treatment other than surgery has been successful in this indication.

A major advantage of combination therapy is clearly that a fungicidal activity can be attained even in difficult medical settings. Further, it certainly lowers the risk of resistance, which was first recognised as a problem in 5-FC monotherapy, but may in future also become a problem for FLU-monotherapy.

The future of therapy of fungal diseases, especially of opportunistic fungi, surely lies in combination therapy. At the moment, the gold standard in Europe is still 5-FC + Amph B, but this may be replaced by 5-FC + FLU or 5-FC + ITRA, depending on the causative fungus and on the localization of the disease. However, it should be mentioned here that the combination between antifungal therapy and the new immune modulating agents may bring even more advantages. For instance, a successful combination of traditional antifungal therapy with G-CSF therapy may revolutionise the therapy of opportunistic fungal infection in leukaemic and cancer patients (preliminary results).

REFERENCES

1. A. Polak, and H.J. Scholer, Mode of action of 5-fluorocytosine, Revue de l'Institut Pasteur de Lyon, 13:, No. 2, 233-244. (1980).
2. A. Polak, Synergism of polyene antibiotics with 5-fluorocytosine, Chemother., 24: 2-16. (1978).
3. A. Polak, H.J. Scholer, and M. Wall, Combination therapy of experimental candidiasis, cryptococcosis and aspergillosis in mice, Chemother., 28: 461-479. (1982).
4. A. Polak, Antifungal combination therapy in localized candidosis, Mycoses (in press). (1990).
5. A. Schaffner, and P.G. Frick, The effect of ketoconazole on amphotericin B in a model of disseminated aspergillosis, J. Inf. Dis., 151 (5): 902-920. (1985).
6. A. Polak, Combination therapy of experimental candidiasis, cryptococcosis, aspergillosis and wangiellosis in mice, Chemother., 33: 381-395. (1987).
7. A. Polak, Combination therapy for systemic mycosis, Infection, 17 (4):, 203-208. (1989).
8. J.E. Bennett, W.E. Dismukes, R.J. Duma, G. Medoff, M.A. Sande, H. Gallis, J. Leonard, B.T. Fields, M. Bradshaw, H. Haywood, Y.A. McGee, Th.R. Cate, C.G. Cobbs, J.F. Warner, and D. W. Alling, A comparison of amphotericin B alone and combined with flucytosine in the treatment of cryptococcal meningitis, New Engl. J. Med., 301 (3): 127-131. (1979).
9. W.E. Dismukes, G. Cloud, H.A. Gallis, T.M. Kerkering, G. Medoff, P.C. Craven, L.G. Kaplowitz, J.F. Fisher, C.R. Gregg, C.A. Bowles, S. Shadomy, A.M. Stamm, R.B. Diasio, L. Kaufman, S.J. Soong, and W.C. Blackwelder, Treatment of cryptococcal meningitis with combination amphotericin B and flucytosine for four as compared with six weeks, New Engl. J. Med., 317 (6(: 334-341. (1987).
10. H. Heidemann, E. Jacqz, E. Ohnhaus, W. Ray, and R. Branch, The importance of Na loading on amphotericin B nephrotoxicity considering the combination with 5-fluorocytosine and ticarcillin, Rec. Adv. Chemother., Antimicrobial Section 3 (Proceedings of the 14th International Congresss of Chemotherapy, Kyoto, 1987), 2628-2629. (1985).

11. D.N. Chernoff, and M.A. Sande, Cryptococcal infections in patients with the Acquired Immunodeficiency Syndrome (AIDS). Paper presented at the Conférence Internationale sur le SIDA, 23-25 June, Paris, Abstract No. 543. (1986).
12. F. Staib, G. Roegler, L. Pruefer-Kraemer, M. Seibold, D. Eichenlaub, and H.D. Pohle, Disseminierte Kryptokokkose bei zwei AIDS-Patienten. Dtsch. Med. Wschr., 111: 1061-1065. (1986).
13. M.A. Viviani, A.M. Tortorano, and P. Antonio et al., European experience with itraconazole in systemic mycoses. J. Am. Acad. Dermatol., (in press). (1990).
14. V. Tozzi, E. Bordi, S. Glagani, G.C. Leoni, P. Narciso, P. Sette, and G. Visco, Fluconazole treatment of cryptococcosis in patients with acquired immunodeficiency syndrome, Am. J. Med., 87 (3): 353. (1989).
15. G. Just-Nübling, C.Laubenberger, E.B. Helm, S. Falk, W. Stille, Diagnose, klinischer Verlauf und Behandlung der Kryptokokken-Meningitis bei AIDS Patienten. Forschg. Praxis 9 (No. 106): VI-VII. (1990).
16. M.C. Bottineau, J.C. Roze, and A. Mouzard, Candidoses néonatales systémiques. Ann. Pediatr., 35 (4): 235-243. (1988).
17. D. Armstrong, Problems in the treatment of opportunistic fungal infections. In: Diagnosis and Therapy of Systemic Fungal Infections (K. Holmberg and R.D. Meyer, ed.), p. 149-158. (1989).
18. M. v. Eiff, M. Essink, N. Roos, W. Hiddemann, Th. Buechner, and J. van de Loo, Hepatosplenic candidosis, Zeitschr. f. Antimkrob. Antineoplast. Chemother., Suppl. 1: 1. (1989).
19. I.K.P. Cheng, G.X. Fang, T.M. Chan, P.C.K. Chan, and M.K. Chan, Fungal peritonitis complicating peritoneal dialysis: report of 27 cases and review of treatment. Quart J. Med., New Series, 71, 265: 407-416. (1989).
20. A. Slingeneyer, B. Laroche, F. Stec, B. Canaud, J.J. Beraud, and C. Mion, Oral ketoconazole plus intraperitoneal 5-fluorocytosine as the sole treatment of fungal peritonitis (abstract). Perit Dial. Bulletin, 4 (Suppl.): S.60. (1984).
21. B. Dupont, and E. Drouhet, Cutaneous, ocular, and osteoarticular candidiasis in heroin addicts: new clinical and therapeutic aspects in 38 patients, J. Inf. Dis., 152, 577-591. (1985).

22. P.A. Burch, J.E. Karp, W.G. Mery et al., Favourable outcome of invasive aspergillosis in patients with acute leukemia, J. Clincl Oncol., 5: 1985-1993. (1987).
23. T. Walsh, and P.A. Pizzo, Fungal infections in granulocytopenic patients: current approaches to classification, diagnosis and treatment, Diagnosis and Therapy of Systemic Fungal Infections (K. Holmberg and R.D. Meyer, ed.), pp. 47-70. (1989).
24. D.A. Borelli, A clinical trial of itraconazole in the treatment of deep mycoses and leishmaniasis. Rev. Inf. Dis., 9 (Suppl. 1): S.57. (1987).
25. G. Moulin, Th. Cognat, E. Ferrier, and H. Alligier, Chromomycose: efficacité de l'association itraconazole + 5-fluorocytosine, Journal de dermatologie de Paris, 14: 54. (1989).

PART II

THERAPY OF DERMATOPHYTOSES, SUPERFICIAL MYCOSES, AND SUBCUTANEOUS MYCOSES

8

Dermatophytoses, Superficial Mycoses, and Subcutaneous Mycoses: Historical Perspectives and Future Needs

Dieter Berg, Manfred Plempel, and Karl-Heinz Büchel

Bayer AG, 5090 Leverkusen-Bayerwerk, FRG

A systematic overview on medicinal fungicides is given by classifying the componds by their chemistry (Table 1).

Table 1: Classes of Antimycotic Structures

1) modified nucleoside bases (5-F-Cytosine), 2) polyketides (Griseofulvin), 3) glutarimides (Cycloheximide), 4) polyenes (special case of polyketides, e.g. Nystatin), 5) allylamines (Naftifine, Terbinafine), 6) azoles, 7) morpholines

The first group is represented by 5-fluorocytosine and can be headed as modified nucleosides and nucleoside-bases. The second example is Griseofulvin, a secondary metabolite derived from the polyketide pathway. The third compound is cycloheximide, representative of a number of analogs from the chemical group of glutarimides. The 4th group - the polyenes - in fact, is a special case of naturally occurring products from the polyketide pathway, examples being nystatin, amphotericin B, and pimaricin. The next two groups originate from pure synthetic chemistry and include the allylamines like naftifine or terbinafine and the large group of azole-derivatives. Together they are representatives of the ergosterol-biosynthesis-inhibitors, (EBI's), short.

The modes of action of these most important chemical classes for chemotherapy are described in the following and discussed with respect to their possible risks in therapy.

It is well known that 5-fluorocytosine was discovered within a screening program for antitumor compounds. It acts selectively against yeasts and some aspergillus species and chromomycetes (1). First it was assumed that the efficacy depended on deamination of 5-FC to 5-Fluoro-uracil which then should be incorporated into nucleic acids. In 1983 it was described (2) that a prior deamination is not necessarily responsible for activity. From these data it is derived that 5-fluorocytosine is glycosylated with 2-deoxyribose, afterwards incorporated into DNA and thus acts as a suicide-inhibitor on SAM-dependent methyltransferase, which is responsible for thymidine-synthesis. During that suicide-inhibition the substrate is activated by a covalent binding to the enzyme in 6-position and the SAM-dependent methylation leads to the 5-methyl-5-fluoro-derivative, that remains covalently linked to the enzyme. That means in total that the methyltransferase is trapped covalently and hence inactivated.

From the mode of action of 5-fluorocytosine one might expect a broad spectrum of biological activity. In fact its antimycotic efficacy is mainly limited to yeasts. Additionally, this is the only compound discussed here against which resistance has developed. Because of the risk of an undesirable inhibition of protein synthesis by blocking DNA-synthesis (and this especially in systems with high turnover) one has to take care that the serum-concentration does not exceed 80 to 100 µg/ml in order to minimize the risk of leucopenia and thrombopenia (Table 2).

Table 2: Possible Risk of 5-F-Cytosine Application

1) leucopenia and thrombopenia, 2) intestinal disturbances, 3) liver disfunctions, 4) allergic reactions, 5) teratogenicity (due to mode of action)

After 5-fluorcytosine administration leucopenia and thrombopenia, intestinal disfunctions, liver disfunctions, allergic reactions, as well as teratogenicity are regarded as possible risks (3). The teratogenicity in particular is directly correlated with the mode of action as inhibitor of DNA-synthesis.

In the case of griseofulvin (Fig. 1) the description of mode of action is not as clear. Several aspects have been studied and described. It is accepted, however, that griseofulvin inhibits RNA-synthesis by interaction with purine bases of polynucleotides (4). As a Result of the disturbed DNA-conformation,translation is simultaneously inhibited. Additionally, morphological observations indicate an inhibition of chitin formation at the same time and studies on inhibition of mitosis by griseofulvin indicate interactions with the microtubule system (5). The proposed mechanisms of griseofulvin action include,

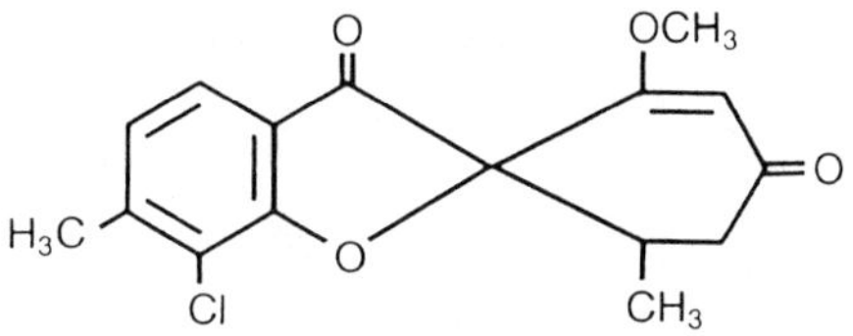

FIG. 1 Mode of action of griseofluvin. Proposed: (a) inhibition of RNA synthesis by interfering with purine bases; (b) inhibition of chitin synthesis (morphological observation); (c) microtubule interaction.

therefore: inhibition of RNA-synthesis by interaction with purine bases, inhibition of chitin synthesis, and microtubule interactions.

Table 3: Possible Risk of Griseofulvin Administration

1) intestinal disfunctions, 2) allergic reactions and photosensibilisation, 3) induction of liver enzymes

Therefore the possible risk of griseofulvin (Table 3) administration can hardly be discussed from the viewpoint of mode of action but can be described by the observed side effects, which are intestinal disfunctions, allergic reactions and photo-sensibilisation, as well as induction of liver enzymes.

The next group to be discussed are the glutarimides (Fig. 2).The most prominent compound from this group is cycloheximide, the mode of action of which has been intensively studied. It is described as an inhibitor of protein synthesis in eucaryotic cells by interfering with the 80S ribosomal subunit with the consequence that the synthesis of peptide linkages is blocked (6).

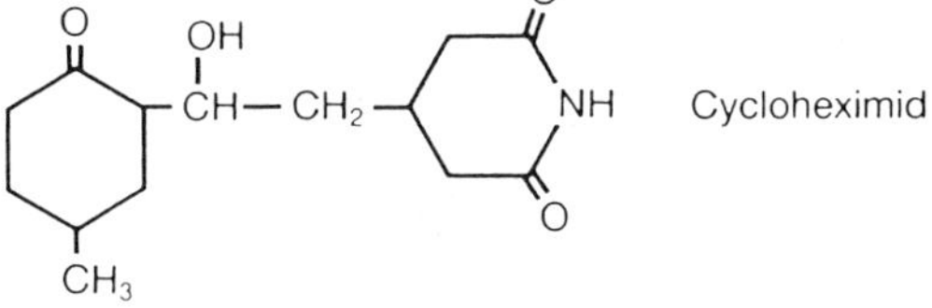

FIG. 2 Mode of action of glutarimides. Proposed: inhibition of protein synthesis in eucaryotes by interfering with 80S-ribosomal subunit, thus preventing synthesis of peptide linkages.

Risk of Glutarimide Administration

high acute mammalian toxicity

This mode of action is directly responsible for the fact that glutarimide administration includes the risk of high acute mammalian toxicity. So this is a classical example of a mode of action which directly leads to pronounced toxicity.

Table 4: Mode of Action of Polyenes
(e.g. amophotericin B, nystatin, pimaricin)

- complexation of ergosterol in plasma membranes of pathogens

  —> changes of membrane permeabilily

  —> leakage of membranes

- antagonism of polyene efficacy by Ca^{++}, Mg^{++} and sterols

The situation is somewhat different within the group of polyenes (Table 4), as, for example, amphotericin B, nystatin, or pimaricin. As mode of action of polyenes a complexation with ergosterol in the plasma membrane of pathogens is accepted (7) . A direct consequence of this complexation reaction is a change in membrane permeability, accompanied by membrane leakage. A positive indication for this mode of action is the antagonism between polyenes on the one hand and calcium, magnesium, and sterols on the other (8) . In principle, this mode of action could be ideal if the tendency for complexation were restricted to ergosterol and would not take place with mammalian sterols. The direct interaction between polyenes and sterols can be quantified by registration of the difference spectra after complexation (Fig. 3).
In Fig. 3 the difference spectra of nystatin/ergosterol and nystatin/cholesterol mixtures are given. Polyene and sterols have each been applied at 5×10^{-5} M. The intensity of interaction between nystatin and sterol is recorded directly by the degree of variation from the baseline. So it can be shown clearly that the complexation between ergosterol and nystatin is more favourable than the one between cholesterol and nystatin. Nevertheless, the tendency for complexation between nystatin and cholesterol has to be regarded as the reason for nystatin's toxicity.

Possible Risk of Polyene Administration (8)

1) nephrotoxicity, 2) CNS-side effects

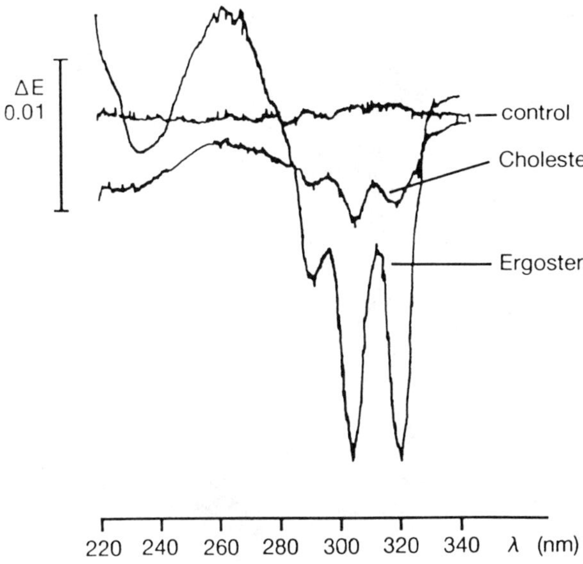

FIG. 3 Difference spectra of nystatin/ergosterol and nystatin/cholesterol complexes.

disadvantage: (9)

photo- and thermolability of polyenes

For this reason nephrotoxicity as well as disfunctions of the central nervous system have been described as side effects after polyene administration. Another additional disadvantage of the polyenes is their pronounced photo- and thermo-lability.
Complexation with membrane sterols is one possibility for disturbing membrane function, the other perhaps more elegant way is to inhibit ergosterol biosynthesis (Table 5).

Table 5: Sterol Biosynthesis Inhibitors (10)

allylamines: Naftifine, Terbinafine

azoles: Bifonazole, Clotrimazole, Itraconazole, Ketoconazole, Miconazole, Oriconazole, Oxiconazole, Tioconazole

morpholines: Amorolfine

Compounds which inhibit sterol-synthesis and which are of interest for mammalian indications can be subdivided into three structural classes. The first group is the allylamines with the example of naftifine and terbinafine. The second and at the moment most important group is the azoles, e.g. bifonazole, clotrimazole, itraconazole, ketoconazole, miconazole, oriconazole, oxiconazole, and tioconazole. The list is not complete by far but should give an impression of the intensity of research activity in that field.

Fungal membranes are physically stabilized by complexation of phospholipids with "quasi-planar" sterols. Under certain structural conditions sterols are relatively planar molecules. In mammalian systems this membrane component is cholesterol, in fungi, however,it is ergosterol. If one looks at the complex between phospholipids and sterols, one can assume that the lipophilic "quasi-planar" part of the sterol interacts with the fatty acid side chains of the phospholipid; the polar OH-group of the sterol, however, is in the neighbourhood of the phosphatidylcholine-residue of the lecithine. This complexation now prevents a phase-transition between quasi-crystalline and liquid phases of phospholipids in the region of the environmental temperature. If the system lacks the sterol complexation-partner or if non-planar sterol precursors accumulate, a fragmentation of the membrane occurs as soon as the critical temperature is exceeded. The phospholipid phase is physically altered and the fungicidal effect can be observed. A series of contributions deals with sterol-biosynthesis inhibitors and therefore should not be discussed mechanistically in detail here.

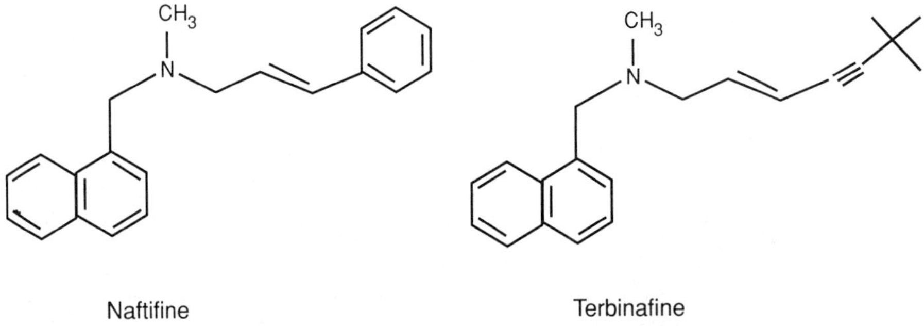

FIG. 4 Mode of action of allylamines: Proposed: inhibition of squalene epoxidation.

The first group of sterol biosynthesis inhibitors (Fig. 4), the allylamines, again act on a step of biosynthesis, which one normally would not expect to be pathogen specific either. After fermentation of pathogens in the presence of naftifine of terbinafine a decrease of ergosterol and a simultaneous accumulation of squalene can be observed, indicating an inhibition of the monooxygenase responsible for epoxidation of squalene, thus blocking the cyclisation reaction to lanosterol.

Due to the relatively narrow spectrum of antifungal activity of the compounds, obviously differences between squalene-epoxidase from different sources do occur. This has been studied intensively by colleagues from Sandoz (12).

The second and at present the most important group of sterol synthesis inhibitors is the so-called azoles. As primary mode of action (13) of azoles an inhibition of C-14-demethylation of trimethylsterols is accepted (Fig. 5). The first step of the C-14-demethylation reaction catalyzed by a cytochrome P_{450}-system involves a hydroxylation of the 14-methylgroup to form the hydroxymethyl-derivative. A second hydroxylation and loss of water leads to the C-14-formyl compound which is then hydroxylated a third time to yield the corresponding carboxylic acid. Decarboxylation does not proceed directly but by withdrawing a proton from C-15, formic acid is eliminated and a Δ^{14}-double bond appears as an intermediate. An NADPH-dependent reduction of the Δ^{14}-double bond then finalizes the demethylation reaction. This final step may be inhibited by various amines, e.g. morpholines (14).

In fungi the demethylation reaction normally takes place after side-chain alkylation (15). The monooxygenase responsible is inhibited by azoles by direct binding of the 3-nitrogen atom of the azole to the iron-atom within the iron-porphyrin-complex of cytochrome P_{450}. The specificity of inhibition depends on the interaction of the lipophilic azole substituents to the binding site of the enzyme which is specifically responsible for the demethylation of 24-methylene-dihydrolanosterol, the pathogen specific intermediate in ergosterol synthesis.

How do these properties of azoles as inhibitors of ergosterol synthesis in fungi fit with their possible risk upon administration ?

<u>Possible Risk of Topical Treatment with Azoles (16)</u>

- high resorption rates and by this expression of possible aromatase or liver P-450 inhibition

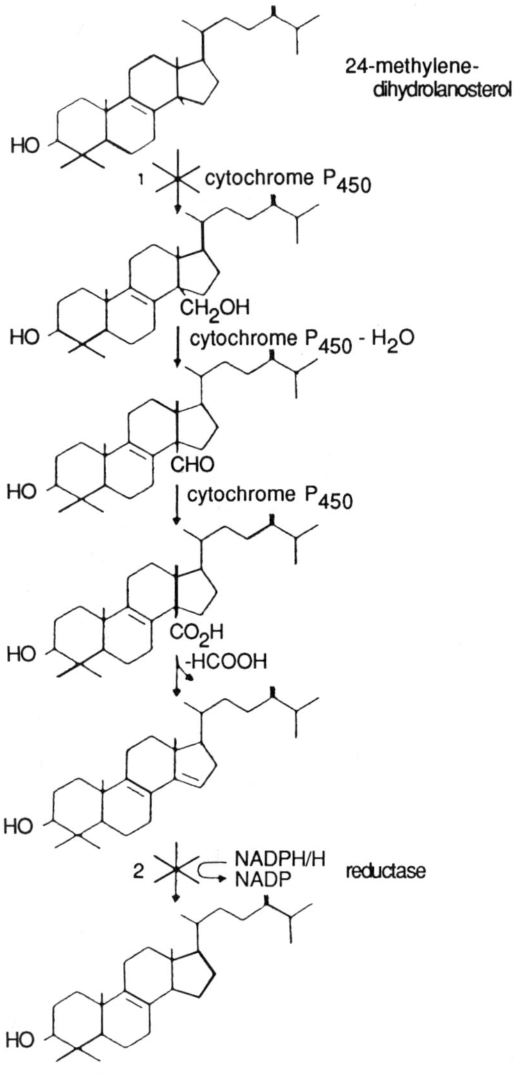

FIG. 5 Mode of action of azoles (generalized). Proposed: inhibition of C_{14}-demethylation of trimethylsterols.

To answer this question we have to separate topical and oral treatment. During topical treatment the main risk of azole application is found in a high skin absorption rate which might be expressed by a possible inhibition of aromatase, that is the steroid-19-hydroxylase, or by unspecific blocking of liver cytochrome P_{450}.

Possible Risk of Oral Administration of Azoles (17)

- non-specific inhibition of monooxygenases
  a) liver P-450
  b) aromatase (steroid-19-hydroxylase) in estradiol production

What can be excluded during topical treatment just by lowering the skin-absorption rate is on the other hand, the main risk during oral administration, namely a minor specificity for sterol synthesis and hence a non-specific inhibition of mono-oxygenases, that means additional effects on liver cytochrome P_{450} and on aromatase, the essential enzyme in estradiol-production.

Consequences for Topical Treatment with Azoles (16)

1) azoles that are not absorbed to a high extent, 2) azoles that remain in the upper parts of the skin dermae, 3) one day treatment

So, as a consequence of topical treatment with azoles one has to state that sterol biosynthesis inhibitors may be applied when they do not exclusively inhibit C-14-demethylation of 24-methylene-dihydrolanosterol, but possess side-effects on other enzyme systems. In this case one has to be sure that the azoles are not absorbed to a great extent, that the azole remains in the upper parts of the skin dermae, and the aim should be a short term treatment, if possible a one-day-treatment.

The conditions to be fulfilled by an orally administered sterol synthesis inhibitor, of course, have to be much greater. For these compounds the substrate specificity for C-14-demethylation of 24-methylene-dihydrolanosterol should be extremely high (18). If additional effects occur these should be limited only to **later specific steps in ergosterol synthesis.** There should be no inhibition of hydroxylation of sterols in C-18- and C-17-positions, which are neccessary for testosterone synthesis. At the same time, aromatase, that is steroid-19-hydroxylase, should not be affected and again the aim should be a short term-treatment.

This discussion of sterol biosynthesis inhibitors and their mode of action may be summarised (Fig. 6) by

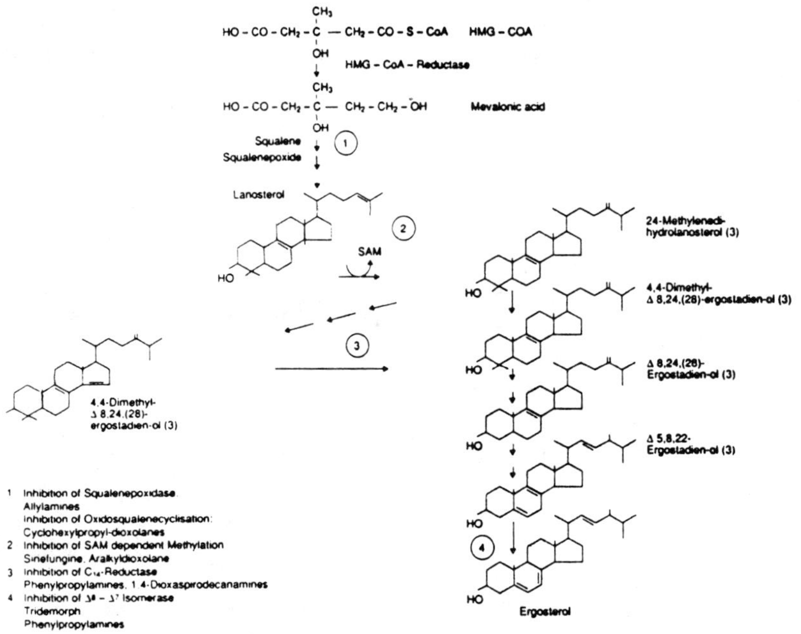

FIG. 6 Mode of action of sterol biosynthesis inhibitors.

pointing out the various mechanisms described so far using a scheme of ergosterol synthesis (19).

There are four prominent sites of inhibition. The first is the conversion of squalene to lanosterol with the allylamines as inhibitors of squalene-epoxidase and the cyclohexylpropyl-dioxolanes which block oxidosqualene-cyclization. We did not refer to this group of compounds as they only exhibit interesting activity as agrochemicals, however, special paper on this is in press (19).

The second point of attack is the SAM-dependent side chain alkylation. A standard inhibitor can be seen in the natural product sinefungin which is a classical SAM-antagonist (20). We additionally found a series of aralkyldioxolanes with that primary mode of action. Again, these compounds primarily are of interest for plant protection. Besides the so called azoles, accumulating 24-methylenedihydrolanosterol compounds have been detected that block Δ^{14}-reduction. These are mainly the phenylpropylamines like amorolfine, fenpropimorph and partly fenpropidine. Finally, $\Delta^{8} \longrightarrow \Delta^{7}$-isomerization reaction is inhibited by tridemorph and partly by fenpropidine(21).

Summing up the history of antimycotic fungicides from a more biochemical point of view there is a series of different chemical classes available, focussing within the last few decades on sterol biosynthesis inhibitors. This development could make us proud as a solution to combat a broad spectrum of pathogens is nowadays available. As pointed out, some side effects are connected with all these classes of compounds so that there is still a need for future innovation.

Where do future developments lead? One important development is the oral application of azoles and allylamines. In this respect terbinafine has to be observed carefully. And again the discovery of a series of natural products should give impact at least as lead structures (Fig. 7).

Nikkomycin Z is representative of a whole series of compounds and is a competitive inhibitor of chitin synthetase (22). Unfortunately, the biological spectrum is mainly limited to yeasts and dimorphic fungi (23),but remarkably enough Richard Hector from San Francisco found a pronounced synergistic effect in vivo with azoles (24). Possibly this is due to the fact that chitin synthetase is located in sterol rich regions of the fungal membrane.

Another example of a promising discovery is the antimycotic LY 121019 (Fig. 8), (25) which shows remarkable in vivo efficacy against Candida albicans. The echinocandin B analogue with the common name cilofungin

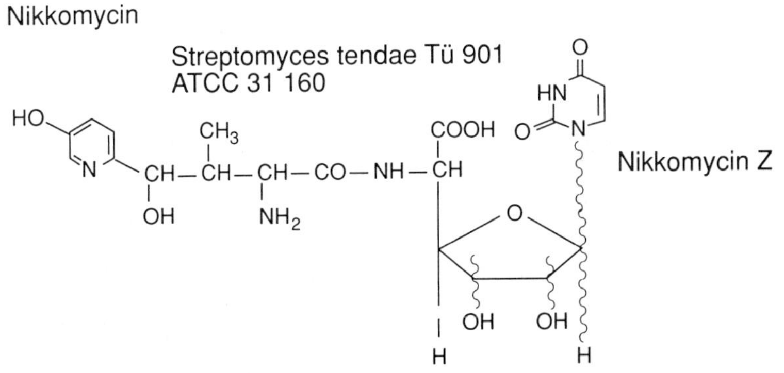

FIG. 7 Structure of nikkomycin Z.

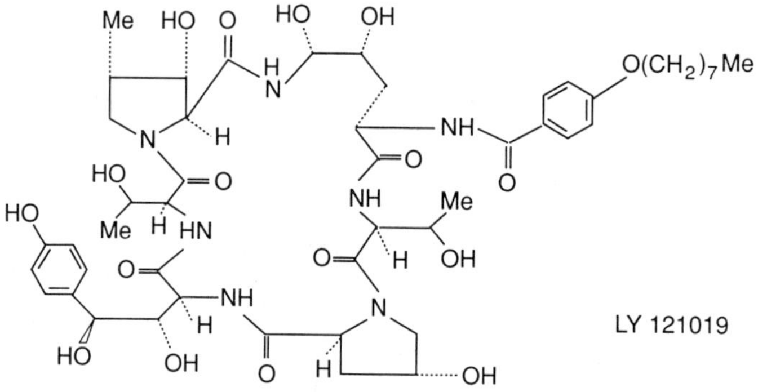

FIG. 8 Structure of cilofungin (Ly 121019).

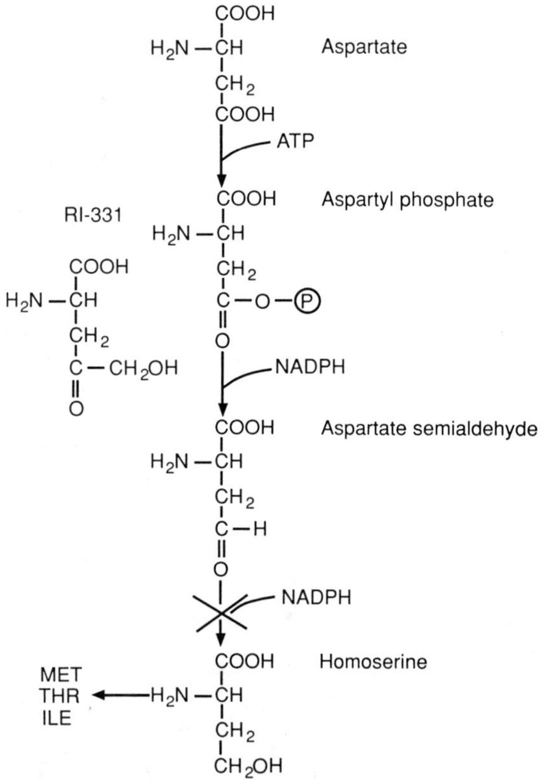

FIG. 9 Structure and mode of action of RI-331. [Source: Yamaki, H. et al. Biochem. Biophys. Res. Commun. 168:2 (1990), 837-843.]

is produced from echinocandin B by enzymatic deacylation using an actinoplanes utahensis culture, followed by acylation with p-octyl-oxo-benzoic acid. It is at least 20-fold less toxic than amphotericin B, exerting synergistic activity between the two antifungals at the same time (26).
The mode of action of cilofungin has been described as an inhibition of 1,3-ß-glucan synthase (27).

Another exciting natural product, RI-331 (Fig. 9) has been described by H. Yamaki et al. (28) and exhibits an unique mode of action by inhibiting homoserine dehydrogenase thus blocking homoserine formation from aspartate semialdehyde. This inhibition of biosynthesis of the essential amino acids from the threonine-family principally promises a broader spectrum of activity which should not be connected with mammalian toxicity.

A final example is cispentacin, FR 109615 (Fig. 10), a new antifungal antibiotic from Streptomyces setonii (29). The compound is almost missing in vitro efficacy but shows remarkable in vivo-effects against Candida albicans in both lung and vaginal infections in mice as well as pronounced efficacy in a systemic infection with Cryptococcus neoformans (30). Its mode of action has not yet been published but from the structure an interference with amino acid pathways would not be surprising.

Future needs in antifungal research:

1) consequent developments of azoles and allylamines, 2) new lead structures, e.g. RI-331 and Cispentacin, 3) inhibition of factors determining pathogenicity

In conclusion, future needs in antifungal research involve consequent developments in the azole and allylamine field as well as chemical synthesis using natural products like RI-331 and cispentacin as leads.

Furthermore, we must gain deeper knowledge about host-pathogen-interactions. If we knew the factors

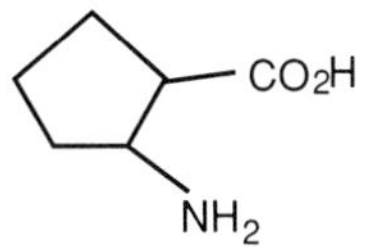

Cispentacin
FR 109615

FIG. 10 Structure of cispentacin. [Source: Iwamoto, F. J. Antibiot. 43:1 (1990), 1-7.]

determining pathogenicity we should be able to inhibit these factors specifically. These might include exo-proteolytic activities of the pathogen as well as recognition of and attachment to the host cell surface.

References:

(1) Sneader, W., "Drug Discovery: The evolution of modern medicines, John Wiley & Sons (1985), 350

(2) Waldorf, A.R., Polak, A., Antimicrob. Agents Chemother. (1983) 23, 79-85

(3) Scholer, H.J., in W.Meinhoff, H. Seeliger, T. Wegmann, H. Schoenfeld (eds): Hahnenklee-Symposium 1982, Roche: Genzach (1983), 169-194

(4) El-Nakeeb, M.A., Mc Lellan, W.C., Jr. Lampen, J.O., J. Bacteriol. (1965) 89, 557-563

(5) Kappar, A., Georgopoulos, S.G., J. Bacteriol (1974), 334-335

(6) Siegel, M.R., Sisler, H.D. Biochim. Biophys. Acta (1965) 103, 558-567

(7) Lampen, J.O., Arnow, P.M., Saffermann, R.S., J. Bacteriol. (1960) 80, 200-206

(8) Gosh, A., Gosh, J.J., Ann. Biochem. Exptl. Med. (Calatta), (1963),23, 606-610

(9) Dekker, J., Ark, P.A., Antibiot. Chemother. (1959), 9, 327-332

(10) Berg., D., Plempel, M. (eds):"Sterol Biosynthesis Inhibitors, Pharmaceutical and Agrochemical Aspects Verlag Chemie/ Ellis Horwood 1988

(11) Ryder, N.S., in (10), 151-167

(12) Petranyi, G., Ryder, N.S., Stütz, A. Science (1984) 224, 1239-1241

(13) Vanden Bossche, H. in (10), 79-119

(14) Mercer, E.I., in (10), 120-167

(15) Jarmann, R.R., Gunatilaka, A.A.I., Widdowson, D.A., Bioorg. Chem. (1975) 4, 202-211

(16) Lücker, P.W. Beubler, E., Kukovetz, W.R., Ritter, W., Dermatologica (1984) 169, 51-56

(17) Schlüter, G., Schmidt, U. in (10), 185-209

(18) Berg, D., Plempel, M., Büchel, K.-H., Holmwood, G., Stroech, K., Ann. N.Y. Acad. Sci. (1988) 544, 338-348

(19) Berg, D., Krämer, W., Weissmüller, J., Pestic. Chem., Pesticide Chemistry in press

(20) Vedel, M., Lawrence, F., Robert-Gero, M., Lederer, E., Biochem. Biophys. Res. Commun. (1978), 85, 371-376

(21) Baloch, R.I., Mercer, E.I., Wiggins, T.E., Baldwin, B.C. Phytochem. (1984) 23, 2219-2226

(22) Gow, L.A., Selitrennikoff, C.P., Current Microbiol. (1984) 11, 211-216

(23) Hector, R., Pappagianis, D. submitted for publication

(24) Hector, R., personal communication

(25) Gordee, R.S., Zeckner, D.J., Ellis, L.F., Thakkar, A.L., Howard, L.C., J. Antibiot. (1984) 37 (9), 1054-1068

9

New Topical Imidazoles Under Development in Japan

TJN-318 (NND-318): Evaluation of Antifungal Activities and the Result of Clinical Open Study on Dermatomycoses

Hisashi Takahashi

Department of Dermatology, Teikyo University School of Medicine
11, Kaga-2, Itabashi-ku, Tokyo 173, Japan

I. INTRODUCTION

A variety of antifungal agents of imidazole derivatives have been developed since 1980. These are known to show antifungal activities by inhibiting cytochrome P-450, which result in a suppression of cell wall conformation.

TJN-318 (NND-318, (±)-(*E*)-(4-(2-chlorophenyl)-1,3-dithiolan-2-ylidene)-1-imidazolylacetonitrile, with a Japanese Accepted Name (=JAN) latoconazole) is a new antifungal imidazole compound with a unique structure, 1,3-dithiolanylidenemethylimidazole (Fig. 1) showing a mode of action similar to and efficacy far more potent than that of existing imidazoles. It originated from Nihon Nohyaku's research laboratories and is now under clinical

Chemical structure :

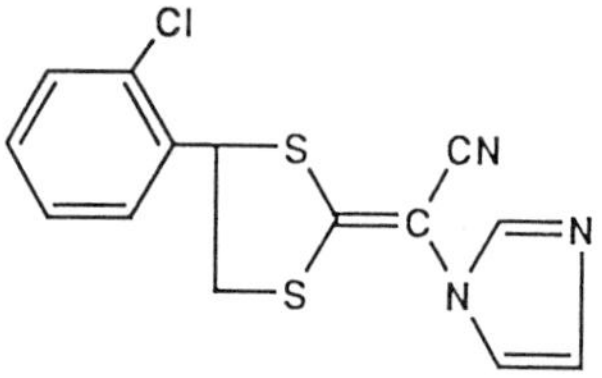

Molecular weight : 319.84

Nonproprietary name : latoconazole (JAN)

Code No. : TJN-318 (Tsumura & Co.)
NND-318 (Nihon Nohyaku Co., Ltd.)

Fig. 1 Chemical name and structure of TJN-318 (NND-318)

development as a drug for superficial dermatomycoses under collaboration with Tsumura & Co..

This article deals with the preclinical and clinical aspects of this material.

II. PRECLINICAL STUDIES

A. *ANTIFUNGAL ACTIVITY(IN VITRO, IN VIVO)*

The spectrum of antifungal activity of TJN-318 is typical of imidazoles, being very broad and composing dermatophytes *Penicillia, Aspergilli, Paracoccidioides brasiliensis, Blastomyces dermatitidis, Foncecaea* and yeasts. MIC (Minimum Inhibitory Concentration) values of TJN-318 against pathogenic fungi were compared with those of 3 major topical agents on the market (Table 1)[3]. The MIC values on dermatophytes ranged from 0.004 - 0.031 μg/ml. TJN-318 was 2-500 times more active than the reference compounds, demonstrating itself to be one of the most potent antifungal agents thus far reported.

Table 1 Antifungal Activity of TJN-318 (NND-318) on Pathogenic Fungi

Species of pathogen	No. of strains tested	MIC (μg/ml)			
		TJN-318	Imidazole (A)	Imidazole (B)	Tolnaftate
T. mentagrophytes	7	0.004-0.031	0.25-1.0	0.25-4.0	0.031-0.5
T. rubrum	6	0.008-0.016	0.25-0.5	1.0 -2.0	0.031-0.125
C. albicans	7	1.6 -50	0.8-12.5	—	—
M. furfur	7	0.63 -2.5	20 -40	1.25-5.0	—
M. pachydermatis	4	0.16 -0.32	20	0.63-2.5	—

Agar plate with olive oil: *Malassezia* — : Not determined

By adding 10^{-7} - 10^{-9}M TJN-318 into the suspension of homogenated mycelium, 80% of 2-^{14}C-acetic acid incorporation to 4-desmethylsterol was inhibited, showing it to be very strong in the inhibition of ergosterol biosynthesis[3].

Tinea pedis model was prepared basically according to the procedures of Fujita et al.[1,2,3]. Active formulations or vehicle were topically applied to the whole sole of the foot once a day for 10 consecutive days. Five days after the last application, skin blocks from planta pedis and tarsus were cultured to detect fungi (Fig. 2). In animals of infected control group (without treatment), 96% and 85% of skin blocks from the planta pedis and tarsus were positive by culture (Fig. 3).

The treatment of 1% TJN-318 polyethylene glycol (PEG) 300 solution eliminated completely the inoculated fungus. By contrast, treatment with 1% PEG 300 solution reduced the rate of fungus-positive skin blocks to 52-66%.

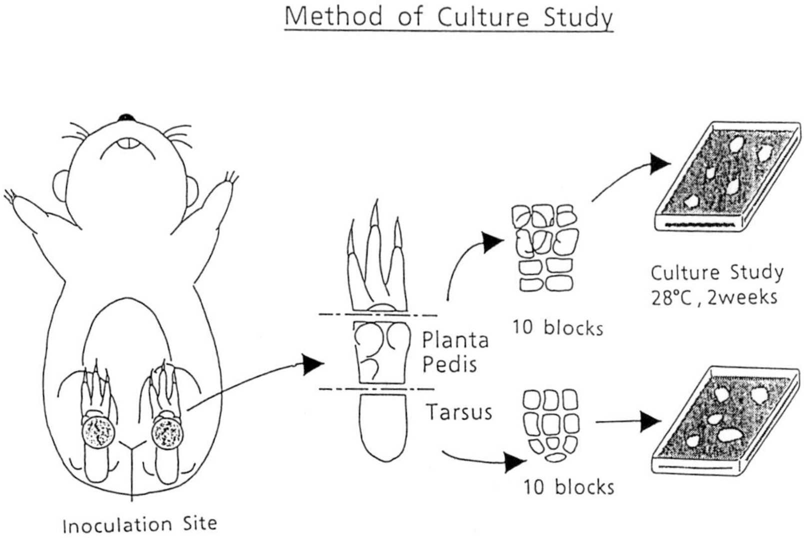

Fig. 2 Method of culture study in tinea pedis model using guinea pigs

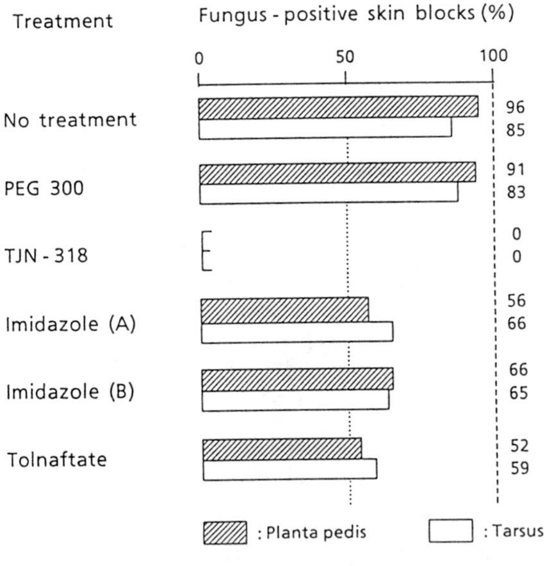

Fig. 3 Results of culture study in tinea pedis model using guinea pigs

Duration of protective effect of TJN-318 on Tinea corporis in guinea pigs after the application was examined[2]. When 1% TJN-318 PEG 300 solution was applied 1-3 days prior to the inoculation, the rate of fungus- positive skin blocks from the loci was reduced to 3 - 8% (Fig. 4). Even though *T. mentagrophytes* was inoculated 4 days after the pretreatment by TJN-318, the rate of fungus-positive skin blocks from the loci was reduced to 21%, showing a long duration of antifungal activity of TJN-318.

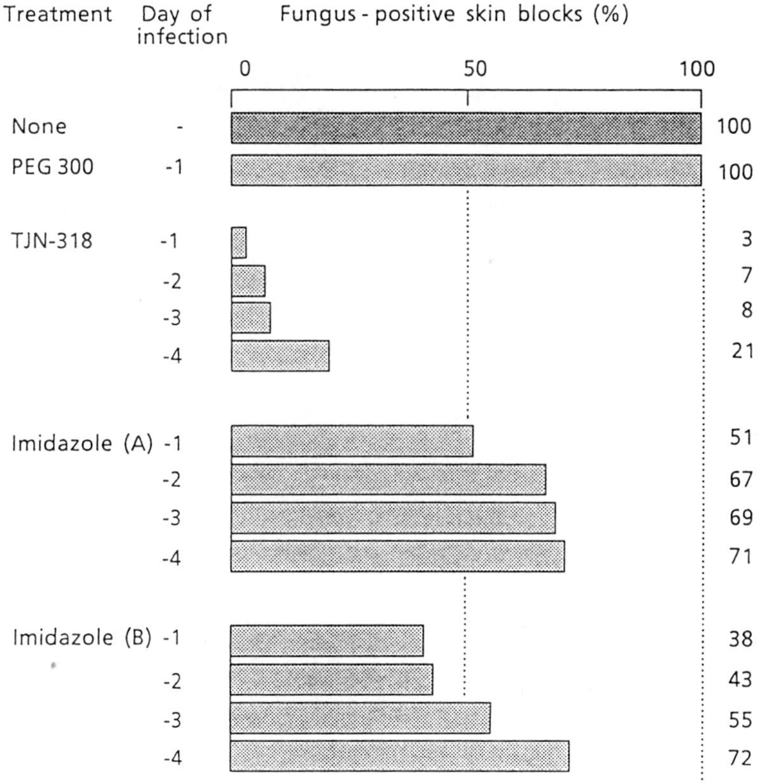

Fig. 4 Results of protective effect studies in tinea corporis model using guinea pigs

B. *TOXICITY AND PHARMACOKINETICS*

In acute toxicity tests, LD_{50} of percutaneous administration was more than 5,000 mg/kg. In 4-week subacute toxicity and reproduction studies administered subcutaneously, no observable effect levels (NOEL) were considered to be 1 - 5 mg/kg/day. When TJN-318 was administered under percutaneous route, which is the same application route as clinical use, NOEL was 10 mg/kg/day in the 4-week subacute toxicity test for rats.

TJN-318 showed negative results in mutagenicity tests. Nor did TJN-318 have primary irritating potency or cause allergic reaction when administered percutaneously.

When ^{14}C-TJN-318 was administered percutaneously to rats, blood concentration of radioactivity reached the maximum level after 9-12 hours. The maximum concentration of radioactivity was 0.044 μg eq. of TJN-318/ml in plasma. Ninety-two percent of the administered ^{14}C-TJN-318 was recovered from the skin surface, and 6.2% in both urine (2.0%) and feces (4.2%). These findings suggest that the percutaneous absorption rate of TJN-318 is around 6 percent.

As described above, there were no findings to cause anxiety for topical application to humans in toxicity studies.

III. CLINICAL STUDIES

A. *PHASE I STUDIES (SKIN IRRITATION TEST)*

Test substances spread on the patch test discs were applied on the backsof healthy male volunteers for 48 hours. Almost all volunteers patched by TJN-318 cream showed negative skin reactions (Table 2). TJN-318 cream also did not show phototoxicity, nor any flare-up suggesting allergic reactions.

Five grams of 1% TJN-318 cream was applied on the backs (20 x 25 cm) of 6 volunteers for 8 hours daily for 7 consecutive days. In toxicological examination such as blood biochemistry and physiology tests, no abnormal findings attributable to TJN-318 were observed.

Table 2 Skin irritation study of TJN-318 (NND-318)

Test substance	Score of irritation*						Total score
	0	0.5	1.0	2.0	3.0	4.0	
0.5% TJN-318 cream	12	1	1	0	0	0	1.5
1.0% TJN-318 cream	13	1	0	0	0	0	0.5
2.0% TJN-318 cream	14	0	0	0	0	0	0.0
TJN-318 cream base	12	2	0	0	0	0	1.0
1% Imidazole (C) cream	2	4	8	0	0	0	10.0
Control	7	6	1	0	0	0	4.0

* 0: no response, 0.5: slight erythema, 1: erythema, 2: erythema and edema, 3: papules and small blister, 4: blister, erosion and necrosis

Volunteers tested: n=14, each 12 patches

B. *EARLY PHASE II STUDY*

An early phase II study, which was an open, non-comparative study, was carried out in 15 hospitals to evaluate efficacy and tolerability of 1% TJN-318 cream in 1989. Patients with tinea pedis, tinea corporis, tinea cruris, tinea versicolor or candidiasis were treated with a single daily application of 1% TJN-318 cream for 2 or 4 weeks. The clinical assessment of efficacy was based on signs of itching, redness, scale, papulation, blister and pustule, and mycological examinations. Evaluation of the improvement of clinical symptoms is summarized in Table 3. The total rate of "remarkably improved" and "improved" was 90% in tinea pedis, 98% in tinea corporis and tinea cruris, 91% in candidiasis and 92% in tinea versicolor. Only 3 patients with tinea pedis failed to respond to 1% TJN-318 cream treatment. The result of mycological

Table 3 Improvement rate of clinical symptoms by TJN-318 (NND-318)

	No. of patients	Remarkably improved	Improved	Fairly improved	Unchanged	Aggravated
Tinea pedis	78	45	25	5	3	0
		58%	32% (90%)	6%	4%	0%
Tinea corporis Tinea cruris	65	50	14	1	0	0
		77%	22% (98%)	2%	0%	0%
Candidiasis	33	23	7	3	0	0
		70%	21% (91%)	9%	0%	0%
Tinea versicolor	25	20	3	2	0	0
		80%	12% (92%)	8%	0%	0%

( ) : The total rate of "Remarkably improved" and "Improved"

examinations is shown in Fig. 5. The rate of negative mycological findings in tinea pedis, which is known for its resistance to treatment against antifungal agents, was 74% after the treatment for 4 weeks by TJN-318. More than 95% of patients with tinea corporis, tinea cruris, candidiasis and tinea versicolor showed the remission of fungi after the treatment for 2 weeks.

According to the clinical symptoms, mycological findings and adverse reactions, utility was classified into 5 grades (Table 4). In 49% and 28% of the patients, the utility for tinea pedis was "very useful" and "useful", respectively. The utility of 1% TJN-318 cream was almost complete in tinea corporis, tinea cruris, candidiasis and tinea versicolor. Four patients (1.8% of total patients) with tinea pedis showed slight adverse reactions with the symptoms of erythema, dryness of the skin, contact dermatitis and vesicles. The tolerance study by local use of 1% TJN-318 cream revealed favorable results.

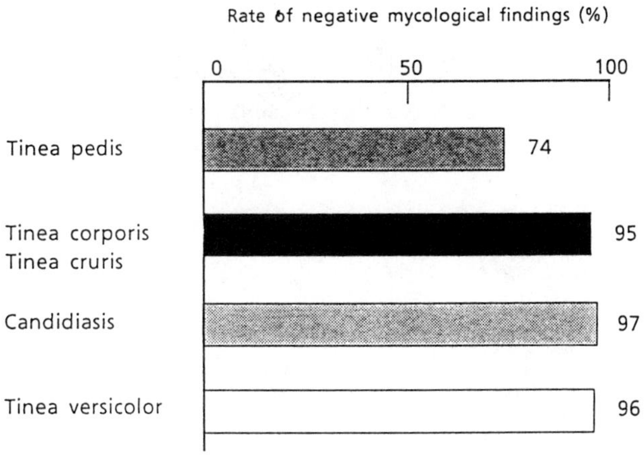

Fig. 5 Mycological findings after TJN-318 (NND-318) treatment

Table 4 Utility of TJN-318 (NND-318)

	No. of patients	Very useful	Useful	Fairly useful	Not useful	Harmful	Adverse reactions
Tinea pedis	78	38	22	15	3	0	4/92
		49%	28% (77%)	19%	4%	0%	
Tinea corporis Tinea cruris	65	49	13	3	0	0	0/71
		75%	20% (95%)	5%	0%	0%	
Candidiasis	33	23	9	1	0	0	0/37
		70%	27% (97%)	3%	0%	0%	
Tinea versicolor	25	20	3	2	0	0	0/26
		80%	12% (92%)	8%	0%	0%	
	201						4/226 1.8%

( ) : The total rate of "Very useful" and "Useful"
Adverse reactions : Erythema, dryness of the skin, contact dermatitis and vesicles

IV. SUMMARY

A newly developed antimycotic imidazole preparation TJN-318 (NND-318) was evaluated for its preclinical and clinical potencies. The results were summarized as follows:

1. A broad antifungal spectrum and extremely low MIC values against pathogenic fungi were noted.

2. Excellent therapeutic efficacy and prolonged protective effect were shown in animal models.

3. In phase I study, skin irritation was very slight and no phototoxicity was detected.

4. In early phase II study by 1% cream, significant clinical improvement, mycological efficacy and very slight adverse reactions (1.8%) resulted.

These results suggest that TJN-318 is a promising agent in treating superficial mycoses.

REFERENCES

1. Fujita, S. and Matsuyama, T., Experimental tinea pedis induced by non-abrasive inoculation of Trichophyton mentagrophytes arthrosporea on the plantar part of a guinea pig foot, J. Med. Vet. Mycol., 25: 203-213 (1987).

2. Ohmi, T., Uchida, M. and Yamaguchi, H. et al, 32nd Meet. Jpn. Soc. Med. Mycol (Niigata), 1988

3. Ohmi, T., Uchida, M. and Yamaguchi, H. et al, 29th ICAAC, Houston, Tex., 1989

Neticonazol (SS 717): Clinical Evaluation of Its Activities

S. Kagawa[1], T. Nishikawa[2]*, H. Takahashi[3],
S. Takahashi[4], S. Watanabe[5]

1) *Department of Dermatology, Tokyo Medical and Dental University School of Medicine, 1-5-45 Yushima, Bunkyo, Tokyo 113, Japan.*
2) *Department of Dermatology, Keio University School of Medicine, 35 Shinanomachi, Shinjuku, Tokyo 160, Japan.*
3) *Department of Dermatology, Akita University School of Medicine, 1-1-1 Hondo, Akita, Akita 010, Japan.*
4) *Department of Dermatology, Teikyo University School of Medicine, 2-11-1, Kaga, Itabashi, Tokyo 173, Japan.*
5) *Department of Dermatology, Shiga University of Medical Science, Tsukinowa, Seta, Otu, Shiga 520-1, Japan.*

I. INTRODUCTION

SS717 is a new antifungal agent of the imidazole group with a unique structure, (E)-1-[2-methylthio-1-[2-(pentyloxy)phenyl] ethenyl]-1-H-imidazole hydrochloride (Fig.1). It is characterized by the absence of halogen group and the presence of S-methyl group[1]. SS717 shows a mode of action similar to that of existing imidazoles[2] and was synthesized and developed as a drug for superficial dermatomycoses by SS Pharmaceutical Co., Ltd.. This article deals with its preclinical and clinical aspects.

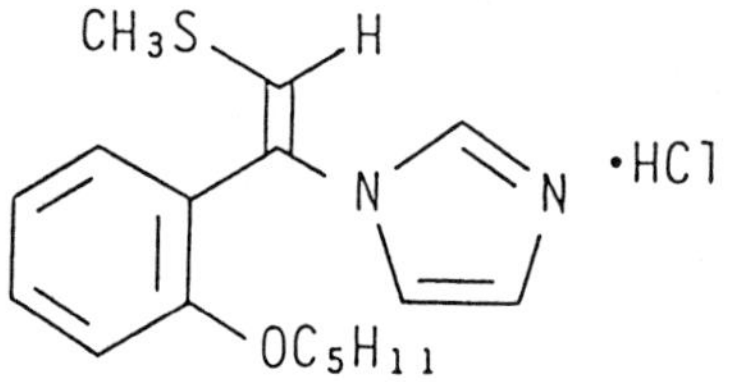

Fig. 1 Chemical Structure of SS717: (E)-1-[2-methylthio-1-[2-(pentyloxy)pentyloxy)]ethenyl]-1*H*-imidazole hydrochloride

II. PRECLINICAL STUDIES: *IN VITRO* ANTIFUNGAL ACTIVITY

MIC (minimum inhibitory concentration) values of SS717 against standard strains of pathogenic fungi were compared with those of 3 major topical agents on the market using Sabouraud dextrose agar plate (Table 1). The MIC against *C. albicans* was lowest for clotrimazole (CTZ), followed by SS717, cloconazole (CCZ) and bifonazole (BFZ). The MIC against *T. mentagrophytes* and *T. rubrum* was lowest for SS717 at 0.01 to 0.20 ug/ml; SS717 exhibited 4 to 15 times stronger antifungal activities of BFZ. The MIC and the minimum fungicidal concentration (MCC), of SS717 and other imidazoles against standard strains using broth dilution methods were compared (data not shown). No major differences were observed between the MIC obtained by the broth dilution and the plate dilution methods. Although the MCC against *C. albicans* was moderate to high for all 4 imidazole drugs, the MCCs against the dermatophytes were lower and those for SS717 and CTZ were notably the lowest. The effects of the addition of serum on the antifungal activity of SS717 and the other imidazole drugs were examined, and the antifungal activity of SS717 and CCZ was less affected, while that of CTZ and BFZ was decreased 1/2 to 1/8. From the above results together with other data not shown here, among the 4 imidazole derivatives, SS717 proved to be the most potent against *T. mentagrophytes, T. rubrum* and *M. canis*. Furthermore, SS717 was more potent in *in vitro* antifungal activity than CCZ and BFZ on MIC, and almost as potent as CTZ on MCC. The antifungal activity of SS717 was little affected by the addition of the serum.

Table 1 Antifungal activity of SS717 and other imidazole antimycotics against some standard strains as measured on Sabouraud dextrose (2%) agar

Organism	Number of strains	MIC range (μg/ml)			
		SS717	CTZ	CCZ	BFZ
Candida albicans	6	3.12-50	1.56-25	3.12-100	6.25->25
Trichophyton mentagrophytes	3	0.10-0.20	0.20-0.39	0.39-1.56	1.56-3.12
Trichophyton rubrum	3	0.10-0.20	0.39	0.20-1.56	0.39-3.12
Microsporum canis	1	0.78	0.78	1.56	>25

Inoculum size: 10^6 cells/ml, Incubation: 3 to 7 days at 27°C
CTZ: Clotrimazole, CCZ: Cloconazole, BFZ: Bifonazole
MIC: Minimum inhibitory concentration

III. CLINICAL STUDIES

A. PHASE I STUDIES (SKIN IRRITATION TEST AND TOLERANCE STUDY)

The skin irritation test in 28 healthy male volunteers showed that 0.5%, 1.0% and 2.0% SS717 cream had less irritating potency than 1.0% BFZ and 1.0% econazole (ECZ), the former two being completely non-irritating. A tolerance study using 2.0% SS717 cream showed no abnormalities in skin symptoms, general symptoms, electrocardiography or laboratory tests, and thus, was considered safe for human application. A skin irritation study using 24 patients with skin diseases showed 0.5% and 1.5% SS717 to be extremely less irritating than 1.0% ECZ, 1.0% BFZ and 2.0% SS717 (data not shown).

B. PHASE II STUDY

An open clinical trial was then conducted to determine efficacy, safety and usefulness of SS717 cream. Based upon the results of the phase I study, 1.0% was chosen as an appropriate concentration for the phase II study. Tinea pedis, tinea corporis, tinea cruris, intertrigo type candidiasis, erosio interdigitalis and tinea versicolor with positive KOH preparations were the subjects. Prior informed consent of the patient was obtained, and 1.0% SS717 was applied to the affected site once daily, after bathing or before retiring. The application period was 4 weeks in patients with tinea pedis and 2 weeks in those with other conditions. Observations were made at one week intervals. The minimum observation time for tinea pedis was at 1, 2 and 4 weeks after application and 1 and 2 weeks for the other conditions. Skin changes were assessed arbitrarily with five grades, i.e. 'remarkably improved', 'improved', 'slightly improved', 'no change' and 'wosened'. Detailed case cards were collected from 25 institutions and evaluation was made by a committee. Out of 454 total cases, 415 were analyzed for overall efficacy, and 448 for safety. The clearance rate of fungi at final examination was 73.8% for tinea pedis, 88.9% for tinea corporis, 92.7% for tinea cruris, 96.3% for intertrigo type cutaneous candidiasis, 87.5% for erosio interdigitalis, and 85.7% for tinea versicolor. Final overall efficacy of more than 'effective' was 72.8% for tinea pedis, 88.9% for tinea corporis, 92.7% for tinea cruris, 95.1% for intertrigo type cutaneous candidiasis, 84.4% for erosio interdigitalis, and 85.7% for tinea versicolor. Side effects were observed in only 1.8% of the total cases. With respect to safety, 98.0% of the total cases were evaluated as 'completely safe' (Table 2).

Table 2 Safety as assessed according to the complaint and clinical observation

Safety / case	Completely safe	Almost safe	Safety is suspected	Not safe	Total cases
No. cum.%	439 98.0	3 98.7	4 99.6	2 100.0	448

cum.%: cumulative percent

Table 3 Usefulness of 1.0% SS717 cream

Disease	Usefulness / case	Extremely useful	Useful	Slightly useful	Not useful	Undesirable	Total cases
Tinea pedis	No. cum.%	32 31.1	44 73.8	18 91.3	6 97.1	3 100.0	103
Tinea corporis	No. cum.%	52 64.2	18 86.4	11 100.0	0	0	81
Tinea cruris	No. cum.%	38 69.1	13 92.7	4 100.0	0	0	55
Intertrigo type cutaneous candidiasis	No. cum.%	53 65.4	23 93.8	4 98.8	0 98.8	1 100.0	81
Erosio interdigitalis candidomycetica	No. cum.%	14 43.8	13 84.4	4 96.9	1 100.0	0	32
Tinea versicolor	No. cum.%	44 69.8	10 85.7	9 100.0	0	0	63

cum.%: cumulative percent

The usefulness showing evaluation rate of more than 'useful' was 73.8% for tinea pedis, 86.4% for tinea corporis, 92.7% for tinea cruris, 93.8% for intertrigo type cutaneous candidiasis, 84.4% for erosio interdigitalis, and 85.7% for tinea versicolor (Table 3). From these results, it was considered that 1.0% SS717 cream, when applied once daily, was as effective and safe as other imidazole drugs in the treatment of dermatomycosis.

C. PHASE III STUDY

A phase III study was performed to determine the efficacy, safety and usefulness of 1.0% SS717 cream in the treatment of tinea, candidiasis, and tinea versicolor through a randomized well controlled comparative study using 1.0% bifonazole cream as the control drug. Six dermatomycoses were selected as the subjects. The control drug was 1.0% BFZ cream which was kindly supplied by Bayer Pharmaceutical Co.. These drugs looked very much alike, and randomized allocated samples were distributed to the participating 37 institutions. The application period and other details of the test were the same as the phase II study. The detailed case cards were collected from 37 participating institutions and their suitability for evaluation was judged by a committee. The usefulness of this compound was evaluated on the double blind basis on the results of efficacy, safety and side effects. After the test was over, the key code was opened and a comparison of SS717 with the reference drug BFZ was made statistically. Statistical analysis was done by Wilcoxon rank order summation test and χ^2 test or Fisher's direct probability calculation method. The significance standard was 5%, and reference was also made to a 10% significance tendency. The homogeneity between the two groups in terms of background factors was considered. When a bias was found, stratum analysis of the affecting factors was performed by Mantel-Haenszel or other tests. Out of 830 total cases, 720 were evaluated for efficacy and 779 for safety. Again final selection of the cases were made by a committee. The clearance rate of fungus at the final examination is shown in Table 4. It varies from 78.5% to 95.2% in the SS717 group and from 64.5% to 88.1% in the BFZ group. There was a trend toward difference in the SS717 group for tinea pedis by the χ^2 test, but no significant difference in other conditions.

Table 4 Final fungal examination by KOH preparation *

Disease	Drug	Negative	Positive	Total cases	Disappearance rate (%)	χ^2 rating
Tinea pedis	SS717	103	28	131	78.6	$\chi^2(1)=3.251$△
	BFZ	93	42	135	68.9	P =0.071
Tinea corporis	SS717	51	14	65	78.5	N.S.
	BFZ	49	17	66	74.2	
Tinea cruris	SS717	43	5	48	89.6	N.S.
	BFZ	37	9	46	80.4	
Intertrigo type cutaneous candidiasis	SS717	40	2	42	95.2	N.S.
	BFZ	37	5	42	88.1	
Erosio interdigitalis candidomycetica	SS717	26	7	33	78.8	N.S.
	BFZ	20	11	31	64.5	
Tinea versicolor	SS717	38	7	45	84.4	N.S.
	BFZ	29	7	36	80.6	

N.S.: Not significant △:10% Significant

* : The application period was 4 weeks in Tinea pedis and 2 weeks in other conditions.

The overall efficacy of SS717 and BFZ for the 6 dermatomycoses is summarized in Table 5, and including cases more than 'effective' varies respectively from 77.1% to 92.9% and 58.1% to 85.7%. By statistical analysis, both Wilcoxon rank sum test and χ^2 test indicated a significant difference in SS717 for tinea pedis. Furthermore, the Wilcoxon test indicated a trend toward difference in SS717 for tinea cruris, significant difference for intertrigo and erosio interdigitalis, and the χ^2 test showed a trend toward difference in SS717 for erosio interdigitalis. For other conditions, however, there were no significant differences.

Table 5 Final overall efficacy of 1.0% SS717 and BFZ cream

Disease	Drug	Efficacy / case	Very effective	Effective	Slightly effective	Not effective	Aggravated	Total cases	Wilcoxon signed ranking	χ^2 rating (more than 'effective')
Tinea pedis	SS717	No.	51	50	22	5	3	131	Z=2.208 *	χ^2(1)=5.137*
		cum. %	38.9	77.1	93.9	97.7	100.0		P=0.027	P =0.023
	BFZ	No.	39	48	39	5	4	135		
		cum. %	28.9	64.4	93.3	97.0	100.0			
Tinea corporis	SS717	No.	30	21	13	1	0	65	N.S.	N.S.
		cum. %	46.2	78.5	98.5	100.0				
	BFZ	No.	30	18	17	1	0	66		
		cum. %	45.5	72.7	98.5	100.0				
Tinea cruris	SS717	No.	30	13	5	0	0	48	Z=1.657 △	N.S.
		cum. %	62.5	89.6	100.0				P=0.098	
	BFZ	No.	22	14	8	1	1	46		
		cum. %	47.8	78.3	95.7	97.8	100.0			
Intertrigo type culaneous candidiasis	SS717	No.	26	13	2	1	0	42	Z=1.968 *	N.S.
		cum. %	61.9	92.9	97.6	100.0			P=0.049	
	BFZ	No.	17	19	5	0	1	42		
		cum. %	40.5	85.7	97.6	97.6	100.0			
Erosio interdigitalis candidomycetica	SS717	No.	15	11	7	0	0	33	Z=1.992 *	χ^2(1)=3.195△
		cum. %	45.5	78.8	100.0				P=0.046	P =0.074
	BFZ	No.	9	9	8	3	2	31		
		cum. %	29.0	58.1	83.9	93.5	100.0			
Tinea versicolor	SS717	No.	32	6	7	0	0	45	N.S.	N.S.
		cum. %	71.1	84.4	100.0					
	BFZ	No.	24	5	7	0	0	36		
		cum. %	66.7	80.6	100.0					

cum. %: cumulative percent

N.S.: Not significant
* : 5% siginificant
△ : 10% siginificant

We found a significant difference in the duration of the disease between the two groups in tinea pedis. In differential analysis, the Wilcoxon rank sum test indicated differences, and the Mantel-Haenszel test indicated a trend to significant differences in SS717 group in cases with 1 to 3 months duration of the diseases, but no significant differences in other levels.

Side effects were observed in only 1.8% of the SS717 group and 2.9% of BFZ; there were no significant differences between the groups. The drugs were 'completely safe' in 98.2% of the SS717 group and 97.1% of the BFZ group, and, again, there were no significant differences (Table 6).

Table 6 Safety of 1.0% SS717 and BFZ creams

Drug	Safety / case	Completely safe	Almost safe	Safety is suspected	Not safe	Total cases	Wilcoxon signed ranking
SS717	No.	389	3	3	1	396	N.S.
	cum.%	98.2	99.0	99.7	100.0		
BFZ	No.	372	3	7	1	383	
	cum.%	97.1	97.9	99.7	100.0		

cum.%: cumulative percent

N.S.: Not significant

The evaluations of more than 'useful' were, for SS717 and BFZ, respectively; 77.1% and 65.2% for tinea pedis, 78.5% and 72.7% for tinea corporis, 89.6% and 78.3% for tinea cruris, 92.9% and 83.3% for intertrigo, 75.8% and 58.1% for erosio interdigitalis, and 86.7% and 80.6% for tinea versicolor (Table 7). Significant differences were observed for the SS717 group by both Wilcoxon and χ^2 test in tinea pedis; the Wilcoxon test indicated a trend toward differences for SS717 in tinea cruris and erosio interdigitalis and also significant difference for SS717 in intertrigo. There were no significant differences in other disorders.

Table 7 Usefulness of 1.0% SS717 and BFZ cream

Disease	Drug	usefulness case	Extremeiy useful	Useful	Slightly useful	Not useful	Undesirable	Total cases	Wilcoxon signed ranking	χ^2 rating (more than 'useful')
Tinea pedis	SS717	No.	50	51	22	5	3	131	Z=2.069*	χ^2(1)=4.588*
		cum. %	38.2	77.1	93.9	97.7	100.0		P=0.039	P =0.032
	BFZ	No.	39	49	38	6	3	135		
		cum. %	28.9	65.2	93.3	97.8	100.0			
Tinea corporis	SS717	No.	29	22	13	0	1	65	N.S.	N.S.
		cum. %	44.6	78.5	98.5	98.5	100.0			
	BFZ	No.	30	18	17	0	1	66		
		cum. %	45.5	72.7	98.5	98.5	100.0			
Tinea cruris	SS717	No.	30	13	5	0	0	48	Z=1.657△	N.S.
		cum. %	62.5	89.6	100.0				P=0.098	
	BFZ	No.	22	14	8	1	1	46		
		cum. %	47.8	78.3	95.7	97.8	100.0			
Intertrigo type culaneous candidiasis	SS717	No.	26	13	2	1	0	42	Z=2.042 *	N.S.
		cum. %	61.9	92.9	97.6	100.0			P=0.041	
	BFZ	No.	17	18	6	0	1	42		
		cum. %	40.5	83.3	97.6	97.6	100.0			
Erosio interdigitalis candidomycetica	SS717	No.	15	10	8	0	0	33	Z=1.871△	N.S.
		cum. %	45.5	75.8	100.0				P=0.061	
	BFZ	No.	9	9	8	3	2	31		
		cum. %	29.0	58.1	83.9	93.5	100.0			
Tinea versicolor	SS717	No.	32	7	6	0	0	45	N.S.	N.S.
		cum. %	71.1	86.7	100.0					
	BFZ	No.	24	5	7	0	0	36		
		cum. %	66.7	80.6	100.0					

cum. %: cumulative percent

N.S.: Not significant
* : 5% siginificant
△ : 10% siginificant

IV. DISCUSSION

Since the development of clotrimazole, many kinds of imidazoles have been synthesized as antifungal agents. The new imidazole group agent, SS717, created as an antifungal agent against superficial dermatomycoses[1,3] was the subject of a preclinical study and phase I, II, and III studies. Its antifungal activity, safety, and usefulness was compared with those of several other popular imidazole antifungal compounds.

From our results, we concluded that 1.0% SS717 cream was equally as effective or superior to 1.0% BFZ cream in a single daily application for tinea, candidiasis, and tinea versicolor and thus a useful drug for the treatment of superficial dermatomycoses. Its benefits are largely due to the facts that its antifungal activity is little affected by the addition of serum protein and that it exhibits stronger antifungal activity than other imidazole derivatives against dermatophytes. Further, it is easily accumulated in the horny layer for a longer period. The fact that the drug is applied in cream form may also play a role in its effectiveness.

REFERENCES

1. Maebashi K, Hiratani T, Uchida K, Asagi Y, Yamaguchi H. *In vitro* antifungal activity of SS717, a new imidazole antimycotic. *Jpn. J. Med. Mycol., 31*:333-342, 1990. (In Japanese)
2. Maebashi K, Hiratani T, Asagi Y, Yamaguchi H. Studies on the mechanism of antifungal action of a new imidazole antimycotic SS717. *Jpn. J. Med. Mycol., 31*:343-354, 1990. (In Japanese)
3. Asaoka T, Kawahara R, Iwasa A. Antifungal activity of SS717, a new imidazole antimycotic I. *In vitro* antimicrobial activity. *Chemotherapy, 38*:105-120, 1990. (In Japanese)

10

Amorolfine, Ro 14-4767/002, Loceryl

PD Dr. A. Polak

Pharmaceutical Research, F. Hoffmann-La Roche Ltd
CH-4002 Basel/Switzerland

Amorolfine is a new antifungal drug (4-(3-(P(1,1-dimethylpropyl)-phenyl)2-methyl-propyl[-2,6-cis-dimethylmorpholine hydrochloride]), which is active against fungi pathogenic to plants, animals and humans.

I. IN VITRO ACTIVITY OF AMOROLFINE

I.1 Fungistatic . Amorolfine possesses remarkable antifungal activity against a broad spectrum of medically important fungi (Table 1) (1, 2). The highest activity is exerted against dermatophytes, but it is also active against yeasts and the molds *Alternaria, Hendersonula* and *Scopulariopsis,* although aspergilli are resistant. The fungistatic activity against yeasts, especially *Candida albicans,* is strongly dependent on the constituents of the medium, its pH, aeration, inoculum size and incubation time. Great interspecies and intraspecies variations in the MIC values are observed, the same phenomenon as with another class of sterolbiosynthesis inhibitors, the azoles (2).

Table 1 Antifungal spectrum of Amorolfine

Species	Number of strains	MIC µg/ml geometric mean	MIC µg/ml range
Dermatophytes	200	0.020	0.001 - 0.13
Pityrosporum spp.	10	0.075	0.005 - 2
Candida albicans	155	0.55	0.001 - >100
Candida spp.	125	0.79	0.001 - >100
Cryptococcus neoformans	55	0.033	<0.0001 - 8
Dematiaceous fungi	70	0.08	0.001 - 2.5
Dimorphic fungi	65	0.12	0.01 - 10
Aspergillus spp.	68	100	30 - >100
Zygomycetes	25	30	30 - >100
Fusarium spp.	8	30	0.3 - 100
Hendersonula sp.	6	0.3	0.1 - 1
Alternaria sp.	5	0.35	0.05 - 1
Scopularopsis	3	0.8	0.2 - 3

I.2 Fungicidal Amorolfine is also fungicidal against yeasts, dermatophytes, dimorphic fungi and dematiaceae. This fungicidal activity is dependent on the time of contact and the concentration of the drug, and in degree is similar to that of oxiconazole or terbinafine (in the case of dermatophytes). 99 % of the cells are killed after 48 hours contact with amorolfine at a concentration of 1 µg/ml for C. *albicans*, 0.003-0.01 µg for dermatophytes, 0.25 µg for dematiaceae and 1.7 µg/ml for *Histoplasma capsulatum* (1, 2).

II. MODE OF ACTION

Amorolfine interferes with the sterol biosynthesis of fungal cells. In all species tested the bulk sterol (ergosterol in C. *albicans*, ergosta-5-22dienol in *H. capsulatum*) disappears from treated cells in a time and concentration-dependent manner. There is a definite correlation between the observed changes in the sterol pattern and growth inhibition (3, 4, 5, 6). Ignosterol, a sterol containing a Δ14 double-bond, is accumulated in *C. albicans*, leading to the conclusion that amorolfine inhibits the Δ14 reduction step in the biosynthesis of ergosterol, which follows C_{14}demethylation. The Δ7-Δ8 isomerization step is also inhibited in presence of amorolfine. Thus, this drug inhibits two steps in the pathway of ergosterol biosynthesis. In crude extracts of *Saccharomyces cerevisiae* the IC_{50} value of amorolfine for the Δ14-reductase is 2.93 μM, and for the Δ7-Δ8-isomerase 0.0018 μM (7).

The high efficacy of amorolfine is most probably due to the fact that two consecutive enzymatic steps in the same pathway are inhibited, which may be viewed as a built-in synergistic effect. Whether inhibition of sterol biosynthesis is responsible for the antifungal action of such compounds as amorolfine has been the subject of much discussion. Recent work by Karst's group (8) on fenpropimorph, an amorolfine analog, made elegant use of mutants of *Saccharomyces cerevisiae* not only to show that this is so, but also to provide strong evidence that it is the lack of ergosterol rather than the accumulation of other sterols that causes cessation of growth in the unbudded G1-phase of the cell cycle. However, electron microscopic studies show an abnormal accumulation of chitin in the membrane, indicating that chitin synthesis is also disturbed. The cell wall thickness is increased, electron transparent areas appear in the cytoplasm and extracytoplasmic vesicles are formed and deposited in the cell wall. These are the same observations as made in azole-treated cells, but it is not clear to what extent these phenomena are responsible for antifungal activity or if they are also a result of ergosterol depletion of the membrane (9, 10).

III. THERAPEUTIC EFFICACY IN ANIMAL MODELS

The therapeutic efficacy of amorolfine is limited to superficial fungal infections. After oral application the drug is practically inactive against deep-seated mycosis, probably due to strong protein-binding and metabolization in rodents.

In vaginal candidosis as little as 0.01 % locally applied resulted in a two order of magnitude reduction in viable candida cells recovered from the vagina of rats. 0.3 % amorolfine cleared the vagina completely (2).

Amorolfine also exerted excellent activity in a model of trichophytosis in the guinea pig, independently of whether therapy was started simultaneously (6 hours after the infection) or therapeutically (3 days after the infection). The duration of the treatment was 11 days and the mycotic foci read at day 12. A simultaneous therapy with 0.01 % amorolfine cream kept 100% of the treated animals mycosis-free. This is lower than the naftifine dosage required and only slightly higher than that used with terbinafine (2). The therapeutic treatment schedule starts on day 3, when mycotic foci are already seen in all animals. In this experiment 0.03 % amorolfine cleared the mycotic foci within 3 weeks. None of the azole derivatives tested (ketoconazole, oxiconazole, itraconazole) have such good efficacy, and only terbinafine at 0.1 % cleared the foci in a shorter period of time (2 weeks) (2, 4).

The cutaneous retention time test has been used to evaluate the persistence of active amorolfine in the skin. Lesions of trichophytosis were scored in guinea pigs following a single application of 0.1 % amorolfine on days 4, 3, 2 and 1 before infection. The severity of the lesions was directly proportional to the length of time elapsed between prophylactic treatment and experimental infection. An effective concentration of amorolfine apparently remained for at least 3 days in the horny layer of guinea pig skin (2, 4). The same long persistence was seen in human skin.After treatment of volunteers with a 0.5 % amorolfine cream or alcoholic solution, tape stripings were taken at various intervals and applied to the surface of microculture slices which had previously been inoculated with a dermatophytic fungus. The persistence in the epidermis was assessed by the degree of inhibition. Amorolfine had a persistent antimycotic effect for at least 48 hours and some inhibition was still seen up to day 3 (11).

Thus from the preclinical data it could be predicted that amorolfine would offer a logical alternative to existing therapies for vaginal candidosis and dermatomycosis. And indeed, clinical trials have shown that all the results obtained in our animal models can be transferred to human chemotherapy.

IV. TOLERANCE AND THERAPEUTIC EFFICIENCY

IV.1 Tolerance. The local tolerance of 0.125, 0.25 and 0.5 % cream was tested in a double-blind trial in two models, the During chamber and a scarification test. Tolerance was judged to be good and the few minor side effects were not dose dependent.

The tolerance of 50 mg vaginal tablets was tested after a single, 3 or 6-day treatment in a double-blind, placebo-controlled study. Amorolfine was well tolerated in all cases (12, 13).

IV.2 Chemotherapeutic efficacy

IV.2.1 Vaginal candidosis. Efficacy against vulvovaginal candidosis was assessed in three series of comparative trials using different single doses of amorolfine in the form of a vaginal tablet or ovulum. Dose-finding studies and comparative trials were performed. Cure was defined as clinical cure with negative mycological findings at the first and second follow-up (7 days and 4-5 weeks after treatment) or positive mycology at the first but negative findings at the second follow-up. Improvement was defined as improvement of signs and symptoms and mycology as above. Failures were defined as positive mycological findings at the first and at the second follow-up.

The best (statistically proven) efficacy was seen at a dose of 50 mg in a vaginal tablet. In an overall clinical and mycological assessment 76 % of the patients were cured by this dose but only 59 % of those treated with 25 mg. Patients treated with the vaginal ovula also responded well to the therapy regardless of the dose. The cure/improvement rate ranging from 75-90 %.

In a further study 50 and 100 mg vaginal tablets and 500 mg clotrimazole vaginal tablets were comparatively tested in a double-blind trial. There was no statistical difference between the efficacy of amorolfine and clotrimazole, although the clotrimazole had more failures (Figure 1) (12, 13).

IV.2.2 Dermatomycosis. Patients with dermatomycosis such as foot and cutaneous infections were treated with various doses of amorolfine cream for 2-6 weeks. Mycological and clinical examinations were performed before, at the end of, and 1 to 3 weeks after treatment. 735 patients were evaluated and infecting species included *T. rubrum* as the most frequent,

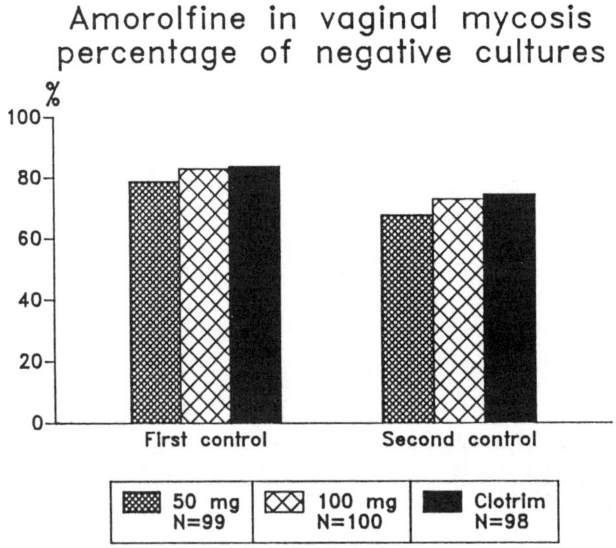

Fig. 1

followed by *T. mentagrophytes, E. floccosum, M. canis, T. terrestre, Candida* spp., aspergilli and *Rodutorula* spp. Of the patients treated with the 0.25 % cream 91.7% had a negative culture 1 week after therapy. The overall clinical results after once daily application showed a 81.3 % cure rate with 0.25 % amorolfine cream, improvement in 10.4 % and failure only in 8.3 %. This high efficacy of amorolfine compared favourably with therapy with 1 % bifonazole, where 84.3 % cure and 7.8 failures were seen.

In these trials it was shown that there was no difference in efficacy between amorolfine concentrations from 0.125% to 0.5% in the cream. Various galenic forms of amorolfine, 0.5 and 2 % spray (double-blind) and a 0.5 % cream (open) were compared in a further trial with *Tinea pedis.* All galenic forms were applied once daily for 3 weeks. Clinical symptoms were observed at the beginning, once during treatment period, at the end of therapy and 2 weeks thereafter. In this localization *T. rubrum* was again the most frequent species isolated (65), *T. mentagrophytes* (25) and *E. floccosum* (10) were also found, in two cases *M. canis* and in 4 cases *Candida* spp. The 2 % spray had a 97.4 % cure, 0.5 % spray lead to an efficacy of 94.1 % and the lowest effect was seen with 0.5 % cream (86.6 % cure) (Figure 2) (12, 13).

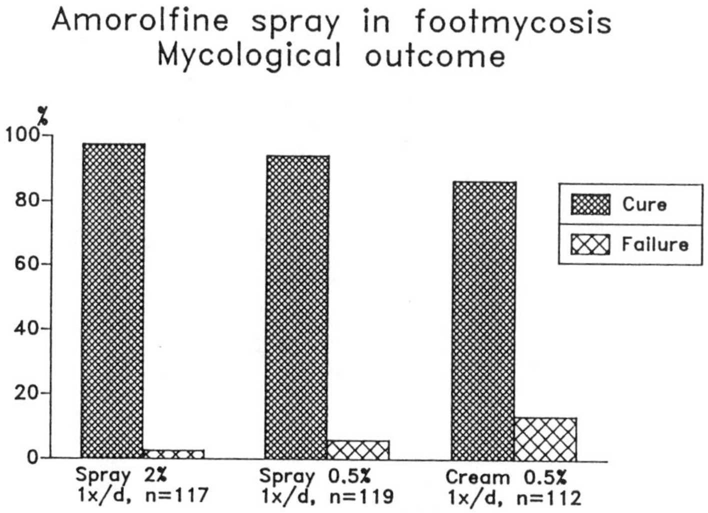

Fig.2

IV.2.3 Onychomycosis. During the clinical studies in this indication it became apparent that the degree of activity of topical treatment is strongly dependent on the size of the infected area of the nails. Those 20 % infected were cured within a 6 months treatment schedule and remained free of fungus even after the treatment was stopped. However, nails with an area of infection of 50 %, although clearly improved, are not cured by 6 months of treatment but require longer to achieve complete cure. Areas of infection of over 70 % showed no improvement and had to be treated with an oral therapy. So for an evaluation of the efficacy of a topical treatment this strong dependence on the area of infection has to be kept in mind and patients with nail infections covering more than 80 % should be excluded from the study (4).

Several studies were performed comparing a 2 % with a 5 % amorolfine lacquer the results of which have been published in various reports (4, 12, 13). In a double-blind randomized study the 5 % nail lacquer applied once weekly was compared with twice weekly application. The therapy lasted 6 months. Clinical and mycological examinations were per-

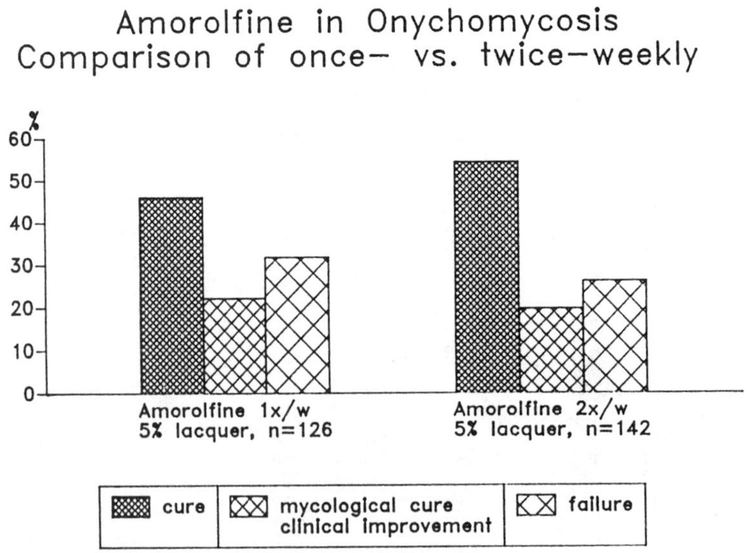

Fig.3

formed before the therapy started, the mycological examinations were repeated 1 and 3 months after the end of therapy, and the clinical symptoms were evaluated monthly. 126 patients were treated once, 142 were treated twice weekly. The efficacy was better with a therapy schedule of twice weekly application, 54.2 % of the patients being mycologically and clinically cured, 19.7 % showing significant improvement and 26.1 % not responding to the therapy (Figure 3) (12, 13).

In summary, amorolfine has been proven to be highly efficaceous in vaginal candidosis and in dermatomycosis of various locations. In addition, it has shown good efficacy after topical treatment of onychomycosis. This therapy is a real milestone in antimycotic therapy, as amorolfine provides for the first time a simple topical treatment for nail infections without surgical removal of the nail or treatment with urea.

REFERENCES

1. A. Polak, Antifungal activity in vitro of Ro 14-4767/002, a phenyl-propyl-morpholine, Sabouraudia 21: 205-213. (1983).
2. A. Polak, and D. Dixon, Antifungal activity of amorolfine (Ro 14-4767/006) in vitro and in vivo, In Recent Trends in the Discovery, Development and Evaluation of Antifungal Agents (R.A. Fromtling, ed.), J.R. Prous, Barcelona, p. 575-582. (1986).
3. A. Polak-Wyss, H. Lengsfeld, and G. Oesterhelt, Effect of oxiconazole and Ro 14-4767/002 on sterol pattern in *Candida albicans*, Sabouraudia, 23: 433-442 (1985).
4. A. Polak, Morpholines in clinical use, In Sterol Biosynthesis Inhibitors (Berg/Plempel, ed.), Ellis Horwood Limited, Weinheim, Cambridge, p. 430-448 (1988).
5. A. Polak, Mode of action of morpholine derivatives, Ann. NY Acad. Sci., 544: 221-228 (1988).
6. A. Polak, Mode of action studies, In Handbook of Experimental Pharmacology; Chemotherapy of Fungal Diseases (J.F. Ryley, ed.), Springer-Verlag Berlin, Heidelberg, Vol. 96, 153-182 (1990).

7. A. Polak, Amorolfine: Résultats précliniques, Bull. Soc. Fr. Mycol. Méd., 1: 9-16 (1989).
8. C. Marcireau, M. Guilloton, and F. Karst, In vivo effects of fenpropimorph on the yeast *Saccharomyces cerevisiae* and determination of the molecular basis of the antifungal property, Antimicrob.Agents Chemother., 43 (6): 989-993 (1990).
9. J. Müller, A. Polak, and R. Jaeger, The effect of the morpholine derivative amorolfine (Roche 14-4767/002) on the ultrastructure of *Candida albicans*, Mykosen, 30(11): 528-540 (1987).
10. A. Polak, W. Melchinger, and J. Müller, The effects of amorolfine and oxiconazole on the ultrastructure of *Trichophyton mentagrophytes*. A comparison, Mykosen (in press). (1990).
11. L. Gip, In vitro studies of the antifungal activity of amorolfine, a phenylpropyl morpholine, Adv. Ther., 6: 26-38 (1989).
12. E. Rhode, M. Zaug, and D. Hartmann, Preliminary clinical experience with Ro 14-4767/002 (amorolfine) in superficial mycoses, In Recent Trends in the Discovery, Development and Evaluation of Antifungal Agents (R.A. Fromtling, ed.), J.R. Prous, Barcelona, p. 575-582 (1986).
13. A. Polak, and M. Zaug, Amorolfine, In Handbook of Experimental Pharmacology; Chemotherapy of Fungal Diseases (J.F. Ryley, ed.), Springer-Verlag Berlin, Heidelberg, Vol. 96, 505-520 (1990).

11

Terbinafine: Clinical Efficacy and Development

H. Mieth and V. Villars*

Department of Dermatology, SANDOZ FORSCHUNGSINSTITUT, A-1235 Vienna, Austria

*Clinical Research, SANDOZ PHARMA LTD., Basle 4002 Switzerland

I. INTRODUCTION

Terbinafine is a member of the chemical class of allylamines. It is structurally related to naftifine, the first representative of this group of antifungals. The promising antifungal profile of naftifine, particularly its primary fungicidal action against a variety of fungal pathogens and its rapid onset of action in skin mycoses after topical application motivated us to study structure-activity relationships of allylamine derivatives in order to find a compound more active *in vitro* and also with superior properties *in vivo*. The result of these efforts is terbinafine (1). This paper provides evidence that the preclinical results obtained with terbinafine with regard to its rapid onset of fungicidal action *in vitro* and *in vivo* are of relevance also under clinical conditions.

II. EXPERIMENTAL ANTIMYCOTIC ACTIVITIES OF TERBINAFINE

A. ANTIFUNGAL PROFILE *IN VITRO*

Minimum inhibitory concentrations (MICs) have been determined for terbinafine by several investigators. The compound is highly active against a wide spectrum of human fungal pathogens including dermatophytes, moulds, yeasts, dimorphic and dematiaceous fungi (2). Dermatophytes are most susceptible to terbinafine, and the MICs found by using various test media are uniformly in the range of nanograms per ml. The susceptibility of yeasts varies widely between the various species, but the mycelial growth form of *Candida albicans* which is considered to be of importance for the pathogenicity of this yeast is consistently susceptible to terbinafine in concentrations of less than 1 µg per ml (3).

At drug concentrations equal to the MIC for the test strain, terbinafine has primary fungicidal action against dermatophytes, moulds and dimorphic fungi, whereas its action against yeasts can be either fungicidal (e.g. *C.parapsilosis*) or fungistatic; thus, its fungicidal effect against *C.albicans* is present only at concentrations higher than the MIC (4, 5).

B. ANTIFUNGAL PROFILE *IN VIVO*

Terbinafine proved to be highly effective in various models of dermatomycoses after topical or oral administration (6). Results obtained with terbinafine in the hair root invasion test (6, 7) and in the skin temperature test (8) suggest that its fungicidal action is also evident *in vivo* after topical or oral treatment of dermatophytoses.

III. CLINICAL EFFICACY OF TERBINAFINE

In clinical studies particular attention was paid to proving the antifungal efficacy of the compound microscopically as well as by culture (weekly intervals for dermatomycoses and monthly intervals for onychomycoses). Patients were rated as effectively treated only if they were free of fungal infections as proved by negative microscopy and culture and had no or only mild, clinical symptoms of erythema and desquamation. In onychomycoses, effective treatment included negative mycology and reversion to normal growth and appearance of the previously infected nails (9).

A. RESULTS AFTER TOPICAL TREATMENT WITH 1% TERBINAFINE CREAM

Standard treatments of 2 weeks (*T.corporis*, skin candidosis, pityriasis versicolor) and 4 weeks (*T.pedis*, interdigital) were carried out. A high percentage of patients with negative mycological results and significant reduction of the mean sum of the symptom score (erythema, desquamation, pruritus, pustules, vesiculation, and incrustation) were observed already after one week of treatment. At the end of treatment and at follow-up two weeks later the percentage of effectively treated patients ranged from 70 to 90%. In view of the rapid onset of the fungicidal action of terbinafine, clinical trials with treatment schedules shortened to half of the standard procedure have been carried out in *T.corporis*, *T.pedis* and skin candidosis in order to test whether this fungicidal activity would lead to clinical cure without further treatment.

The results comparing mycology and effective therapy after topical short-term and standard treatment once daily and follow-up are shown in Table 1. In *Tinea corporis* the high cure rates achieved after 1 or 2 weeks of treatment were maintained after a follow-up period of 3 or 2 weeks, respectively. Comparable results were obtained in skin candidosis after treatment for one or two weeks.

In the pilot study for the 2 week treatment of *T.pedis* in 35 patients the mycological parameter improved until follow-up, similarly to the short term treatment of *T.corporis* and skin candidosis. The result (effective treatment of 66% of the patients) was slightly inferior to that achieved in 277 patients treated for 4 weeks, but the difference was not statistically significant.

TABLE 1 Terbinafine (1% cream)

Percentage of negative mycology and effective therapy after standard and short term treatment in T. corporis, T. pedis (interdigital) and skin candidosis

Indication	Treatment duration	End short Rx (%)	End standard Rx (%)	Follow-up (%)	
T. corporis	1 week n= 67	61/36		90/84	at week 4
	2 weeks n=130		91/81	92/83	
T. pedis	2 weeks n= 35	65/40		83/66	at week 6
	4 weeks n=277		88/78	91/78	
Candidosis	1 week n= 63	58/33		80/72	at week 4
	2 weeks n= 90		88/74	89/79	

B. RESULTS AFTER ORAL TREATMENT WITH TERBINAFINE 250 MG DAILY

Results similar to that of topical treatment with regard to the rapid onset of fungicidal action of terbinafine were obtained in T.pedis (plantar), T.corporis and skin candidosis after oral administration of 250 mg daily. As shown for T.pedis in Figure 1, during the treatment scheduled for 6 weeks already 40% of the patients became mycologically (KOH and culture) negative at week 4 and about 80% at week 6 the end of treatment. At follow-up two weeks later the percentage of mycologically negative patients increased further to about 90%.

The mean sum of clinical scores (Figure 1) declined continuously, reaching a minimum at follow-up 2 weeks after the last dose. The further improvement of both the mycological and the clinical parameters indicates that fungicidal drug concentrations were still present at the site of infection after the end of treatment.

The advantage of the fungicidal activity of terbinafine is evident when comparing its cure rate of 74% with that of a fungistatic drug like griseofulvin, which cured only 45% of the patients (Figure 2).

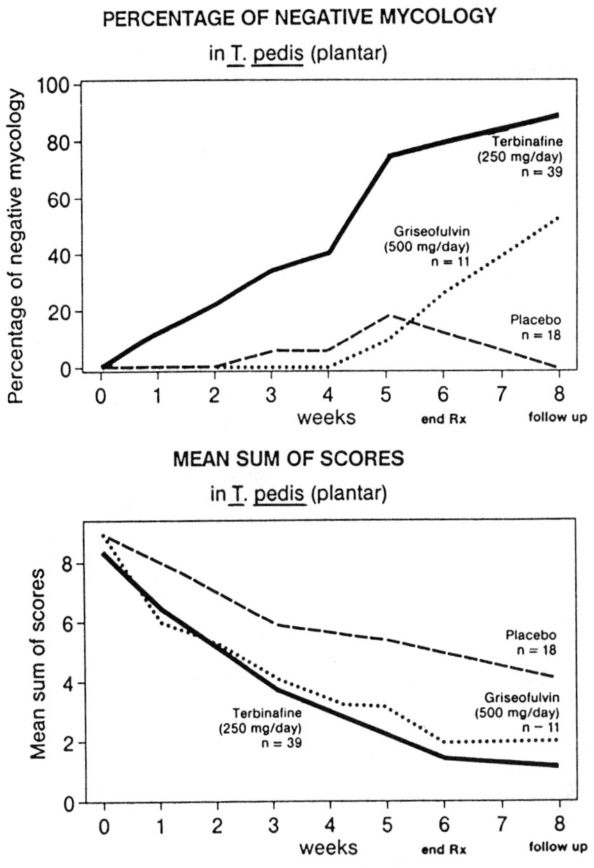

FIG. 1: Results after oral treatment with terbinafine (250 mg/day), griseofulvin (500 mg/day) and placebo during 6 weeks of treatment (end Rx) and 2 weeks follow-up.

This favourable result and the expectation that a short-term treatment would positively influence patient compliance suggested testing the efficacy of 250 mg terbinafine once daily in the same indication but treated only for 2 weeks.

As shown in Figure 3, the 2 week treatment also led to a continuous eradication of the fungi and to a decrease of the mean sum of scores even during the follow-up period of 6 weeks after the last dose.

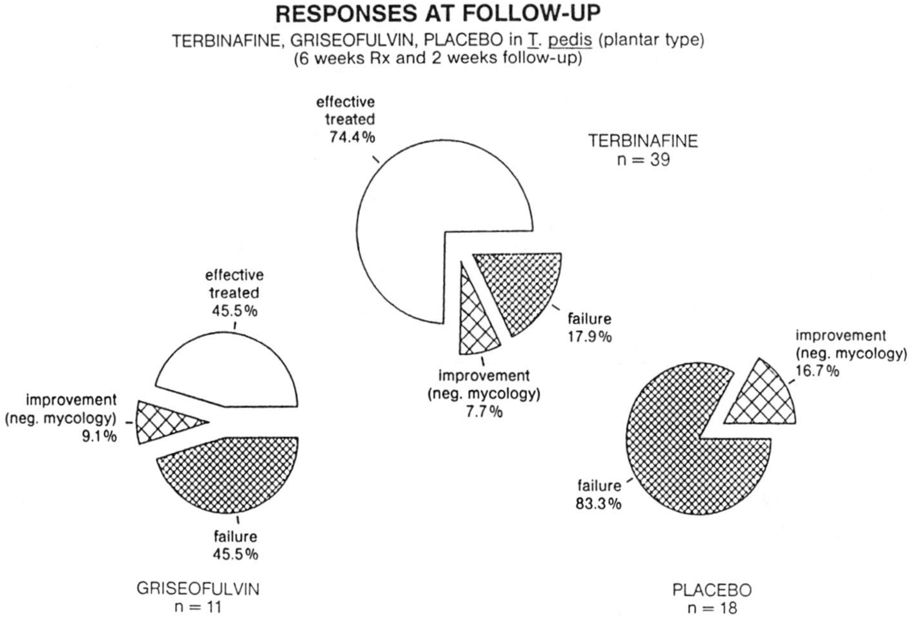

FIG. 2: Percentage of effectively treated patients after 6 weeks of treatment with terbinafine (250 mg/day), griseofulvin (500 mg/day) and placebo at follow-up 2 weeks after the last dose.

At follow-up 6 weeks after the 2 week treatment, 71% of the patients were classified as effectively treated (Figure 4). This is comparable to the results obtained in patients treated for 6 weeks and evaluated 2 weeks later (Figure 2).

The rapid onset of action and the long lasting effect of terbinafine encouraged us to evaluate its efficacy also in onychomycosis, effective treatment of which is known to be problematic. Its response to current available drugs is unsatisfactory, even after long treatment schedules of more than one year. In addition, high relapse rates are observed at follow-up (10).

The efficacy of oral terbinafine, 250 mg daily, was tested in onychomycosis (11). Of the evaluated patients, 22 had dermatophytic infections of the fingernails and 69 patients of the toenails. Twenty-one (95%) out of 22 evaluable fingernail infections became

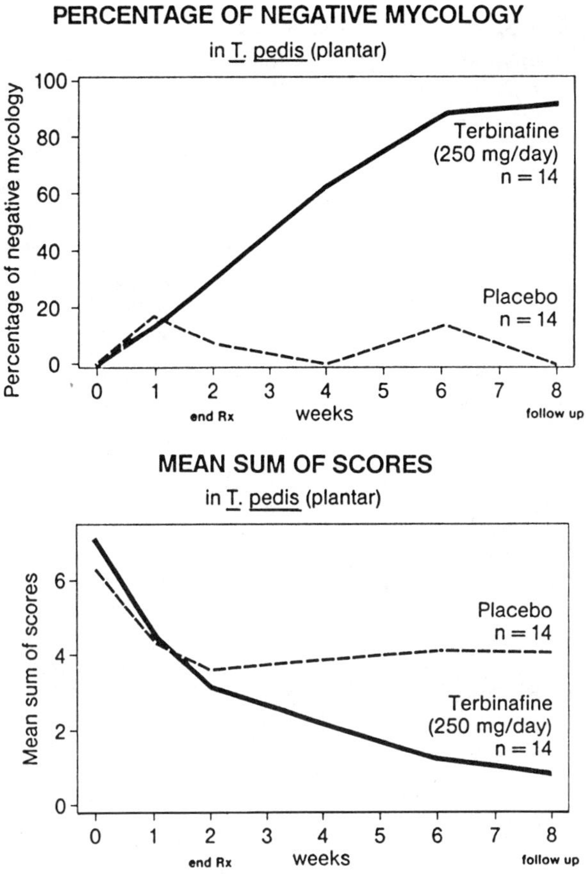

FIG. 3: Results after oral treatment with terbinafine (250 mg/day) during 2 weeks of treatment (end Rx) and 6 weeks follow-up.

mycologically negative after a daily treatment of up to 6 months, and 20 (91%) of the patients were effectively treated. Fifty-three (77%) out of 69 evaluable dermatophytic toenail infections treated up to 12 months became mycologically negative and 50 (72%) were effectively treated at the end of treatment (Table 2). However, of 11 toenail infections rated as failures at the end of treatment by our strict criteria, 7 were cured during the follow-up period; this

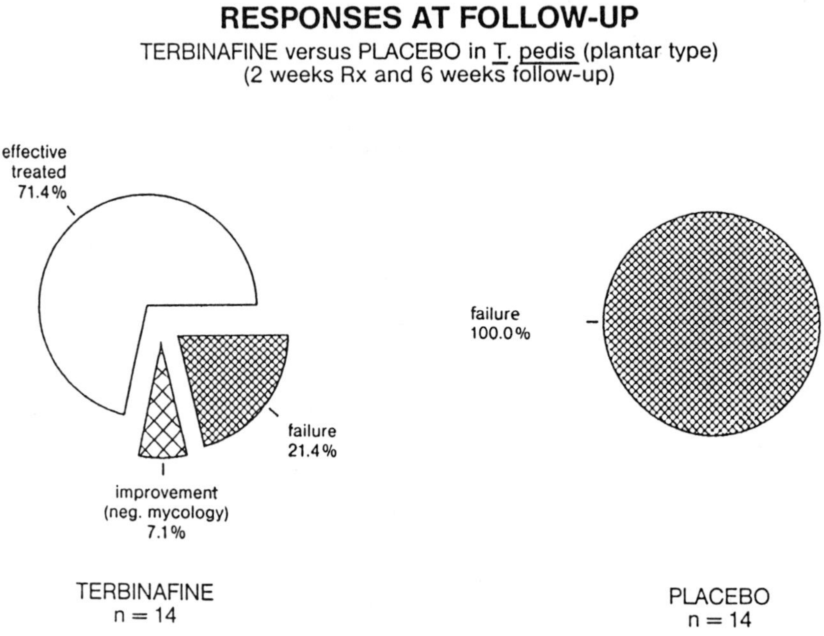

FIG. 4: Percentage of effectively treated patients after 2 weeks of oral treatment with terbinafine (250 mg/day) at follow-up 6 weeks after the last dose.

TABLE 2 Terbinafine

Efficacy in onychomycoses
Oral treatment with 250 mg/patient/day

	Treatment	Results at end Rx		Median time
		mycological negative	effectively treated	to achieve negative mycological results
Fingernails n = 22	up to 6 months	21 (95%)	20 (91%)	12.5 weeks
Toenails n = 69	up to 12 months	53 (77%)	50 (72%)	28 weeks

TABLE 3 Percentage of Patients Treated Orally and Relapse at Follow-Up

	Treatment duration	Terbinafine follow-up Short term (2-4 wks)	Terbinafine follow-up Long term (10 mts)	Comp. Drug follow-up Short term (2-4 wks)	Comp. Drug follow-up Long term (10 mts)
T. pedis	6 weeks	0% n=121	6% n=16	10% n=87	40% n=12
T. corporis	4 weeks	0% n=481	n.d. –	3% n=232	n.d. –
Onychomycoses	6-12 months	0% n=131	10 - 20% expected	---	> 50%*

*(from literature)

finally improved the rate of mycologically and clinically cured toenail infections to 87% and 83%, respectively.

The median time calculated to achieve persistently negative mycology was 12.5 weeks for fingernails and 28 weeks for toenails.

In order to evaluate whether a fungicidal effect will be reflected by the rate of relapse after treatment, a follow-up period of 12 months has been planned in this study. These data are, however, not yet available.

Long term follow-up evaluation of T.pedis patients (10 months after treatment) comparing relapse rates after terbinafine and griseofulvin therapy indicates that the fungicidal action of terbinafine favourably affects the rate of relapse (Table 3). Clear differences in favour of terbinafine, particularly at long-term follow-up were seen in T.pedis and are also expected in onychomycoses considering the results of patients analysed so far. Whether the skin or nail infections observed at long term follow-up after treatment are relapses or reinfections is difficult to evaluate and remains an open question.

IV DISTRIBUTION OF TERBINAFINE IN VARIOUS SKIN COMPARTMENTS

The excellent results after oral treatment of dermatomycoses with terbinafine are consistent with the pharmacokinetics of the compound. The determination of terbinafine levels during and after treatment of volunteers with 250 mg of terbinafine once daily for 12 consecutive days revealed that the compound concentrated rapidly in the stratum corneum with about 9 µg/g tissue, in sebum with about 45 µg/ml and in hair with about 2.5 µg/g of tissue. The concentrations in the dermis-epidermis without stratum corneum were similar to the plasma levels, ranging from 0.1 to 1 µg/ml at the beginning of the treatment, but increased gradually during the 12 day treatment to up to three times the serum levels. Elimination of the drug from tissues occurred with a half-life of 4 to 5 days, keeping drug levels above fungicidal concentrations (as determined in vitro) for more than 3 weeks (12). This slow decrease of drug concentration in target tissues of dermatomycoses is certainly responsible for the prolonged antimycotic activity of terbinafine after discontinuation of treatment.

V CONCENTRATIONS OF TERBINAFINE IN FINGER- AND TOENAILS

Drug levels have been studied in normal and target nails (infected by dermatophytes) of 12 patients treated for onychomycosis by oral administration of 250 mg daily for up to 48 weeks (13). Nail clippings were taken every 4 weeks from the distal end of target and normal nails, weighed and analysed by HPLC for terbinafine concentrations. Terbinafine was first detected 4 weeks after starting therapy and rapidly reached stable mean drug levels of 0.25 to 0.55 µg per g tissue. No difference was found between drug concentrations in toe- and fingernails, or in infected and normal nails. This early record of drug concentrations in the distal part of nail tissue and the steady state of drug levels during therapy indicates that terbinafine probably diffuses through the nail tissue. The rate of nail growth of 1 or 2 mm per month (determined for toenails and fingernails, respectively) was not fast enough to account for the presence of the drug as a result of being incorporated into newly formed nail at the proximal nail bed.

VI TOLERABILITY OF TERBINAFINE IN MAN

Topically applied 1% terbinafine cream is well tolerated, as only 1.8% of 1757 patients evaluated so far had mild side effects such as burning, irritation or erythema. This side effect profile is comparable to that of currently marketed drugs.

Orally administered terbinafine is also well tolerated (14). In 1388 patients the overall percentage of 10.4% and 11.5% of side effects observed in patients treated with 250 or 500 mg of the compound daily was only slightly higher than observed with placebo and compared favourably with griseofulvin and ketoconazole. Most adverse but mainly mild events concerned the gastro-intestinal tract and included gastritis, abdominal pain, diarrhoea, nausea and fullness. Other reactions reported included skin rash and urticaria, headache or tiredness. Careful evaluation of haematopoetic, hepatic and renal function during all clinical studies showed no evidence of drug-related, clinically significant abnormalities.

VII SUMMARY

The antifungal profile of terbinafine is characterized by its primary fungicidal action _in vitro_ and _in vivo_ against dermatophytes and various other fungal pathogens. This antifungal property becomes clinically evident after topical and oral treatment of dermatomycoses by:

- the rapid eradication of fungi at the site of infection
- the high cure rates even in chronic hyperkeratotic forms and onychomycoses and
- the low rate of relapse even at long term follow-up

Terbinafine is well tolerated in man and is at present the only antimycotic with fungicidal activity proved after topical and oral treatment of dermatophytoses.

References:

1. G. Petranyi, N. S. Ryder and A. Stütz, Allylamine derivatives, a new class of synthetic antifungal agents inhibiting fungal squalene epoxidase, Science, 224: 1239 (1984).
2. I. Schuster, M. Schaude, F. Schatz and H. Mieth, Preclinical characteristics of allylamines, Sterol Biosynthesis Inhibitors, Pharmaceutical and Agrochemical Aspects (D. Berg and M. Plempel, eds.) Ellis Horwood, Chichester, p. 449 (1988).
3. M. Schaude, H. Ackerbauer and H. Mieth, Inhibitory effect of antifungal agents on germ tube formation in Candida albicans, Mykosen, 30: 281 (1987).
4. G. Petranyi, J. G. Meingassner and H. Mieth, Antifungal activity of the allylamine derivative terbinafine in vitro, Antimicrob. Agents Chemother., 31: 1365 (1987).
5. S. Shadomy, A. Espinel-Ingroff and R. J. Gebhart, In-vitro studies with SF 86-327, a new orally active allylamine derivative, Sabouraudia, 23: 125 (1985).
6. G. Petranyi, J. G. Meingassner and H. Mieth, Activity of terbinafine in experimental fungal infections of laboratory animals, Antimicrob. Agents Chemother., 31: 1558 (1987).
7. G. Petranyi, I. Leitner and H. Mieth, The hair-root invasion test, a semi-quantitative method for experimental evaluation of antimycotics in guinea-pigs, Sabouraudia, 20: 101 (1982).
8. H. Mieth and G. Petranyi, Preclinical evaluation of terbinafine in vivo, Clin. Exp. Dermatol., 14: 104 (1989).
9. T. C. Jones and V. V. Villars, Terbinafine, Handbook of Exp. Pharmacol. Vol.96, Chemotherapy of fungal Diseases (J. F. Ryley, ed.) Springer, Berlin, p. 483 (1990).
10. Editorial, Onychomycosis and terbinafine, Lancet, 335: 636 (1990).
11. M. J. D. Goodfield, Clinical results with terbinafine in onychomycosis, J. Dermatol. Treatment, 1 (Suppl. 2): 55 (1990).
12. J. Faergemann, H. Zehender, T. Jones and H. I. Maibach, Terbinafine levels in serum, stratum corneum, dermis-epidermis (without stratum corneum) hair, sebum and eccrine sweat, J. Investig. Dermatol., 94: 523 (1990).
13. A. Y. Finlay, L. Lever, R. Thomas and P. J. Dykes, Nail matrix kinetics of oral terbinafine in onychomycosis and normal nails, J. Dermatol. Treatment, 1 (Suppl.2): 51 (1990).
14. V. Villars and T. C. Jones, Present status of the efficacy and tolerability of terbinafine (Lamisil) used systemically in the treatment of dermatomycoses of skin and nails, J. Dermatol. Treatment, 1 (Suppl. 2): 33 (1990).

12

Butenafine Hydrochloride, a New Antifungal Agent: Clinical and Experimental Study

Ryoichi Fukushiro[1], Harukuni Urabe[2], Saburo Kagawa[3], Shohei Watanabe[4], Hisashi Takahashi[5], Shinya Takahashi[6], and Hiroshi Nakajima[7].

1 Emeritus Prof., Kanazawa University, Kanazawa City 920, Japan
2 Emeritus Prof., Kyushu University School of Medicine, Fukuoka City 812, Japan
3 Emeritus Prof., Tokyo Medical and Dental University, Bunkyo-ku, Tokyo 113, Japan
4 Prof., Dermatology, Shiga University of Medical Science, Otsu City 520-21, Japan
5 Prof., Dermatology, Teikyo University School of Medicine, Itabashi-ku, Tokyo 173, Japan
6 Prof., Dermatology, Akita University School of Medicine, Akita City 010, Japan
7 Prof., Dermatology, Yokohama City University School of Medicine, Yokohama City 232, Japan

I. INTRODUCTION

Butenafine hydrochloride is a benzylamine derivative which has a potent antifungal activity. The chemical structure of butenafine hydrochloride is shown in Fig. 1.

We have studied this compound aiming at its development as

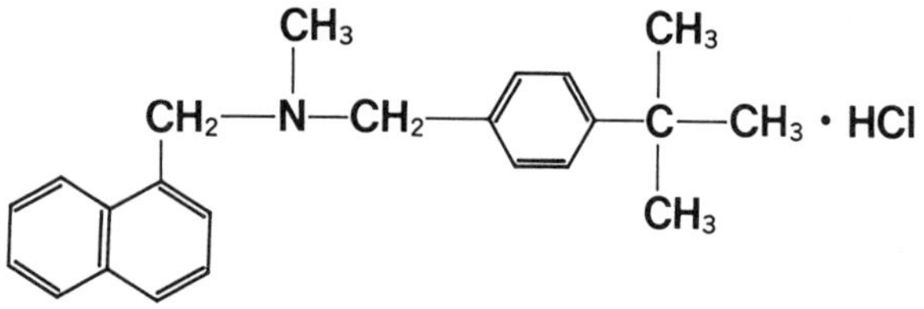

$C_{23}H_{27}N \cdot HCl$: 353.93
N-4-*tert*-butylbenzyl-*N*-methyl-1-naphthalenemethylamine hydrochloride

Fig. 1 The structure of butenafine hydrochloride

an antifungal agent. The results of preliminary studies, both in vitro and in vivo, and clinical studies of this drug are reported.

II. EXPERIMENTAL STUDY

A. *SAFETY TEST*

Percutaneous administration of the drug was confirmed to be safe.[1] No remarkable changes were observed concerning the local irritation, reproduction, mutagenicity and other toxicity tests of butenafine.[2)-7)]

B. *IN VITRO ANTIFUNGAL ACTIVITY*

The minimum inhibitory concentration (MIC) of the drug against dermatophytes is shown (Table 1).

Butenafine demonstrated growth inhibition at the concentration of 0.05 µg/ml or less. Its activity was 7 - 38 times stronger than that of the comparative drugs, tolnaftate and clotrimazole.[8]

Butenafine also demonstrated excellent antifungal activity against Aspergillus fumigatus, Sporothrix schenckii and so forth.

The drug did not inhibit the growth of Candida albicans even at the concentration of 100 µg/ml on Sabouraud's dextrose agar medium. But, in Sabouraud's dextrose broth medium adjusted to pH

Table 1 In vitro Antifungal Activity

Microorganism	No. of Strains	MIC (μg/mℓ)		
		Butenafine	Tolnaftate	Clotrimazole
T. mentagrophytes	22	0.012 (0.006-0.025)	0.133 (0.05-0.2)	0.255 (0.2-0.78)
T. rubrum	41	0.007 (0.0015-0.025)	0.061 (0.006-0.39)	0.267 (0.1-0.78)
M. canis	14	0.024 (0.0125-0.05)	0.181 (0.05-0.39)	0.266 (0.1-0.78)

Cultured on Sabouraud's dextrose agar medium at 27°C for 7 days.

5.0 by the addition of 5 N-HCl, the MIC of butenafine was 27 μg/ml. From this, it was found that the anti-Candida albicans activity of butenafine was affected by pH of the medium. It was considered due to the water-solubility of the drug.[13]

The MIC of butenafine against Malassezia furfur was 3.13 μg/ml, almost equal to that of clotrimazole.

C. *IN VIVO ANTIFUNGAL ACTIVITY*

1. *The therapeutic effects on cutaneous Trichophyton mentagrophytes infection in guinea pigs* We studied the in vivo antifungal activity against cutaneous T.mentagrophytes infection in dorsal skin of guinea pigs according to the method of S. Sakai et al.[9]

The activity of butenafine was superior to that of comparative drugs, tolnaftate and clotrimazole (Table 2).[10]

2. *The therapeutic effects on tinea pedis by T. mentagrophytes in guinea pigs* We studied the in vivo antifungal activity against experimental tinea pedis in guinea pigs by the method of S. Fujita & T. Matsuyama.[11]

Butenafine showed the highest efficacy among the tested drugs. The eradication rates of both of the 1% cream and solution were about 90% (Table 3).[12]

Table 2 In vivo Antifungal Activity against Cutaneous *T.mentagrophytes* Infection in Guinea Pigs

Drug	Dose×Times	Negative/Total (%)
Butenafine	0.01%×10	30/50 (60.0)
	0.1 %×10	47/50 (94.0)
	1.0 %× 4	50/50 (100)
	1.0 %×10	50/50 (100)
Tolnaftate	0.01%×10	5/50 (10.0)
	0.1 %×10	20/50 (40.0)
	1.0 %× 4	32/50 (64.0)
	1.0 %×10	50/50 (100)
Clotrimazole	1.0 %×10	14/50 (28.0)
Infected untreated control	—	0/50 (0)

Topical treatments were applied once daily for 4 or 10 consecutive days, starting 2 days after infection.
10 sections were cut out from each treated site.

Table 3 In vivo Antifungal Activity Against Tinea Pedis in Guinea Pigs (by Fujita's Method)

	Drug	Dose	Negative/Total (%)	Negative foot pads/Total foot pads
Cream	Butenafine	1.0%	170/192 (88.5)	9/16
	Bifonazole	1.0%	60/192 (31.3)	0/16
	Clotrimazole	1.0%	52/192 (27.1)	0/16
	Infected untreated control	—	18/192 (9.4)	0/16
Solution	Butenafine	1.0%	214/240 (89.2)	9/20
	Tolnaftate	2.0%	153/240 (63.8)	4/20
	Clotrimazole	1.0%	95/240 (39.6)	0/20
	Infected untreated control	—	40/240 (16.7)	0/20

Topical treatments were applied once daily for 20 consecutive days, starting 10 days after infection.
12 sections were cut out from each treated foot pad.

D. *THE PROPHYLACTIC ACTIVITY AGAINST CUTANEOUS T.mentagrophytes INFECTION*

We studied the prophylactic activity against cutaneous T. mentagrophytes infection in guinea pigs according to the method of M. Plempel et al.[14]

Under the test conditions, the prophylactic activity of 1% butenafine solution was superior to that of comparative drug, 1% bifonazole solution. (Fig. 2)[10]

E. CONCENTRATION IN THE SKIN OF GUINEA PIGS

1% ^{14}C-labelled butenafine was applied to the dorsal skin of guinea pigs according to the method of H. Takahashi et al.[15]

High concentration of butenafine (>50 µg/g) was observed within the depth of 300 µm of the skin (Fig. 3)[16]. It was estimated that butenafine remained for 24 hours at the treatment site.

(n=5)

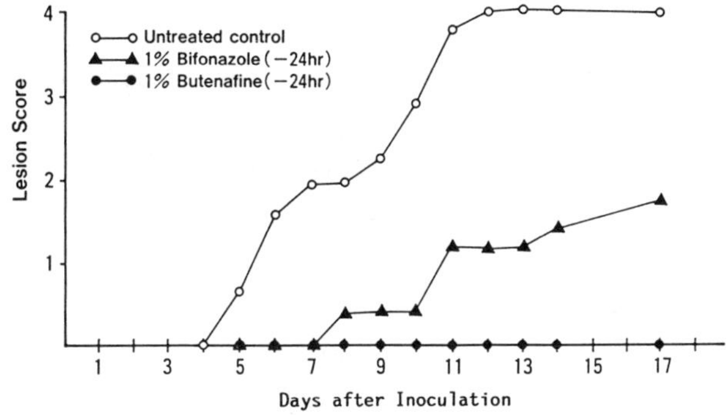

The drugs were treated 24 hours before inoculation.

Fig. 2 Prophylactic Activity against Cutaneous *T.mentagrophytes* Injection in Guinea Pigs.

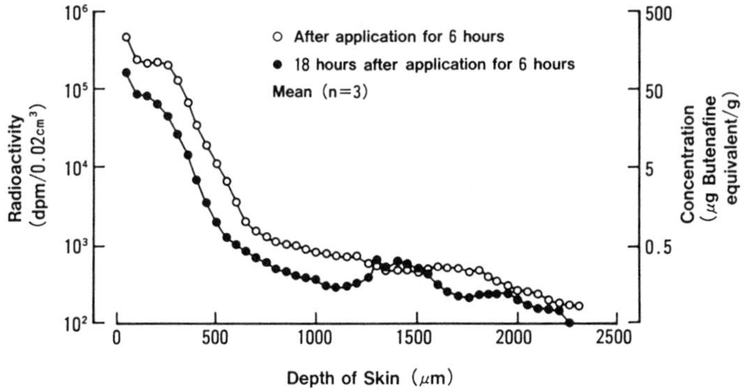

Fig. 3 Concentration Change of ^{14}C-labelled Butenafine Hydrochloride

F. MECHANISM

The mechanism of butenafine was considered to inhibit the biosynthesis of ergosterol inactivating squalene epoxidase, which is a concerting enzyme from squalene to squalene epoxide. This was similar to that of thiocarbamates and allylamines. The mechanism was different from that of imidazoles, which inhibit 14-α-demethylation of lanosterol.

III. CLINICAL STUDY

A. PHASE II STUDY[17)]

A total of 521 subjects were employed in the 1% butenafine cream and 177 in the butenafine solution. Among these, evaluable subjects for efficacy were 456 in cream and 158 in solution, and evaluable subjects for safety were 492 in cream and 166 in solution.

Drugs were applied once daily to the infected sites. But, in interdigital erosive candidiasis and perionychial candidiasis, twice or more daily application was admitted.

The duration of application was 4 weeks for tinea pedis, tinea manus and perionychial candidiasis and 2 weeks for other infections.

Observation was conducted on the starting day, the 14th day and the 28th day of treatment in tinea pedis, tinea manus, and perionychial candidiasis and on the starting day, the 7th day and the 14th day of treatment in other infections.

The overall efficacy was evaluated based on the overall judgement of the skin and mycological findings conforming to the rating scale shown in Table 4.

The final overall efficacy in the phase II study (Table 5) and the incidences of side effects (Table 6) are shown below. In side effects classified by the kinds, contact dermatitis and irritation were 1.22% in butenafine cream and 0.60% in butenafine

Table 4 Evaluation Criteria of Overall Efficacy

Overall Evaluation of Skin Findings	Mycological Findings	
	Negative (−)	Positive (+)
Markedly Improved	1. Excellent	3. Fair
Improved	2. Good	3. Fair
Slightly Improved	2. Good	3. Fair
Unchanged	4. Poor	4. Poor
Aggravated	5. Aggravated	5. Aggravated

Table 5 Final Overall Efficacy

Diagnosis		"Excellent"+"Good"/Total (%)	
		Cream	Solution
Tinea	T. pedis & T. manus	145/175 (82.9)	61/77 (79.2)
	T. cruris	49/53 (92.5)	18/22 (81.8)
	T. corporis	76/90 (84.4)	12/15 (80.0)
Candidiasis	Intertriginous candidiasis	55/68 (80.9)	2/3 (66.7)
	Interdigital erosive candidiasis	8/11 (72.7)	6/7 (85.7)
	Perionychial candidiasis	5/6 (83.3)	4/5 (80.0)
	T. versicolor	43/53 (81.1)	25/29 (86.2)

Table 6 Side Effects

Diagnosis		No. of Cases with Side Effects (%)	
		Cream	Solution
Tinea	T. pedis & T. manus	7/198 (3.54)	1/85 (1.18)
	T. cruris	2/59 (3.39)	0/22 (0.00)
	T. corporis	0/90 (0.00)	0/15 (0.00)
Candidiasis	Intertriginous candidiasis	6/72 (8.33)	0/3 (0.00)
	Interdigital erosive candidiasis	1/11 (9.09)	1/7 (14.29)
	Perionychial candidiasis	0/9 (0.00)	0/5 (0.00)
	T. versicolor	0/53 (0.00)	0/29 (0.00)
Total		16/492 (3.25)	2/166 (1.20)

(%) except unevaluable cases

solution. Redness 1.22%, itching 0.41%, papule 0.20% and enlarged rash 0.20% were observed in cream.

B. *PHASE III COMPARATIVE STUDY*[18)]

A total of 304 subjects were employed in the 1% butenafine (K) group and 307 in the 1% bifonazole (B) group. Among these, evaluable subjects for efficacy were 261 in the K-group and 263 in the B-group and evaluable subjects for safety were 285 in the K-group and 279 in the B-group.

Drugs were applied once daily for 4 weeks for tinea pedis and for 2 weeks for other infections.

Observations were conducted on the starting day, the 14th day and the 28th day of treatment in tinea pedis and on the starting day, the 7th day and the 14th day of treatment in other infections.

The evaluation criteria of overall efficacy in this study were the same as those in the phase II study.

The final overall efficacy is shown in Table 7. The effectiveness rates were calculated as the number of "Excellent" plus "Good" case per total cases. There were no significant differences in the effectiveness rates between the two drugs.

The incidences of side effects are shown in Table 8. In side effects classified by the kinds, irritation was 0.35% in K-group and 0.36% in B-group, redness 0.70% in K-group and 1.79% in B-group, itching 1.05% in K-group and 0.72% in B-group, contact dermatitis 0.35% in K-group and 1.08% in B-group, scale 0.72% in B-group, vesicle-pustule 0.35% in K-group and 0.72% in B-group, maceration 0.35% in K-group, papule 0.35% in K-group and 0.36% in B-group, flush, erosion, swelling and erythema were observed each 0.36% in B-group.

IV. SUMMARY

1. No remarkable changes were observed in the safety tests on

Table 7 Final Overall Efficacy

Diagnosis		"Excellent" + "Good" /Total	Effectiveness Rate: "Excellent" (%)	Effectiveness Rate: "Excellent" + "Good" (%)	
T. pedis	K	77/99	46.5	77.8	N.S.
	B	74/103	39.8	71.8	
T. cruris	K	36/43	65.1	83.7	N.S.
	B	36/39	56.4	92.3	
T. corporis	K	38/44	63.6	86.4	N.S.
	B	41/51	51.0	80.4	
Intertriginous candidiasis	K	30/33	51.5	90.9	N.S.
	B	27/32	62.5	84.4	
T. versicolor	K	36/42	83.3	85.7	N.S.
	B	33/38	78.9	86.8	

K : Butenafine, B : Bifonazole
▨ : "Excellent", ☐ : "Good" (Figures are accumulated %)
Data of "Excellent" + "Good" were analyzed by χ^2-test.

Table 8 Side effects

Diagnosis	No. of Cases with Side Effects(%)	
	Butenafine	Bifonazole
T. pedis	4/119 (3.36)	8/116 (6.90)
T. cruris	0/44 (0.00)	1/41 (2.44)
T. corporis	0/44 (0.00)	0/15 (0.00)
Intertriginous candidiasis	2/36 (5.56)	2/33 (6.06)
T. versicolor	0/42 (0.00)	1/38 (2.63)
Total	6/285 (2.11)	12/279 (4.30)

(%) except unevaluable cases

local irritation, reproduction, mutagenicity and other toxicity of butenafine.

2. Butenafine had potent antifungal activity against pathogenic fungi, particularly against dermatophytes _in vitro_.

3. The effect of butenafine was superior to that of the comparative drugs, tolnaftate, clotrimazole and bifonazole in _in_

vivo tests against cutaneous *T.mentagrophytes* infection and intractable tinea pedis infection in guinea pigs.

4. Butenafine well permeated into the horny layer and remained for 24 hours, and showed highly prophylactic activity.

5. The results described demonstrate that butenafine showed sufficient efficacy at 1% concentration and by once daily treatment.

6. The mechanism of butenafine was estimated to inhibit the biosynthesis of ergosterol by way of inactivating squalene epoxidase.

7. In the phase II study, 1% butenafine cream or solution given once daily was useful in the treatment of superficial fungal diseases (dermatophytosis, superficial candidiasis and tinea versicolor).

8. In the clinical efficacy study comparing 1% butenafine cream with 1% bifonazole cream, no significant differences were observed in the final overall efficacy between the two drugs. Side effects were minimal in both of them.

9. Butenafine hydrochloride thus proved to be a useful antifungal agent in the treatment of superficial fungal diseases.

REFERENCES

1) Iwagaya, Y., et al.: Chronic toxicity study of butenafine hydrochloride in dogs. Clin. Rep. 24:1664-1695, 1990.
2) Daidohji, S., et al.: Fertility study of butenafine hydrochloride in Rats. Clin. Rep. 24:1697-1707, 1990.
3) Shibuya, K., et al.: Teratogenicity study of butenafine hydrochloride in rats. Clin. Rep. 24:1709-1723, 1990.
4) Shimomura, K. and Hatakeyama, Y.: Reproduction study by percutaneous administration of butenafine hydrochloride during the fetal organogenesis period in rabbits. Preclin. Rep. Cent. Inst. Exp. Anim. 16(2):1-12, 1990.
5) Daidohji, S., et al.: Peri and post-natal study of butenafine hydrochloride in rats. Clin. Rep. 24:1725-1740, 1990.
6) Yoshida, J., et al.: Mutagenicity test of butenafine hydrochloride --Reverse Mumation test in bacteria and chromosome aberration test in CHL cells --. Clin. Rep. 24:1753-1761, 1990.
7) Maruyama, K., et al.: Dermal and ocular irritation study of butenafine hydrochloride in rabbits. Clin. Rep. 24:1763-1776, 1990.

8)Maeda, T., et al.: Synthesis and antifungal activity of butenafine hydrochloride(KP-363), a new benzylamine antifungal agent. Chem. Pharm. Bull. (in press).
9)Sakai, S., et al.: Studies on chemotherapy of Trichophyton infection. l. anti fungal properties of halogen phenol esters. J. Sci. Res. Inst. 46:113-117, 1952.
10)Arika, T., et al.: Effects of butenafine HCl(KP-363), a new benzylamine derivative, on experimental dermatophytosis in guinea pigs. Antimicrob. Agents Chemother. (in press)
11)Fujita, S. and Matsuyama, T.: Experimental tinea pedis by non-abrasive inoculation of Trichophyton mentagrophytes athro-spores on the plantar part of guinea pigs. J. Med. Vet. Mycol. 25:203-213, 1987.
12)Arika, T., et al.: Effects of butenafine HCl (KP-363), a new benzylamine derivative, on experimental tinea pedis in guinea pigs. Antimicrob. Agents Chemother. (in press)
13)Arika, T., et al.: In vitro and in vivo anti-Candida albicans activity of butenafine hydrochloride. Jpn. J. Med. Mycol. (in press)
14)Plempel, M., et al.: Antimycotic efficacy of Bifonazole in vitro and in vivo. Arzneim.-Forsch./Drug Res. 33(I):517-524, 1983
15)Takahashi, H., et al.: The percutaneous absorption of salicylic acid. J. Dermatol.(Tokyo) 3:135-138, 1976
16)Hase, T., et al.: Metabolic fate of butenafine hydrochloride (KP-363) (1st Report) --Absorption, distribution and excretion in rats, guinea pigs and dogs after a single administration of ^{14}C-KP-363--. Clin. Rep. 24:1778-1799, 1990.
17)Kagawa, S., et al.: Clinical results of KP-363 (butenafine hydrochloride) cream and solution, a new antifungal agent, on dermatophytosis in phase II study. Nishinihon J. Dermatol. 52:586-595, 1990.
18)Nakajima, H., et al.: Clinical evaluation of butenafine hydrochloride (KP-363) cream in dermatophytosis --Comparison with bifonazole cream in a well-controlled comparative study--. Nishinihon J. Dermatol. 52(5) (in press)

13

Hyperthermic Treatment of Chromomycosis

M. Hiruma

Department of Dermatology
National Defense Medical College
Tokorozawa, Saitama, Japan

INTRODUCTION

Ever since the report by MacKinnon and Conti-Diaz [1] on their success with hyperthermic treatment of sporotrichosis, several attempts have been made to employ this therapy against chromomycosis [2-4]. In Japan, Yanase and Yamada [5] used hyperthermic treatment in a patient with chromomycosis erroneously diagnosed as sporotrichosis. In spite of this error, the treatment was found to be effective and the patient was cured within 9 weeks. Since then, this treatment has attracted attention in Japan and is often used to combat chromomycosis. In this report, I will describe our results of hyperthermic treatment in a case of chromomycosis of the breast, and summarize the data on Japanese patients who underwent the same treatment.

REPORT OF ONE CASE

The patient was a 59-year-old housewife with a history of asthma, goiter, and pulmonary emphysema. Her current complaint dated back to about July 1988, when an eczematous lesion appeared on her right nipple. She had no memory of any minor trauma in this area. Since there were no subjective symptoms, she at first ignored the lesion, but it gradually enlarged, so that the nipple itself could hardly be seen. In July 1989, she was suspected of having mammary Paget's disease, and was referred to our department.

Examination of the skin disclosed an oval, well-defined, infiltrated erythematous plaque with a small amount of scales and crusts, measuring 28 × 18 mm. The configuration of the nipple itself could not be distinguished. Neither axillary nor cervical lymph nodes were palpable. Direct microscopy of KOH preparation of the crusts revealed many sclerotic cells.

Microscopic examination of a biopsy specimen from the lesion, stained with hematoxylin and eosin, showed proliferation of the epidermis and granulomatous infiltrates in the upper and middle dermis, consisting of neutrophils, histiocytes, giant cells and lymphocytes. Sclerotic cells were observed within giant cells and in microabscesses (Fig. 1a). The results of laboratory examinations were within normal range.

Cultures from a part of the biopsy specimen and crusts yielded a dematiaceous fungus. Colony growth was found to be relatively rapid. The colonies appeared black and their surfaces were covered by short, gray aerial hyphae. Slide culture revealed abundant *Cladosporium*-type sporulation and a certain amount of *Rhinocladiella*-type growth. These findings led to identification of the isolate as *Fonsecaea pedrosoi*.

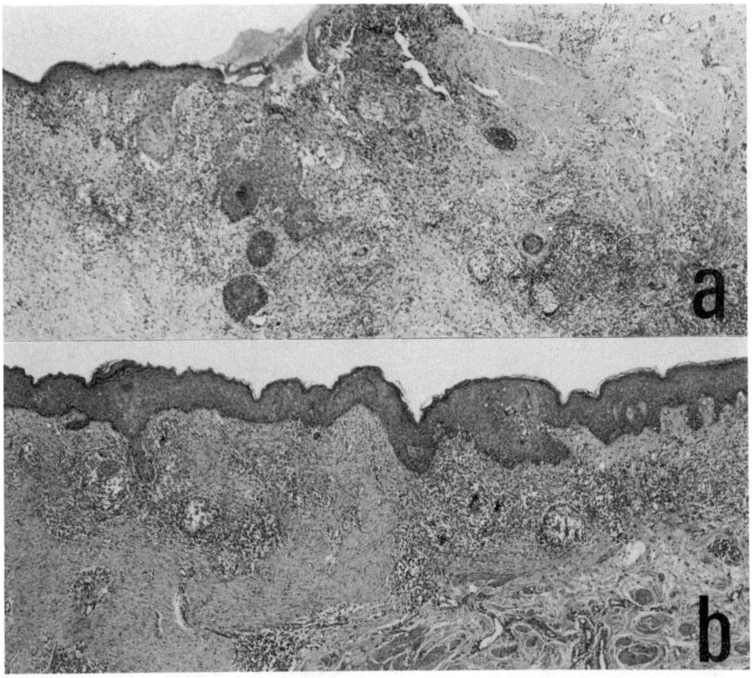

Fig. 1a and b. Light micrographs from biopsy specimens a: at the start of treatment, b: After 3 months

Hyperthermic treatment and clinical course: The patient was initially treated with hyperthermia using home equipment providing far-infrared rays, however, she found this too time-consuming for her busy schedule. Therefore the mean was abandoned in favor of total excision of the lesion in the third month following the start of treatment.

So, this is an example of therapeutic failure in the application of hyperthermia for a case of chromomycosis. The treatment consisted of warming the skin surface to approximately 42°C for one hour once daily. The isolate could grow at 32°C and 37°C, but not at 40°C.

The clinical findings one month after the start of treatment revealed that infiltration had subsided. At this stage, the patient was instructed to apply the treatment twice daily in the morning and at night, each time for one hour. After 3 months, improvement was noted, but scales and crusts were still present. The results of a direct examination and culture were both positive. Owing to the patient's dissatisfaction with the time requirements of hyperthermic therapy, the lesion was then excised totally. Microscopic examination of a biopsy specimen from the lesion after 3 months showed that cell infiltration had abated but the fungi were observed in the micro-abscesses and in the giant cells. No invasion of the mammary gland had taken place (Fig. 1b). The culture from the biopsy specimen proved to be positive. However, as the clinical symptoms had improved, I judged the hyperthermic treatment to have brought improvement.

SUMMARY OF REPORTED CASES TREATED WITH HYPERTHERMIC TREATMENT ALONE IN JAPAN

In Japan, a total of 24 cases of chromomycosis, including the present case, have reportedly been treated by hyperthermia alone. This therapeutic modality has been combined with therapeutic agents such as 5-flourocytosin in 8 reported cases to date. In this report, I will summarize the data on cases treated with hyperthermia alone as detailed in Table 1.

Half of the lesions treated with hyperthermia were on the trunk. In chromomycosis, most lesions are found on exposed areas, and occurrences on the trunk are rare. Among the devices used for hyperthermic treatment, an electrical or infrared foot warmer was necessary because the lesions are more extensive in chromomycosis than in sporotrichosis. Many treatment sessions lasted all day, while others were as short as 2 hours. Tagami et al. [6] stated that a stricter regimen is necessary for chromomycosis than for sporotrichosis, and recommended that hyperthermic treatment be applied for as long as possible at the maximum temperature the patient can stand. In this sense, hyperthermic treatment of chromomycosis is more difficult than that of sporotrichosis.

Table 1. Reported cases of chromomycosis treated with hyperthermic treatment alone in Japan

Sex	Male	13
	Female	11
Age	Range	23-80 yrs
Site of lesion	Face	2
	Trunk	12
	Limbs	11
Etiologic agents	*F. pedrosoi*	17
	E. jeanselmei	4
	Unknown	3
Hyperthermic devices		
	Benzene pocket warmer	14
	Chemical pocket warmer	3
	Hot bath	2
	Electrical foot warmer	1
	Infrared foot warmer	1
	Far-infrared warmer	1
	Moxibustion	1
Daily duration of treatment		
	All day	12
	12 hours	4
	6 hours	2
	2 hours	3

The therapeutic results were as follows: complete cure in 15, improvement in 6, relapse in 2, and no change in one. The mean duration of treatment among the cured patients was approximately 3 months. As for the clinical course, some improvement in the symptoms was noted within 2 to 3 weeks after the start of treatment. This result appears to illustrate the efficacy of this means; however, it is possible that authors fail to mention hyperthermic treatment when it is found to be ineffective. We feel that further studies are necessary to determine the effectiveness of hyperthermic treatment on chromomycosis.

The present case is considered to belong to the "improvement" category. One of the reasons for the failure to achieve a complete cure is explained that: an electrical device was used as the heat source and the attached cord placed undue restriction on the patient's daily activities during treatment. Therefore, in my opinion, the most important task in relation to this type of treatment of chromomycosis is the development of a more effective and convenient device.

There are several clinical problems related with this method of treatment of chromymycosis. First, depending on the invading species, the prognosis may be grave and the selected treatments must be carefully applied ; second, the surface area of the lesion is often too extensive for a pocket warmer to raise the skin temperature sufficiently, so that heating equipment adequate for the size of the foci must be carefully selected ; third, the etiologic agents are not always of a single species; some may be able to grow at 42°C, and in such an instance, a satisfactory result cannot be expected from hyperthermia ; and fourth, the daily duration of treatment is long: if the mean period is 3 months, poor patient compliance will severely limit the number of cases that can be cured.

In regard to the mode of action of hyperthermic treatment in sporotrichosis and chromomycosis, two mechanisms have been speculated: one is a direct fungicidal or fungistatic action of heat on the organism, and the other, the effect of a rise in skin temperature on the defense mechanisms of the host [6,7]. In sporotrichosis, direct action appears plausible to a certain extent [8,9]. On the other hand, *Fonsecaea pedrosoi* has been reported to grow at a temperature up to 37°C, with growth arrested at 39°C, and death within 18 days at 42°C [10,11]. This organism is thus considerably more heat resistant than *Sporothrix schenckii*. Therefore, the concept of direct hyperthermic action alone is insufficient to explain the result.

Recent advances in the development of new antifungal agents have been remarkable. However, the success of hyperthermic treatment is also very encouraging. We look forward to further developments of this therapeutic modality.

REFERENCES

1. Mackinnon JE, Conti Diaz IA: The effect of temperature on sporotrichosis. Sabouraudia 2: 56-59, 1962.
2. Conti Diaz IA, Vignale RA, Pena De Pereira ME: Cromoblastomicosis tratada con termoterapia local. Med. Cutan 4: 383-386, 1969.
3. Akagi M: Moxibustion and chromomycosis. Hifu 16: 364, 1974.
4. Oka K: A case of mycotic abscess caused by Phialophora gougerotii. Rinsho Hifuka 28: 209-216, 1974.
5. Yanase K, Yamada M: Pocket-warmer therapy of chromomycosis. Arch Dermatol 114: 1095, 1978.
6. Tagami H, Ginoza M, Imaizumi S, Urano S: Successful treatment of chromomycosis with topical heat therapy J Am Acad Dermatol 10: 615-619, 1984.
7. Takahashi Y: The influence of the temperature and its exposure time on the growth of pathogenic dematiaceous fungi. Yokohama Igaku 38: 715-721, 1987.
8. Hiruma M, Kagawa S: The effects of heat on *Sporothrix schenckii in vitro* and *in vivo*. Mycopathologia 84: 21-30, 1983.
9. Hiruma M, Kagawa S: Effects of hyperthermia on phagocytosis and intracellular killing of *Sporothrix schenckii* by polymorphonuclear leukocytes. Mycopathologia 95: 93-100, 1986.
10. Silva M: The saprophytic pahse of the fungi of chromomycosis: Effect of nutrients and temperature upon growth and morphology. Trans NY Acad Sci 21: 46-57, 1965.
12. Conti Diaz IA: Temperatures maximales de agentes de micetomas y cromoblastomicosis. An Fac Med Montev 50: 190-196, 1965.

14

Hyperthermic Treatment of Sporotrichosis

I. A. Conti Díaz and M. Hiruma*

Department of Parasitology, School of Medicine, Institute of Hygiene, Montevideo, Uruguay.
** Department of Dermatology, National Defense Medical College, Tokorozawa, Saitama, JAPAN.*

INTRODUCTION

Sporotrichosis is commonly presented as a chancriform lesion with multiple lymphangitic nodules, affecting mainly one upper limb. In Uruguay, 80.5% of cases follow armadillo scratches (1)

Although some cases would cure spontaneously, most cases need treatment. Lesions from untreated cases may persist for years.

Oral iodides have been used successfully since 1906. However, frequent iodism makes it necessary to stop the therapy. Also, during pregnancy iodide use is contraindicated for avoiding neonatal hypothyroidism and thyromegaly (2).

The purpose of this paper is to emphasize the importance of local heat therapy in sporotrichosis and its usefulness when used together with other treatments for the disease.

HISTORICAL

Treatment of sporotrichosis by local heating was devised on the basis of experimental results in rats by Mackinnon and Conti Díaz, in 1962 (3). A successful first result in a patient with sporotrichosis mentioned in the above paper was promptly confirmed by Galiana and Conti Díaz (4), by other American authors (5-8) and mainly by Japanese researchers (9-13). Indeed, more than 15 reports on the use of local hyperthermia in sporotrichosis have appeared in Japan including a successful cure obtained in 8 weeks by treatment with pocket warmers twice a day for 30 minutes each time (13).

In 1980, Roberts affirmed: "If oral iodides fail or have to be withdrawn because of side effects, a second line of treatment which consists of raising the temperature of the affected limb may be employed" (14).

Classical methods for local hyperthermia such as dry or wet dressings, rubefacients, pocket warmers, etc. take time and the patients' daily activities may be restricted during treatment. For these reasons it becomes necessary to look for better new local heating methods.

Recently, Hiruma et al. (15) have tried local hyperthermia by means of infrared and far infrared rays. Lesions in children or on the face are difficult to treat but when lesions on the limbs were selected, infrared treatment enabled the duration of treatment to be shortened by two thirds in comparison with that of pocket warmer treatment, and excellent results were obtained.

MECHANISMS OF ACTION OF LOCAL HEAT THERAPY

The effects of heat on *Sporothrix schenckii* both *in vitro* and *in vivo* were studied by Hiruma and Kagawa (16). They demonstrated very well that spores *in vivo* are much more heat-sensitive than those *in vitro*. Only one hour of heating at 42·C, was enough to reduce the germination rate to 10%.

Anyway, we agree with Roberts (14) when he says: "It is rather doubtful if inhibition of *S. schenckii* by high temperatures is the only explanation for the success of the method."

In this regard we think that inhibition of the fungus *in vivo* by high temperature would be the result of its direct effect on the parasite and also by an improvement of the local defensive response of the host.

Local heat acts as a stimulus for thermoreceptors involved in the mechanisms of thermoregulation. The rise of the skin temperature is followed by vasodilatation of the vessels of the subcutaneous plexes in order to "carry off" local heat. The same thing happens with rubefacients which act directly on the smooth muscle of the vessels of the subcutaneous plexus (4). Vasodilatation means, of course, a local increase in the number of white blood cells (leucocytes).

At the same time it is very well known according to Van t'Hoff Arrhenius' law that the thermal coefficients (Q.10) up to 38°C. for the majority of biological processes are two or more; that is to say that defensive mechanisms would improve with the rise in temperature of the tissues (4) (17). So, the basic processes of the primary, secondary and tertiary anti-infectious mechanisms such as immune complex formation, opsonic adherence, immune adherence via C3 receptor on macrophages followed by phagocytosis, etc. would be helped and improved in efficacy by the increase of skin temperature.

It is also known that PMN leucocytes are present in the beginning of an inflammatory reaction immediately after injury. In sporotrichosis, Cunningham et al. (18) demonstrated that the myeloperoxidase, hydrogen peroxidase and iodine (MPO-H_2O_2-I) system in PMN of normal people is important in the intracellular killing of *S. schenckii*. The system is characterized by oxidation of iodide by the myeloperoxidase and hydrogen peroxide into an iodine form. In this regard we must remember that in 1969, Urabe and Nagashima postulated that the therapeutic effect of potassium iodide might be mediated through the direct antifungal action of molecular iodine (19).

Very interestingly, González Mendoza et al. in Mexico (20) found a depressed phagocytic activity in patients with sporotrichosis and suggested that iodine from potassium iodide may contribute to the reinforcement of the microbicidal action of the PMN leucocytes.

Finally, in 1980, Hiruma and Kagawa (21) demonstrated the effects of hyperthermia on phagocytosis and intracellular killing of *S. schenckii* by PMN leucocytes. There was no effect of hyperthermia on the phagocytosis rate but the killing rate increased significantly at 40°C.

In summary, cure by heat therapy in sporotrichosis may be the result of several mechanisms, such as a direct inhibition of *S. schenckii* cells in tissues, local hyperleucocytosis, unspecific improvement of phagocytosis and other defensive mechanisms of the host, and finally through an improvement of the intracellular killing of fungal cells by PMN leucocytes by a better utilization of I originated in the MPO-H_2O_2-I system.

LOCAL HEAT THERAPY AND OTHER TREATMENTS

Treatment of sporotrichosis patients with oral iodides plus simultaneous local hyperthermia has proved to be highly satisfactory (22). It must be pointed out that most cases in Uruguay are treated during the winter months because they become infected in March or April in or around the Holy Week when many hunters go to the countryside to get "mulitas" (armadillos).

Furthermore, in past years, we have treated sporotrichosis with itraconazole. We observed that those patients that followed correctly our recommendations of keeping the affected limbs warm, needed shorter periods of therapy to be cured.

It seems worthwhile recommending local heating when other treatments for sporotrichosis are being used (iodides, itraconazole).

REFERENCES

1. Conti Díaz, I.A.: La esporotricosis en el Uruguay. Aspectos epidemiológicos y clínicos. An. Fac. Med. Montevideo, 4 (2), 137-146, 1981.
2. Romig, D.A., Douglas, W.V. and Chien Liu.: Facial sporotrichosis during pregnancy. Arch. Intern. Med., 130, 910-912, 1972.
3. Mackinnon, J.E. and Conti Díaz, I.A.: The effect of temperature on sporotrichosis. Sabouraudia, 2, 56-59, 1962.
4. Galiana, J. and Conti Díaz, I.A.: Healing effects of heat and a rubefacient on nine cases of sporotrichosis. Sabouraudia, 3, 64-71, 1963.
5. Trejos, A. and Ramírez, O.: Local heat in the treatment of sporotrichosis. Mycopath. & Mycol. Appl., 30, 47-53, 1966.
6. Laca, E.: Esporotrichosis ulcerosa de pierna tratada por el calor. El Tórax, 13, 229-231, 1964.
7. Thomas, C.C., Pierce, H.E. and Labiner, G.W.: Sporotrichosis responding to fever therapy. J.A.M.A., 147, 1342-1343, 1951.
8. Adam, J.E., Dion, W.M. and Reilly, S.: Sporotrichosis due to contact with contaminated sphagnum moss. C.M.A. Journal, 126, 1071-1073, 1982.
9. Watanabe, S., Morita, N.S. and Takasu, T.: Local heat therapy of sporotrichosis. Jap. J. Clin. Dermatol., 25, 1053-1059, 1971.
10. Soh, Y.: Treatment of sporotrichosis : The effect of topical thermotherapy. Jap. J. Med. Mycol., 16, 106-110, 1975.

11. Hiruma, M., Yamamoto, I., Hirose, I. and Kagawa, S.: Topical thermotherapy for sporotrichosis. Rinsho Dermatol., 20, 413-419, 1978.

12. Takahashi, S., Masahasi, T. and Male, O.: Lokale thermotherapie bei sporotrichose. Hautarzt, 32, 525-528, 1981.

13. Hiruma, M., Katoh, T., Yamamoto, I. and Kagawa, S.: Local hyperthermia in the treatment of sporotrichosis. Mykosen, 30, 315-321, 1987.

14. Roberts, S.O.B.: Treatment of superficial and subcutaneous mycoses. In : Antifungal Chemotherapy. Speller ed., John Wiley & Sons, Toronto, 1980.

15. Hiruma, M., Ohata, H., Shimizu, T., Ohnishi, Y., Kawada, A. and Kukita, A. Hyperthermic treatment of sporotrichosis using infrared lamps and far-infrared heaters. In press.

16. Hiruma, M. and Kagawa, S.: The effects of heat on *Sporothrix schenckii in vitro* and *in vivo*. Mycopathologia, 84, 21-30, 1983.

17. Houssay, B.A., Lewis, J.T. Orías, O., Menéndez, E.B., Hug, E., Foglia, V. and Leloir, L.F. : Fisiología humana. "El Ateneo" ed., Buenos Aires, 1952.

18. Cunningham, K.M. et al.: Phagocytosis and intracellular fate of *Sporothrix schenckii*. J. Infect. Dis., 140, 815-817, 1979.

19. Urabe, H. and Nagashima, T.: Mechanism of antifungal action of potassium iodide on sporotrichosis. Dermatologia Internationalis, 8 (1), 36-39, 1969.

20. González Mendoza, A., Meléndez Ruiz, C.E. and Ramos Zepeda, R. : Phagocytic activity of polymorphonuclear leucocytes against yeast cells of *Sporothrix schenckii* in patients with sporotrichosis. Proc. Fifth Conf. on the Mycoses. Scient. Pub. N° 396, P.A.H.O., 1980.

21. Hiruma, M. and Kagawa, S.: Effects of hyperthermia on phagocytosis and intracellular killing of *Sporothrix schenckii* by polymorphonuclear leukocytes. Mycopathologia, 95, 93-100, 1986.

22. Conti Díaz, I.A. Unpublished observations.

PART III

CLINICAL ASPECTS OF SYSTEMIC AZOLES

15

Historical Perspectives of and Projected Needs for Systemic Azole Antifungals

R. J. Hay

Department of Dermatology, Guys Hospital
St. Thomas's Street, London SE1 9RT, U.K.

INTRODUCTION

Work on the antifungal activity of the azole derivatives started in the 1940s with the observation that benzimidazole inhibited the growth of certain yeasts as well as streptococci. While the finding was novel at the time, it was many years before the first antifungal imidazole, chlormidazole, discovered during an investigation of benzimidazole derivatives, was assessed in clinical trials as a topical antifungal agent (1). The drug appeared to be of use principally against dermatophyte infections and pityriasis versicolor and produced good therapeutic responses. However, the majority of the systemic mycoses under treatment were those caused by the endemic pathogens such as Coccidioides immitis or Histoplasma capsulatum for which the newly discovered polyene agents were a potential solution even though the problems associated with the toxicity of amphotericin B were recognized early on. Its failure to cure certain infections such as coccidioidal meningitis had also been noted. The recent rise in the numbers of cases of systemic fungal infections has coincided with the development of techniques of therapy involving immunosuppression which have now revolutionised the treatment of certain cancers such as childhood leukaemia as well as organ grafts. The removal of host immune effector cells as part of the treatment was inevitably followed by complications such as an increased frequency of infection, including those caused by opportunistic fungi such as *Candida* species, *Aspergilli* and zygomycetes. The importance of fungi as pathogens in the neutropenic patient and, more recently, patients with HIV infections is now well recognised. The need for systemically active drugs which offer a safety margin superior to amphotericin B yet which are as active as the latter is, therefore, a recent quest. The search for newer comounds with antifungal efficacy which are systemically active has also been extended to the superficial mycoses where, for instance, there is a need to find alternatives for other drugs, notably griseofulvin. In addition, this has provided the opportunity to improve therapy for infections mainly confined to the tropics including mycetoma.

While many of the azole antifungals are primarily aimed at superficial mycoses and are only available in topical form, there are several which can be used as systemically active therapeutic agents. All are believed to share a common mode of action by inhibition of the conversion of lanosterol to ergosterol at the 14-alpha-demethylase step. The drugs interact with the haem ion of cytochrome P 450 which catalyzes this step.

IMIDAZOLES

CLOTRIMAZOLE

Clotrimazole was one of the first antifungal azoles which had systemic activity. It is active in vitro against a variety of organisms including yeast pathogens, aspergilli and dermatophytes. It is also widely used as a topically active antifungal drug. Although clotrimazole is poorly soluble in water over 90% of the administered dose is absorbed after oral administration [2]. Subsequently it was observed that with continuing administration of the drug beyond about two weeks, drug levels in serum fell indicating enhanced metabolism [3]. This was also borne out by clinical experience and the best approach to therapy with oral clotrimazole was to give the drug intermittently. Oral clotrimazole is now not widely used as a systemic agent although it is available in some countries in troche form. It has been used for the treatment of both oropharyngeal candidosis and aspergillosis [4]. But the inability to sustain adequate blood levels has proved a problem. Transient neurological disturbances as well as nausea and diarrhoea have also been reported in patients taking the drug.

MICONAZOLE

The development of miconazole as a systemic therapy was the first breakthrough in the development of new azole drugs which could be used for the treatment of systemic fungal infections. The drug is broadly active against fungal pathogens including *Candida* species but many mould fungi are inhibited by the drug in vitro, some at high concentrations. Miconazole is topically active and used for the treatment of most superficial mycoses. While miconazole can be given orally, high doses are needed to produce adequate blood levels. For instance, at least 1 gm has to be administered in order to achieve serum levels of 1.16 mg/l 2-4 hours post dose [5].

A more satisfactory method of administering the drug for systemic therapy is by intravenous route at doses of about 50mg/kg 8 hourly. Miconazole does not penetrate the urine, CSF or joints in high concentrations. The drug is generally well tolerated, the main side effects being pruritus, phlebitis but on rare occasions anaphylaxis or ventricular tachycardia have been reported.

Miconazole has been evaluated for both intravenous and oral use although in the latter instance it has mainly been employed as a prophylactic. While the intravenous formulation responses in the management of invasive candidosis have been favourable in patients presenting with candidaemia, but it appears less effective in the presence of neutropenia [6]. In the other systemic mycoses miconazole has been used with some success in coccidioidomycosis [7]. One condition which responds, in many instances, to intravenous miconazole is infection due to *Pseudallescheria boydii* [8], although even here failures have been recorded.

In addition to its use for diagnosed infections miconazole has also been employed as empirical therapy in cancer patients with fever. A small difference in favour of patients receiving miconazole in addition to other antibiotics has been noted in one study [9]. The use of miconazole in the management of mycoses in the seriously ill patient presented investigators with a major problem, as yet unresolved, the evaluation of mycological and clinical responses by objective criteria [10].

KETOCONAZOLE

The development of ketoconazole heralded another change. This was the first imidazole which could produce sustainable therapeutic levels after oral administration [11]. The drug does not penetrate CSF or urine in high concentrations, yet in early clinical studies was found to produce a high recovery rate in a wide range of mycoses. Because it can be given orally it was used for superficial mycoses and was found to be active against all the major pathogens from dermatophytosis to pityriasis versicolor. In fact, in the latter condition responses have been reported after as little as a single 400 mg dose.

As an agent against systemic mycoses ketoconazole was found to produce good responses in both paracoccidioidomycosis and histoplasmosis [12]. Non-meningeal cryptococcosis and some clinical forms of blastomycosis were also found to respond [13]. While there have been fewer studies in systemic candidosis therapeutic successes have been reported, although infections affecting patients with continuing neutropenia do not respond well [14]. Even *Candida* infections affecting sites where the drug would be expected to produce low serum levels such as the urinary tract and joints may respond [15]. Ketoconazole is not active against aspergillosis.

The drug has also been used as an oral prophylactic drug although there appears to be impaired absorption in some neutropenic patients [16]. Unfortunately, in common with other antifungal prophylactics, there is little proof to show that it is effective in preventing systemic candidosis although it works well in suppressing oral infection in compromised patients [17].

The disadvantages of ketoconazole are two fold [18]. In the first place it became clear comparatively late in the development of the drug that it had two important side effects. The first, hepatitis, occurs in about 1:10,000 patients, particularly those receiving treatment for nail infections. While this is a low incidence for an adverse reaction it dampened enthusiasm for its use over long periods in non-life threatening infections. In addition, ketoconazole causes adrenal suppression, although this is dose related. This important observation showed that azoles might affect the human isozyme of the target cytochrome P 450 and subsequent development of this group of drugs has been designed to avoid interaction with the human cytochrome system. One other observation, only clearly established in patients with chronic mucocutaneous candidosis, was the occurrence of resistance amongst *Candida* isolates from patients treated with long term ketoconazole [19]. This is still a rare event but resistance to ketoconazole is usually accompanied by cross resistance to other azole drugs [20].

TRIAZOLE ANTIFUNGAL DRUGS

Compounds with antifungal activity based on 1-substituted 1,2,4-triazoles are important agricultural fungicides. They also form the basis for a series of drugs with activity against human pathogenic fungi.

ITRACONAZOLE

Itraconazole is a member of this new group of drugs amongst the azole series, the triazole antifungals. Poorly soluble in aqueous solution, itraconazole produces low serum levels 2 hours after administration (200-300ng/ml after a single 100mg dose) but is avidly bound to plasma proteins [21]. The drug also penetrates the urine or CSF in low concentrations but is bound to tissue including brain. In vitro its spectrum of activity is broad and covers *Aspergillus* species amongst other pathogens. It also affects dematiaceous fungi including many of the agents of chromomycosis.

In clinical practice itraconazole is used against

dermatophytosis, candidosis and pityriasis versicolor. While it is probably less effective than ketoconazole in the latter infection it can be used to treat many forms of ringworm in a two week period of therapy [22]. It is also effective in a range of subcutaneous infections including chromomycosis and sporotrichosis [23].

Amongst the systemic mycoses itraconazole is used for many of the infections caused by dimorphic fungi such as histoplasmosis, blastomycosis, paracoccidioidomycosis or coccidioidomycosis. This includes long term suppressive therapy in patients with HIV infection. While it is difficult to compare results with ketoconazole, studies of the kinetics of recovery in infections such as paracoccidioidomycosis suggest that it may produce remission in a shorter time than ketoconazole [24]. Amongst the opportunistic pathogens it works in both candidosis and aspergillosis. Evidence for the latter is somewhat anecdotal [25,26] but in one prophylactic study its use was associated with significantly fewer cases of invasive aspergillosis than the comparative group receiving ketoconazole [27]. Itraconazole has been used for the treatment of cryptococcosis either on its own or in combination with flucytosine [25]. In addition, in AIDS patients it can be given as long term suppressive therapy to prevent relapse.

Adverse reactions are not common with itraconazole and at present no serious side effects have been reported. Poor absorption has been seen in both neutropenic and AIDS patients. A newer formulation of the drug in cyclodextrin which can be used either orally or intravenously may offer a solution to this.

FLUCONAZOLE

Fluconazole has strikingly different characteristics to itraconazole. It is well absorbed, over 70% of the orally administered dose being detected in serum [28]. It penetrates peritoneum and CSF in concentrations approaching those achieved in serum. It is also largely excreted via the kidneys, an unusual feature for an azole. Fluconazole has broad spectrum activity against fungi, although *in vitro* it is difficult to assess and appears to have little effect on *Aspergilli.* It can be given both orally and intravenously. Another important feature of the drug, following on from its renal excretion is the fact that the dose has to be modified in patients with renal impairment.

Fluconazole is active in superficial mycoses, particularly oral and vaginal candidosis. In the latter disease it is given in a single 150mg dose [29]. Fluconazole produces rapid clearance of oropharyngeal candidosis in patients with AIDS [30] and neutropenic cancer patients [31]. It is used both for primary therapy and long term suppression of cryptococcal meningitis in patients with AIDS [32,33]. This has many advantages such as earlier discharge from hospital and the recovery rate is high, although at present comparisons with amphotericin B have not been reported. Systemic candidosis is also treatable with this drug [34]. In particular, infections involving sites such as urine or peritoneum appear to respond well fluconazole, although there is still comparatively little experience in the neutropenic patient [35]. There is no reported clinical usage of fluconazole in aspergillosis.

Adverse reactions are uncommom with this drug. To date there has been one report of resistance occurring in a patient with *Torulopsis glabrata* infection [36].

SUMMARY

The azoles form an important part of the group of drugs which can be used systemically to treat fungal disease. They have the advantage of a low incidence of side effects coupled with good therapeutic responses particularly in the nonimmunocompromised patient. They cover most of the superficial mycoses as well as many of the deep infections caused by fungi. They do have certain disadvantages - notably interaction with human cytochrome P 450. At present this does not appear to be a feature of the triazoles. In a very low proportion of cases there is evidence of the development of drug resistance if ketoconazole is administered continuously over a long period in the face of a lack of clinical response. Improvements in the therapeutic spectrum of these drugs are still desirable. For instance, widening the range of activity to include the zygomycte fungi is one such target. In addition, a major goal remains the development of a drug which is effective against fungal infections in the persistently neutropenic patient.

REFERENCES

1. Seeliger HPR (1958). Pilzemmende Wirkung eines neuen Benzimidazol derivates. Mykosen **1** 162-171.

2. Duhm B, Maul W, Medenwald H, Patzchke K, Puetter J and Wagner LA (1974)
The pharmacokinetics of clotrimazole [14]C. Postgraduate Med.J. **50** Supplement 1 13-17.

3. Holt RJ and Newman RL (1972).
Laboratory assessment of the antimycotic drug clotrimazole. J.Clin.Path. **25** 1089-1097.

4. Crompton GK and Milne LJ (1973)
Treatment of bronchopulmonary aspergillosis with clotrimazole. Br.J.Dis.Chest. **67** 301-307.

5. Bolaert J, Daneels R, Van Landuyt H and Symoens J (1976). Miconazole plasma levels in healthy subjects and in patients with impaired renal function. Chemotherapy **6** 165-169.

6. Jordan WM, Bodey GP, Rodrigues V, Ketchel SJ and Henney J (1979).
Miconazole therapy for treatment of fungal infections in cancer patients. Antimicrob.Ag.Chemother **16** 792-797.

7. Sung JP, Grendahl JG and Levine HB (1977).
Intravenous and intrathecal miconazole therapy for systemic mycoses.
West.Med.J. **126** 5-13.

8. Lutwick LI, Rytel MW, Yanez JP, Galgiani JN and Stevens DA. (1976).
Deep infections for *Petriellidium boydii* treated with miconazole. JAMA **241** 272-273

9. Saral R (1981). Prophylactic use of intravenous miconazole in leukaemia and bone marrow transplant patients. In The role of intravenous miconazole in the treatment of systemic mycoses. R.Soc.Med.Int.Congress. Symp.Ser. **45** 37-42.

10. Bennett JE (1981)
Miconazole in cryptococcosis and systemic candidiasis - a word of caution.
Annals of Internal Medicine **94** 708-709.

11. Huang YC, Colaizzi JL, Bierman RH, Woestenborghs R and Heykants J, (1986).
Pharmacokinetics and dose proportionality of ketoconazole in normal volunteers.
Antimicrob.Ag.Chemother. **30** 206-210.

12. Negroni R, Robles AM, Arechavala A, Tuculet MA and Galimberti R (1980)
Ketoconazole in the treatment of paracoccidioidomycosis and histoplasmosis.
Revs.Infect.Dis. 1980 **2** 643-649

13. National Institutes of Allergy and Infectious Diseases Mycoses Study Group (1985)
Treatment of blastomycosis and histoplasmosis with ketoconazole Results of a prospective randomised clinical trial.
Annls.Intern. Med. **103** 861-872.
14. Fainstein V, Bodey GP , Elting L et al (1987)
Amphotericin B or ketoconazole therapy of fungal infections in neutropenic cancer patients.
Antimicrob. Ag.Chemother. **31** 11-15.
15. Dupont B and Drouhet E (1985). Cutaneous, ocular and osteoarticular candidiasis in heroin addicts: new clinical and therapeutic aspects in 38 patients. J.Infect.Dis. 1985 **152** 577-591.
16. Mazzoni A, Fiorentini C, Cevenini R and Nanetti A (1985). Limits of antifungal prophylaxis by ketoconazole in leukaemic patients.
Chemioterapia **4** 299-302.
17. Meunier-Carpentier F (1984). Chemoprophylaxis of fungal infections.
Am.J.Med. **76** 652-656.
18. Clissold SP (1987).
Safety in clinical practice. In Ketoconazole Today. Jones HE (Ed). Addis Press, Manchester. pp77-91.
19. Ryley JF, Wilson RG and Barrett-Bee K (1984).
Azole resistance in Candida albicans.
J Med. Vet. Mycol. **22** 53-63.
20. Kerridge D, Fasoli M and Wayman FJ (1988)
Drug resistance in Candida albicans and Candida glabrata. In ntifungal Drugs. St.Georgiev. V Ed.
Annls N.York Acad.Sci. **544**. 245-259.
21. Heykants J, Van Peer A, Van de Velde V, Van Rooy P, Meuldermans W, Lavrijsen K, Woestenborghs R, Van Cutsem J and Cauwenbergh G (1989).
The clinical pharmacokinetics of itraconazole: an overview. Mycoses 32 (Suppl 1) 67-87.
22. Degreef H, Marien K, de Veylder H, Duprez K, Borhys A and Verhoeve L (1987)
Itraconazole in the treatment of dermatophytoses: a comparison of two daily dosages.
Reviews of Infectious Diseases **9** Supplement 1 104-108.
23. Restrepo A, Robledo J, Gomez I et al. (1986)
Itraconazole therapy in lymphangitic and cutaneous sporotrichosis. Archs Dermatol. **122** 413-417.
24. Negroni R, Palmieri O, Koren K et al. (1987)
Oral treatment of paracoccidioidomycosis and histoplasmosis with itraconazole. Revs Infect. Dis. **9** s47-s50.
25. Viviani MA. Tortorano AM, Langer M et al (1989). Experience with itraconazole in cryptococcosis and aspergillosis. J. Infect **18** 151-165.
26. Denning DW, Tucker RM, Hanson LH and Stevens DA (1989)
Treatment of invasive aspergillosis with itraconazole.
American Journal of Medicine. **86** 791-800.
27. Tricot GE, Joosten MA, Boogaerts MA, Van de Pitte J and Cauwenbergh (1987).
Ketoconazole v itraconazole for antifungal prophylaxis in patients with severe granulocytopenia. Reviews of Infectious Diseases **9** s94-s99.

28. Humphrey MJ, Jevons S and Tarbit MH (1985)
Pharmacokinetic evaluation of UK 49,858, a metabolically stable triazole antifungal in animals and humans.
Antimicrob.Ag.Chemother. **28** 648-653

29. Brammer KW and Lees LJ (1987)
Single dose oral fluconazole in the treatment of vulvovaginal candidiasis: an interim analysis of a comparative study versus three-day intravaginal clotrimazole tablets.
In Recent trends in the Discovery, Development and Evaluation of Antifungal agents. RA Fromtling Ed. JR Prous Publishers, Barcelona pp 151-156.

30. Dupont B and Drouhet E (1988)
Fluconazole in the management of oropharyngeal candidosis in a predominantly HIV antibody positive group of patients.
J. Med.Vet.Mycol **26** 67-71.

31. Meunier F, Gerain J, Snoeck R, Libotte F, Lambert C and Ceuppens AM (1987)
Fluconazole therapy of oropharyngeal candidosis in cancer patients.
In Recent trends in the discovery, development and evaluation of antifungal agents. RA Fromtling Ed. JR Prous Publishers, Barcelona p 169-174.

32. Byrne WR and Wajszczuk CP (1988)
Cryptococcal meningitis in the acquired immunodeficiency syndrome (AIDS): successful treatment with fluconazole after failure of amphotericin B.
Ann.Intern.Med **108** 384-385.

33. Stern JJ, Hartman BJ, Sharkey P, Rowland V, Squires KE, Murray HW and Graybill JR (1988)
Oral fluconazole therapy for patients with acquired immunodeficiency syndrome and cryptococcosis: experience with 22 patients.
Am.J.Med **85** 477- 480.

35. Levine J, Bernard DB, Idelson BA, Farnham H, Saunders C and Sugar AM (1989)
Fungal peritonitis complicating continuous ambulatory peritoneal dialysis (CAPD) - successful treatment with fluconazole, a new orally active antifungal agent.
Am.J.Med **86** 825-827

36. Warnock DW, Burke J, Cope NJ, Johnson EM, Von Fraunhofer NA and Williams EW (1988)
Fluconazole resistance in Candida glabrata.
Lancet **ii** 1310.

16

Therapeutic Results with Miconazole in Japan

Akira Ito

The First Department of Internal Medicine,
Yokohama City University, School of Medicine,
3-46 Urafune-cho, Minami-ku, Yokohama 232, JAPAN

1. CHARACTERISTICS OF MICONAZOLE

Since 1963 Janssen Pharmaceutical Incorporated in Belgium has been synthesizing imidazole derivatives and investigating them biologically. From among about 1500 compounds synthesized and screened for antifungal activity, Miconazole was selected, and is a phenethylimidazole derivative.

The sale of Miconazole injection was permitted in 1976 in Belgium where it was developed, and Janssen sells it under the brand name of Daktarin i.v. Permission has now been obtained in

37 other nations including U.S., West Germany, Denmark and Switzerland. Japan approved its sale in November 1985.

Indications for Miconazole injection in Japan are fungemia pulmonary mycosis, mycosis of the digestive and urinary tract, and mycotic meningitis caused by classical deep-seated mycosis like Cryptococcus neoformans, Candida species, and Aspergillus species and also by Coccidioides immitis, imported from U.S.. In U.S. and European countries, blastomycosis, histoplasmosis, paracoccidioidomycosis and chronic mucocutaneous candidiasis are also approved as indications.

In Japan, an initial dose of 200 mg of Miconazole is dissolved in at least 200 ml of the solvent and drip-infused intravenously over 30 to 60 min. After confirmation of no side effects, 200 to 400 mg is administered by intravenous drip over 30 min. once to three times daily. Since Miconazole is hardly transported to the spinal fluid, it is concomitantly injected to the meningeal cavity in the cases with meningitis.

In U.S. and European countries, the total permitted dose is larger than in Japan and its local administration is also approved. The maximum dose of Monistat sold in U.S. is 3600 mg for coccidioidomycosis, 2400 mg for cryptococcosis and 1800 mg for candidiasis.

According to the package insert of Belgium's Daktarin, local administration for wound infections and infusions into the urinary bladder, cavity, and bronchi are also approved.

Miconazole exerts strong antifungal effects against Candida spp., Cryptococcus spp., and Aspergillus spp., which are principal organisms causing deep-seated mycosis and against a wide fungal spectrum of Torulopsis spp., Trichosporon spp., Mucor spp., Fonsecaea spp., Phialophora spp., Cladosporium spp., Sporothrix spp., Histoplasma spp., Blastomyces spp. and Geotrichum spp.[1]. No resistance to Miconazole has been encountered either in preserved or in clinically isolated strains.

The action mechanism of Miconazole is the inhibition of cell membrane synthesis by its low concentrations and direct injury of cell membrane by its high concentrations[2]. Inhibition of cell membrane enzyme has also been reported[3].

With respect to the pharmacokinetics, serum concentrations were determined by bioassay after an intravenous drip of 200 to 600 mg of Miconazole in patients with deep-seated mycosis. Peaks of 1.0 to 1.6 μg/ml were reached at the end of drip, followed by rapid decreases to 1/4 or less of this after 7 to 8 hrs[4].

When serum concentrations are determined by HPLC after intravenous drip of 600 mg, the values found tend to be higher than those determined by bioassay[5]. This tendency may be attributable to the fact that HPLC detects not only free but also protein-binding Miconazole.

Miconazole is widely distributed in tissues of the body. After an intravenous drip of tritium-labeled Miconazole to rats, high radioactivity is detected in the adrenals, liver, lungs and kidneys[6]. In humans it easily enters the joint fluid and aqueous fluid of the anterior chamber, but little is transported to the spinal fluid[7]~[10].

Although the human pathways of metabolism and excretion are unknown, it is thought to be rapidly metabolized in the liver and 1% or less of the dose is excreted unchanged in the urine[11]. The excretion is not affected even by renal failure[12].

With respect to interaction, there is a report that Miconazole should not be used with amphotericin because its action inhibiting ergosterol synthesis prevents amphotericin from binding to cell membrane and diminishes its effect.

There are conflicting reports about the antagonistic effect of the concomitant use of these two drugs[13]-[18].

2. CLINICAL RESULTS

The clinical effects of Miconazole were based on 69 reports published in Japan.

The subjects were 200 cases diagnosed such as candidiasis,

aspergillosis, cryptococcosis and others. Cases of concomitant use of amphotericin injection were excluded.

Regarding the background factors of patients, this study involved 107 men, 85 women and 8 immature infants infected with fungi. Average age was 49. The underlying diseases were 62 cases of hematologic malignancies and blood disorders and 21 cases of IVH catheterization.

With respect to the efficacy, overall clinical effects evaluated from clinical symptoms, radiological findings and endoscopic findings were classified as Excellent, Good, Poor and Worst. Mycological effects based on mycological examinations were classified as disappeared, decreased, unchanged and increased. Excluding 5 cases impossible to judge, the effective rate was calculated. The drug was effective on candidiasis in 108 of 121 cases (89%), on aspergillosis in 24 of 35 cases (68%), on cryptococcosis in 23 of 29 cases (79%) and on other mycosis in 10 of 10 cases (100%). Overall effective rate was 85%. Fungi disappeared in 55 of 93 cases of candidiasis (59%), in 12 of 18 cases of aspergillosis (67%) and in 12 of 24 cases of cryptococcosis (50%). Overall disappearance rate was 59%.

The effective rate classified by disease was 21 of 27 cases of pulmonary candidiasis (78%), 40 of 42 cases of candidemia (95%) and 47 of 52 other candidiasis. (90%).

In aspergillosis, the effective rate was 16 of 19 cases of pulmonary aspergillosis (84%), 5 of 11 cases of pulmonary aspergilloma (45%) and 3 of 5 other cases (60%).

In cryptococcosis, the effective rate was 16 of 21 cases of meningitis (76%), 5 of 6 cases of pulmonary cryptococcosis (83%) and 2 of 2 cases of cutaneous cryptococcosis (100%).

According to the clinical effects of Miconazole by the relationship between clinical effect and mean daily dose, cases given 600 mg or less accounted for the majority of the 200 cases, and the effective rate was 91 of 106 cases (86%). In 86 of 200 cases mean daily doses were between 601 and 1200 mg, and the effective rate was 71 of 86 cases (83%). Three cases received 1201 mg or more, and the effective rate was 100%.

In candidiasis 92 of 126 cases received 800 mg or less, and the effective rate was 79 of 87 cases (91%). In aspergillosis 23 of 36 cases were given 800 mg or less, and the effective rate was 15 of 22 cases (68%). In cryptococcosis 801 mg or more was injected in 20 of 29 cases, and the effective rate was 16 of 20 cases (80%).

For mycological effect, Candida strains were detected in 125 cases, and the disappearance rate of Candida spp. as a whole was 55 of 93 cases (59%). For the causative organisms, the disappearance rate of C. albicans was 33 of 52 cases (64%), that of C. parapsilosis 5 of 7 cases (71%) and that of C. tropicalis 7 of 14 cases (50%).

The disappearance rate of A. fumigatus was 12 of 16 cases (75%) and that of Cr. neoformans 12 of 24 cases (50%). The present study detected fungi in 186 cases of mycosis as a whole, and the rate of disappearance was 79 of 135 cases (59%).

We studied the clinical effect of Miconazole in cases where previous treatments had been ineffective and found it effective in 11 of 18 cases (61%) where amphotericin had been ineffective. After the failure of 5-FC, Miconazole was effective in 13 of 16 cases (81%), and after the failure of the concomitant use of amphotericin and 5-FC, Miconazole was effective in 23 of 25 cases (92%).

The methods of administration in Japan are limited to intravenous drip and infusion into the meningeal cavity. The literature, however, contains results of treatment by various other methods. These are in many cases used concomitantly with intravenous drip. Their effective rate is considered high.

Miconazole is also used in the pediatric field, but with no recommended dosage established in Japan. American reports show dosage of 20 to 40 mg/kg/day. In the present study, the effective rate was 8 of 12 cases (67%), and there were no side effects which led to discontinuation of the drug's use.

Fungal infections often complicate those immature or newborn infants that require concentrated care because of serious suspended animation or intracranial hemorrhage. Miconazole was effective in all such cases, and especially remarkable in 3 of 8. No side effects were noted. Especially in immature infants, some antimicrobial agents may cause renal disorders which makes it difficult to continue the treatment. Miconazole was considered superior in therapeutic effect and safety compared with existing antifungal agents.

Side effects of Miconazole reported in U.S. and Europe are allergy, phlebitis, itching sensation, nausea, vomiting, eruption, diarrhea, spasm, hypertriglyceridemia and abnormal liver function. In Japan, although the occurrence of side effects is being surveyed as phase IV, the incidence rate is relatively small. The incidence rate of digestive tract disorders such as nausea, vomiting and anorexia was 6%, that of hypersensitivity 3%, and that of increased GOT and GPT 2%. Therefore, Miconazole seems safe to use.

REFERENCES

1. T. Hiratani and H. Yamaguchi: Laboratory assessment of a systemic antimycotic miconazole (base): in vitro activity, Chemotherapy, 32:534-540, (1984).
2. H. Yamaguchi, M. Miyaji and K. Nishimura: Chemotherapy of mycosis. Biology of Pathogenic Fungi, Nanzando Company, Limited, Tokyo. P.319-354, (1987).
3. H. Yamaguchi: Advances in research of mechanism of imidazole-antimycotics action. In Filamentous Microorganisms. (Biomedical Aspects ed.), Japan Scientific Societies Press. Tokyo. PP.355, (1985).
4. K. Uchida and H. Yamaguchi: Bioassay for miconazole and its levels in human body fluids. Chemotherapy. 32:541-546, (1984).
5. A. Ito, "Serum concentrations determined after an intravenous drip of 600 mg of Miconazole" Proceedings of the 37th Chemotherapy. Tokyo. pp.86 (1989).
6. H. Kosuzume, J. Ishiguro, T. Tsuchiya, M. Kurita and H. Ohnishi: Metabolic Fate of Miconazole (1). Iyakuhin Kenkyu. 7:382-391, (1976).
7. J.R. Graybill and H.B. Levine: Successful treatment of cryptococcal meningitis with intraventricular miconazole. Arch. Int. Med., 138:814-816, (1978).
8. D.A. Stevens, H.B. Levine. and S.C. Deresinski: Miconazole in coccidioidomycosis. II. Therapeutic and Pharmacologic studies in man. Amer. J. Med., 60:191-202, (1976).
9. S.C Deresinski, J.N. Galgiani and D.A. Stevens: Miconazole treatment of human cocidioidomycosis. Status report. In Coccidioidomycosis, Current Clinical and Diagnostic Status, ed. by Ajillo, L., Symposia Specialists, Miami, pp. 267 (1977).
10. P.D.Hoeprich and E. Goldstein: Miconazole therapy for coccidioidomycosis. JAMA. 230:1153-1157, (1974).
11. J. Brugmans: Systemic antifungal potential, safety,

biotransport and transformation of miconazole nitrate. Eur. J. Clin. Pharmacol., 5:93-99, (1972).

12. J. Boelaert, R. Daneels, H.V. Landuyt and J. Symoens: Miconazole plasma levels in healthy subjects and in patients with impaired renal function. Chemotherapy (J.D. Williams and A.M. Geddes, ed.) Plenum Publishing Corporation, New York, PP.165, (1976).

13. L.P. Schacter, R.J. Owellen, H.K. Rathbun and B. Buchanan: Antagonism between miconazole and amphotericin B. Lancet, 7:PP.318, (1976).

14. R.F. Cosgrove, A.E. Beezer and R.J. Miles: In vitro studies of amphotericin B in combination with the imidazole antifungal compounds clotrimazole and miconazole. J. Infect. Diseases., 138:681-685, (1978).

15. B. Dupont and E. Drouhet: In vitro synergy and antagonism of antifungal agents against yeast-like fungi. Postgraduate Medical Journal, 55:683-686, (1979).

16. J.R. Graybill, L. Mitchell and H.B. Levine: Treatment of experimental murine cryptococcosis: a comparison of miconazole and amphotericin B, Antimicrob. Agents and Chemother. 13: 277-283, (1978).

17. J. Brajtburg, D. Kobayashi, G, Medoff and G.S. Kobayashi: Antifungal action of amphotericin B in combination with other polyene or imidazole antibiotics. J. Infect. Diseases., 146:138-146, (1982).

18. F.C. Odds: Interactions among amphotericin B, 5-fluorocytosine, ketoconazole and miconazole against pathogenic fungi. Antimicrob. Agents and Chemother, 22:763-770, (1982).

17

Overview of Fluconazole

Dr. J.M. Feczko

Clinical Research Department
Pfizer Central Research
Sandwich, Kent, England, CT13 9NJ

I. INTRODUCTION

Previously available antifungal agents such as amphotericin B, flucytosine and the imidazoles -- miconazole, clotrimazole, tioconazole and ketoconazole -- represented significant breakthroughs for the treatment of superficial and systemic mycotic infections. However, their clinical value has been limited primarily by their relatively high risks of toxicity, pharmacokinetic deficiencies and/or limited options in their methods of administration. Thus, the search has continued for a broad spectrum systemically-effective antifungal which could be administered either orally or parenterally, be at least as effective, and better tolerated than its class predecessors.

Fluconazole, a novel triazole compound, is the culmination of efforts to develop a better tolerated antifungal with greater specificity and more desirable pharmacokinetic properties than existing antifungal agents. Unlike ketoconazole and other azoles, fluconazole is water soluble, allowing for both oral and intravenous dosage forms. It is also the first azole antifungal to be renally excreted primarily as unchanged drug rather than undergoing extensive hepatic metabolism.

A. *MODE OF ACTION*

Fluconazole inhibits the fungal demethylase enzyme required for the conversion of lanosterol to ergosterol, the major sterol in fungal cell membranes. In mammalian cells cholesterol is the major membrane sterol and it is produced from lanosterol by a similar enzymatic conversion. Studies have shown that fluconazole exhibits greater specificity than ketoconazole for the fungal enzyme. It has also been shown that, unlike ketoconazole, fluconazole has no significant effect on endogenous gonadal or adrenal steroidogenesis at therapeutic dosages in humans.

B. *PHARMACOKINETICS*

The intrinsic properties of previously available antifungals have imposed limitations on their overall clinical value, particularly in the treatment of systemic fungal infections.

Fluconazole differs from ketoconazole and other earlier azole antifungals in that the imidazole ring is replaced by a triazole ring. As a result, the metabolic stability of the molecule is increased. The presence of a second triazole ring, a hydroxyl group and the difluorophenyl group results in a much less lipophilic molecule.

In contrast to other antifungals, fluconazole is water soluble and is formulated for both oral and intravenous administration and its pharmacokinetic properties are similar after administration by either route.

In the fasting state, peak plasma concentrations of fluconazole occur between 0.5 and 1.5 hours post dose. Its bioavailability after oral administration is greater than 90%, and it demonstrates a plasma half-life of 25-30 hours. Its volume of distribution is 0.7 - 0.8 L/kg, similar to that of body water.

Table 1
FLUCONAZOLE PHARMACOKINETIC SUMMARY

Rapid and high oral absorption (>90%)
Absorption unaffected by food
Long plasma half-life (approx. 30 hours)
High urinary excretion of unchanged drug
Low plasma protein binding (12%)
Volume of distribution (0.7 - 0.8 L/kg) - similar to volume of body water

Fluconazole is cleared primarily by glomerular filtration. Studies with healthy volunteers show that over 80% of an oral dose is excreted unchanged in the urine and that single and multiple doses of fluconazole result in predictable and linear pharmacokinetics. Clearance of fluconazole is directly related to glomerular filtration rate so that in patients with decreased renal function, either the daily dose or the dosing interval must be altered.

In contrast to previous azole compounds, fluconazole's protein binding is only 12% resulting in high levels of circulating unbound active drug.

C. *PENETRATION INTO BODY FLUIDS AND TISSUES*

Oral or intravenous administration of fluconazole results in rapid and widespread distribution of active compound. High, sustained therapeutic levels are rapidly achieved in a variety of body fluids and tissues (Table 2).

Fluconazole achieves high concentrations in all body fluids and tissue sites commonly subject to fungal infection. In patients with fungal meningitis fluconazole levels in the CSF during therapy have been over 80% of corresponding serum levels. CSF levels exceed 50% of serum levels even in the absence of meningeal inflammation.

Table 2
FLUCONAZOLE LEVELS IN BODY FLUIDS AND TISSUES

Peak concentration in plasma (400mg single dose) : 8mg/l

Peak concentration at steady state (400mg daily) : 20.0mg/l

Cerebrospinal fluid	:	50-90% of plasma
Saliva	:	same as plasma
Sputum	:	same as plasma
Blister fluid	:	same as plasma
Urine	:	10 x plasma
Peritoneal fluid	:	same as plasma
Vaginal tissue	:	same as plasma
Skin scrapings (hand)	:	10 x plasma
Blister skin	:	2 x plasma
Fingernails	:	same as plasma

D. *CLINICAL EFFICACY*

Fluconazole has shown excellent therapeutic activity against various types of superficial and systemic fungal infections in immunocompromised patients. Several reviews of clinical data have been recently published (1,2,3). This paper will only summarize some of the most recently completed trials.

1. *Oropharyngeal/esophageal candidiasis.* Severe oropharyngeal candidiasis (OPC) adds significantly to the morbidity and quality of life deterioration experienced by immunocompromised patients.

One hundred and ninety-three patients with OPC complicating underlying malignancy were randomized 2:1 to 100mg of fluconazole once daily for 7 days versus clotrimazole troche five times daily for 14 days. Mycological evaluations were made pre and post therapy in all patients and clinical observations were performed by a third party observer blinded to therapy. Clinical responses occurred in 80% of fluconazole treated patients compared to 61% on clotrimazole ($p<0.0001$). At 7 days followup of those with persistent clinical lesions only 20/38 (53%) were culture positive in the fluconazole group compared to 71/20 (85%) on clotrimazole ($p=0.014$).

In a similarly designed study in 258 patients with AIDS/ARC, clinical response was noted in 98% of the fluconazole group and 97% of the clotrimazole group. Complete mycological eradication of the oropharynx was achieved in 67% of fluconazole patients and 54% of clotrimazole.

The frequent recurrence of OPC in patients with AIDS/ARC prompted a study evaluating prophylactic treatment. Patients with AIDS/ARC who had OPC were treated in an open trial with 50mg of fluconazole daily until they underwent clinical and mycological cure. They were then randomized in a double blind fashion to 150mg fluconazole given once weekly versus identical placebo for 6 months. One hundred and six patients were so randomized and at six months 22.2% of fluconazole patients had symptomatic relapse compared to 78.7% on placebo ($p<0.001$).

Clinical response in esophageal candidiasis may occur in the presence of persisting mycological involvement as documented by follow-up endoscopy. It is therefore essential that repeat endoscopic evaluations are performed.

A double blind trial evaluated 100-200mg/day of fluconazole compared to 200-400mg/day of ketoconazole in the treatment of endoscopically proven esophageal candidiasis. Sixty-one immunocompromised patients (87% with AIDS) were evaluable.

Clinical response occurred in 66% of fluconazole treated patients compared to 55% or ketoconazole. This overall symptomatic response was not statistically significant though faster responses and therefore shorter duration of treatment was noted in the fluconazole group (p=0.047). Endoscopic confirmation was performed post therapy in all patients, 87% on fluconazole compared to 53% on ketoconazole showed complete endscopic resolution (p=0.04).

A smaller open study in 20 patients with esophagitis randomized to either oral fluconazole or I.V. amphotericin results in clinical responses in 9/10 in each treatment group.

2. *Prophylaxis.* A recently completed trial compared 50mg daily of fluconazole versus oral polyenes given 5-6 times daily prophylactically during chemotherapy induced neutropenia. In the fluconazole group 10/254 were diagnosed with proven fungal infection compared to 31/255 on polyenes (p=0.001). The advantage in favour of fluconazole was mainly a result of the prevention of oropharyngeal disease (4 cases versus 22 in the fluconazole and polyene groups respectively, p=0.001). Though there were only one-half as many candidemias documented in the fluconazole group compared to polyenes (3 versus 6) this result did not reach statistical significance.

Trials are currently in progress examining higher doses of fluconazole in fungal prophylaxis in bone marrow transplant patients and those with chemotherapy-induced neutropenia.

3. *Systemic fungal infections.* In the U.S. a component of the clinical trial programme include an extended access, compassionate protocol in which patients with proven fungal infections who had failed to respond to conventional antifungal therapy or who had a major contraindication or manifested severe toxicity were allowed to receive fluconazole.

Response rates in both systemic candidiasis and acute cryptococcal meningitis were significant (Table 3 & 4).

This included excellent responses in candida peritonitis (32/35) and hepatosplenic candidiasis (15/16).

Results of comparative trials in the therapy of acute cryptococcal meningitis and the maintenance of remission are presented in more detail in this volume by Dr. W. Dismukes. In summary 194 patients with AIDS and acute cryptococcal meningitis were randomized to either fluconazole 200mg-400mg daily or I.V. amphotericin. No significant differences were seen in clinical response, mycological eradication or overall mortality between the two treatment groups though sterilization of the CSF occurred more rapidly with amphotericin. A study of 183 patients with previously treated acute cryptococcal meningitis who were

Table 3

CLINICAL RESPONSE IN CANDIDIASIS

	N	Response (%)
Esophagitis	44	40 (90.9)
UTI	38	30 (78.9)
Candidemia	32	29 (90.6)
Disseminated	31	22 (71.0)
Pneumonia	19	18 (94.7)
Peritonitis	35	32 (91.4)
Multiple Mucocutaneous sites	26	24 (92.3)
Hepatosplenic	16	15 (93.7)

Table 4

ACUTE CRYPTOCOCCAL MENINGITIS

CLINICAL RESPONSE

N	Responders (%)
181	109 (60.2)

MYCOLOGICAL RESPONSE

N	Eradication (%)
123	81 (65.9)

randomized to daily fluconazole (200mg orally) versus weekly I.V. amphotericin for the prevention of relapse was terminated by an independent monitoring committee with 3/106 patients relapsing on fluconazole versus 14/77 given amphotericin ($p<0.001$). Discontinuations due to side effects or laboratory abnormalities also favoured fluconazole with 3/110 discontinuing versus 10/85 on amphotericin ($p=0.03$).

E. *FLUCONAZOLE SAFETY PROFILE*

Fluconazole has been well tolerated as evidenced by its use in controlled clinical trials involving over 4000 patients.

The side effect profile of fluconazole was evaluated in 4,048 patients who received therapy for at least seven days. Those side effects that occurred at an incidence of 1% or more included: nausea (3.7%); headache (1.9%); skin rash (1.8%); vomiting (1.7%); abdominal pain (1.7%) and diarrhoea (1.5%). The incidence of side effects was somewhat higher in HIV-infected patients than in non-HIV-infected patients. However, the patterns were similar in both groups, as was the rate of only 1.5% of the patients in each group who discontinued therapy due to side effects.

In the combined data base, seriously ill patients (predominantly with AIDS or malignancy) rarely have developed serious hepatic reactions or exfoliative skin disorders during treatment with fluconazole. However, the patients who suffered these reactions were also receiving multiple concomitant medications including many known to be hepatotoxic or associated with exfoliative skin disorders which predisposed them to these complications. Thus, the causal association of the adverse hepatic/exfoliative skin reactions with fluconazole therapy is uncertain.

Table 5
MOST COMMON CLINICAL ADVERSE EFFECTS
IN 4,048 SUBJECTS RECEIVING FLUCONAZOLE*

Symptom	Percentage of patients
Nausea	3.7
Headache	1.9
Rash	1.8
Vomiting	1.7
Abdominal pain	1.7
Diarrhoea	1.5
Number discontinued because of side effects 61 =	1.5%

* Incidence $\geq$ 1%

Table 6

LFT Abnormalities

Fluconazole versus Placebo

N = 684 subjects/patients (427 - fluconazole; 257 - placebo)

Prophylactic studies in AIDS and Malignancies

Pharmacokinetic Trials

Dose 50 - 400 mg daily

	Fluc N (% abnormal)		Placebo N (% abnormal)	
SGOT	373	(1.6)	202	(1.5)
SGPT	426	(1.9)	254	(1.6)
Alk Phos	425	(0.7)	253	(1.2)
Bilirubin	427	(0.9)	251	(1.2)
Any LFT	427	(3.3)	254	(4.3)

Table 7

LFT Abnormalities

Fluconazole versus Amphotericin

N = 414 patients (249 - fluconazole; 165 - Amphotericin)

AIDS and Malignancies

Mean daily dose fluconazole = 191 mg

	Fluc N (% abnormal)		AmB N (% abnormal)		% Considered Treatment Related	
					Fluc	AmB
SGOT	195	(7.1)	129	(6.2)	1.0	0
SGPT	172	(8.1)	115	(7.8)	1.2	0
Alk Phos	184	(12.5)	122	(16.4)	1.0	3.3
Bilirubin	185	(3.3)	118	(7.6)	0.6	0
Any LFT	191	(18.8)	126	(27.7)	2.6	2.9

Only 3 subjects discontinued due to LFT abnormalities (2 - fluc; 1 - Ampho)

In combined trials from placebo-controlled pharmacokinetic studies in healthy subjects, and prophylactic placebo-controlled studies in patients with AIDS or malignancy the incidence of abnormalities noted in various liver function parameters was similar in both the fluconazole and placebo groups.

Relation of liver function abnormalities in patients with AIDS or malignancy to any given therapy is difficult to ascertain due to the severely debilitated condition of the patients as well as concomitant medications. In pooled comparative studies versus intravenous amphotericin B no significant incidence of possibly treatment related LFT abnormalities was noted.

F. *DRUG INTERACTION PROFILE*

In formal interaction studies fluconazole administered in multiple doses up to 400mg daily has produced no noticeable effects on testosterone, estrogen, or ACTH-stimulated cortisol concentrations. No significant effects have been documented with cyclosporin A at fluconazole doses of 100mg/day in bone marrow transplant patients.

However, at fluconazole dosages of 100mg daily or more, drug interactions of known or potential clinical consequence may occur with warfarin, sulfonylurea oral hypoglycaemics, phenytoin, rifampin and cyclosporin A (renal transplant patients). The

Table 8
DRUG INTERACTIONS RESULTS
OF STUDIES WITH FLUCONAZOLE

Drug	Effect	Response
Cimetidine	↓ Fluconazole	0
Oral contraceptives	0	0
Antacids	0	0
Cyclosporine	↑ Cyclosporine	Monitor cyclosporine levels
Oral hypoglycemics	↑ Hypoglycemic	Monitor Glucose/adjust hypoglycemic effect
Warfarin	↑ Prothrombin	Monitor Prothrombin
Phenytoin	↑ Phenytoin	Monitor/adjust phenytoin
Rifampin	↓ Fluconazole	Consider increasing fluconazole dose

type of interaction to be expected is indicated in the accompanying table. In most cases the type of interaction seen is a modest increase in the plasma concentrations (and hence AUCs) of the drug in question. Monitoring of plasma levels and/or relevant pharmacological parameters may be necessary if fluconazole is used in patients receiving such drugs so that adverse effects resulting from the interaction may be minimised by an appropriate reduction in drug dosage.

G. *SUMMARY*

Fluconazole is a new triazole antifungal agent which demonstrates near-ideal clinical pharmacokinetics as well as more potent and specific activity against fungal infections than other available azole antifungals. Compared to predecessors in the same class, fluconazole is more water soluble and can be administered orally and parenterally with similar concentrations in plasma achieved via both routes. It is rapidly and completely absorbed in both fasting and fed patients. It has a plasma half-life of 25 to 30 hours and, thus, offers the important advantage of effective round-the-clock antifungal action with once-daily dosing.

The bioavailability of fluconazole after oral administration is greater than 90%, and is minimally bound to plasma proteins (12%) in contrast to the high degree of protein binding observed with other antifungal azoles (99% for miconazole and ketoconazole). Single and multiple doses of fluconazole produce predictable and linear dose-related plasma concentrations and excellent total body distribution, including effective penetration into cerebrospinal fluid, vaginal tissue and other commonly infected sites. Up to 80% of an oral dose is excreted unchanged in the urine.

Fluconazole has demonstrated excellent antifungal efficacy in the treatment of various types of superficial mycoses at doses of 50-100mg daily, and of systemic infections at doses of 200-400mg daily, including those caused by candidal, cryptococcal and other common fungal pathogens. It has achieved high rates of cures in patients whose immune system is compromised due to malignancy, cytotoxic chemotherapy, radiation therapy or HIV infection.

Fluconazole has been extremely well tolerated. In over 4,000 study patients with various predispositions and infectious conditions, the most common side effects attributed to fluconazole have been nausea, abdominal pain, headache and rash. Side effects have been usually of only mild or moderate severity and have only rarely necessitated the withdrawal of treatment.

While occasional alterations in laboratory parameters have been reported, there is little evidence that fluconazole up to 400mg/day causes clinically significant alterations in clinical chemistry parameters even in seriously ill patients.

Bibliography References:

1. S.M. Grant, S.P. Clissold. Fluconazole: A Review of its Pharmacodynamic and Pharmacokinetic Properties, and Therapeutic Potential in Superficial and Systemic Mycoses, Drugs 39 (6): 877-916, 1990.

2. Fluconazole: A Novel Advance in Therapy for Systemic Fungal Infections in Reviews of Infectious Diseases 12 (3): Mar-Apr 1990.

3. Discovery, Development and Evaluation of New Antifungal Agents in Recent Trends in the Discovery, Development and Evaluaion of Antifungal Agents (R.A. Fromtling, ed.), Part 2. Section 2, 77-176.

18

Results of Itraconazole Treatment in Systemic Mycoses in Animals and Man

J. Van Cutsem and G. Cauwenbergh

Janssen Research Foundation, B-2340 Beerse, Belgium

INTRODUCTION

Itraconazole is a broad-spectrum lipophylic antifungal triazole with a Mol Wt of 705.64 (Fig. 1). It is active in vitro against a large number of fungi of medical interest (1,2). Itraconazole has been evaluated successfully in various in-vivo models, using normal and immunodepressed animals, treated topically, orally or parenterally. The animals were infected by several routes with a broad range of antimycotic agents (3,4). Clinical studies have demonstrated marked therapeutic efficacy of itraconazole with the same broad-spectrum (5,6).

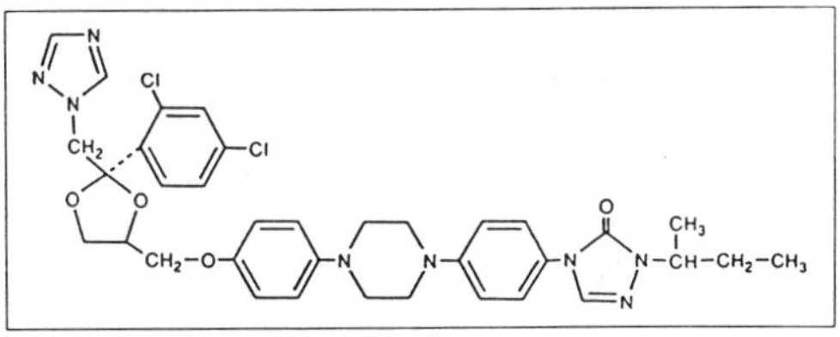

FIG. 1. Chemical structure of itraconazole

IN-VITRO EXPERIMENTS

The in-vitro activity of azoles may be largely influenced by various factors : e.g. the culture medium, its pH and the temperature, inactivation or binding to components of the medium, the drug solubilizer, solubility and the diffusion potency of the compound, the endpoint of the experiment, the fungal species and isolate, the inoculum size, the fungal phase, ...(1). An adequate correlation between in-vitro and in-vivo activity was found for itraconazole in brain heart infusion broth (BHI br). The test medium for Pityrosporum ovale was Dixon broth. Stock solutions of itraconazole were prepared in dimethyl sulphoxide and further diluted serially in the decimal dilution test. Controls were included. The antifungal assay was performed at 25°C for 14 days, except for yeast-phase activity of dimorphic fungi (37°C). Candida and Torulopsis were considered sensitive if growth was inhibited by ≥ 90 % at the end of the test period. For all other fungi, complete absence of growth was the criterion used. The in-vitro results are shown in Table 1 as the % of strains that are sensitive at 0.1 and 1 $\mu g.ml^{-1}$.

ANIMAL EXPERIMENTS

A large number of experiments have been performed (3,4,6,7,8). In this study only a summary is given of some animal experiments that are important in comparison with clinical trials.

For oral treatment itraconazole was dissolved in polyethylene glycol 200 (PEG) or in some experiments in hydroxypropyl-ß-cyclodextrin (HP-ß-CD). For parenteral treatment the itraconazole solution in HP-ß-CD has been used. The commercial preparation of amphotericin B, Fungizone Squibb ® and PEG (oral)- or aqueous (parenteral) solutions were used for fluconazole. Albino guinea-pigs were used in all experiments presented in this study. Vaginal candidosis, however, was induced in hysterectomized and ovarectomized Wistar rats by intravaginal infection with Candida albicans. The rats were in permanent pseudo-oestrus. For dermatophytosis, the skin of the back of the guinea-pigs was scarified before infection with Microsporum canis or with Trichophyton mentagrophytes. Pityrosporum ovale was infected on the intact occluded skin (Table 2). Only the animals with absence of clinical lesions and complete eradication of the fungi were considered cured.

C. albicans was infected IV in guinea-pigs to obtain systemic and disseminated disease. Oral prophylactic treatment with itraconazole or with the excipient for one, two or three days before infection was administered to guinea-pigs (Table 3). The guinea-pigs were infected IV with 1000 or 2000 CFU of C. albicans per g body weight (BW). The animals were observed daily and the skin folliculitis scored as 0 (complete absence of skin lesions), + (pin point eruptions), ++ (folliculitis with erythema and inflammation) or +++ (extensive invasion of the skin surface). Fourteen days after infection the animals were sacrificed . The left kidney and the skin were homogenized and cultured. For evaluation of therapeutic activity the IV inoculum of C. albicans consisted of 8000 CFU per g BW (Table 4). Itraconazole was administered orally or IV to normal and to immunodepressed guinea-pigs. Groups of guinea-pigs were also treated with oral fluconazole or with parenteral amphotericin B. Neutropenia was induced in the guinea-pigs by IP administration of 0.25 $mg.kg^{-1}$ mechlorethamine hydrochloride on day 5 and 4 before infection. The neutropenia persisted for the complete duration of the experiment.

Systemic invasive aspergillosis was obtained by an IV inoculum of 25.000 CFU of Aspergillus fumigatus per g BW (Table 5). All untreated and excipient-treated controls died between day 4 and 7 after infection. Itraconazole was given orally and parenterally to the animals, starting on the day of infection or 24 hours later. Fluconazole was only given orally in early treatment. Amphotericin B was administered parenterally. All survivors were sacrificed 28 days after infection. Cultures were performed from nine organs of all dead and sacrificed animals.

Progressive meningeal, generalized and disseminated cryptococcosis can be obtained in the guinea-pig, infected IV with Cryptococcus neoformans. An inoculum of 200 CFU per g

BW is sufficient to lead to fatal disease, if untreated. Itraconazole and fluconazole were given orally or parenterally for 35 days, starting three days after infection (Table 6). These two triazoles were also given in combination therapy. Combination therapies of itraconazole/5-flucytosine and itraconazole/amphotericin B were also evaluated (Table 7). All survivors were sacrificed one week after the end of treatment. The presence or absence of skin cryptococcomas was evaluated. Brain and meninges and 12 other organs were cultured after homogenization.

Sporotrichosis can be produced in the guinea-pig by various routes. Disseminated sporotrichosis in various organs occurred after IV injection of spores of Sporothrix schenckii (Table 8). The guinea-pigs were treated orally for 14 or for 28 days with itraconazole or with fluconazole. The animals were sacrificed and considered to be cured if all organs were negative by culture and improved if only one out of 6 organs was positive. Guinea-pigs were infected intratesticularly with Histoplasma duboisii and treated orally for 14 days with itraconazole(Table 9). The same parameters were used as in sporotrichosis.

The results of animal experiments are presented in Tables 2 to 12. In general a relatively good correlation is possible between the animal experiments in well established models that allow extrapolation to the human diseases. We have to keep in mind that uniform infections can be produced in small experimental animals and that naturally occurring infections in man are rarely uniform especially in immunocompromised patients. Patients can be infected in various organs with large variations in terms of invasion and severity of the disease, influencing the outcome of treatment.

CLINICAL EVALUATION IN MAN

Large series of clinical trials have been performed worldwide with itraconazole (9-13). Only the results of studies that have been submitted for worldwide registration of itraconazole have been presented in the tables 2, 4-6, 8-12. (Data on file Janssen Res. Foundation). The results of fixed protocols in the treatment of superficial mycoses are presented in Table 2. In tinea corporis or cruris, treated for 15 days with 100 mg itraconazole, clinical and mycological cure were obtained in 88 and 82% respectively of all patients. To obtain comparable results in tinea pedis or manus, itraconazole was administered for 30 days. Cure of vaginal candidosis after oral treatment with itraconazole was possible with a one-day treatment schedule of 200 mg b.i.d., as well as in 2 or 3 days dosage of 200 mg o.d.

Eighty percent of patients suffering from pityriasis versicolor were cured clinically and mycologically with a total dosage of 1000 mg (in 5 or in 10 days).

For 106 patients suffering from various manifestations of infection by Candida spp (81%) or Torulopsis glabrata (19%) the global response rate was defined as cure or marked improvement (Table 4). Itraconazole was well tolerated and appeared to be efficacious in different clinical manifestations of these infections.

A total of 251 evaluable patients with various manifestations of aspergillosis (Table 5) have been treated at a median daily dose of 200 mg itraconazole during 91 days (median). Global response was rated as cure or marked improvement in aspergillosis and in other systemic fungal diseases. Itraconazole may be considered to be effective in the treatment of the entire spectrum of diseases related to Aspergillus spp.

Cryptococcal meningitis is considered as one of the markers of immunodepression, especially in AIDS patients. A dose of 200 mg is efficacious in all patients, but notably better results were obtained with daily intake of 400 mg of itraconazole. In AIDS patients with cryptococcal meningitis only one out of 13 relapsed during maintenance therapy (Table 6).

Impressive results were obtained in the treatment of human sporotrichosis (Table 8). Treatment duration is always variable, but should be extended at least until complete mycological cure.

Histoplasmosis responded well to itraconazole therapy (Table 9). Histoplasmosis is also one of the mycoses that may be found in AIDS patients and that responded very well. Rarely patients relapsed during therapy or during follow-up for several months. Both H. capsulatum and the more difficult to treat H. duboisii reacted favourably. The treatment of blastomycosis has been initiated by Dismukes et al., and Graybill, Stevens et al. (Table 10). The results of treatment with itraconazole are comparable to those obtained in histoplasmosis.

The results obtained in paracoccidioidomycosis in 76 patients with a daily dose of 100 mg of itraconazole (median) for 6 months (median) and a global therapeutic response in 92% of the patients, negative mycology in three months in 71% and 91% after six months proved its high effectiveness.

Chromomycosis by Cladosporium carrionii is more sensitive to itraconazole than if the infection is caused by Fonsecaea pedrosoi (Table 11).

Various other systemic mycoses have been treated with itraconazole : a large number responded to the treatment, (Table 12), also protothecosis caused by an alga.

It is also important to note that itraconazole is active in coccidioidomycosis. Tucker et al. (6) reported the treatment with itraconazole of 39 patients with coccidioidomycosis, including pulmonary-, bone and joint-, lymphatic-, skin and soft tissue-, meningeal- and urogenital involvement. They obtained 63% full response, 30% partial response and 7% no response, in a mean of 213 days of treatment (50 - 400 mg per day). They noted successful itraconazole treatments also in other fungal infections. To illustrate the broad-spectrum efficacy of itraconazole : high percentages of keratitis by various fungal agents responded to itraconazole in patients (14) and in animals (3), as well as Penicillium marneffei disseminated infection (M.A. Viviani, unpubl. results, 15). A study in neutropenic patients had suggested that itraconazole is at least equipotent to amphotericin B in treating invasive fungal diseases (J.W. Van 't Wout et al., unpubl. results).

Low numbers of patients with itraconazole-related side-effects occurred, and these are generally mild and minor.

CONCLUSION

Itraconazole is a lipophilic triazole with an extremely large spectrum of antifungal activity and a pharmacokinetic profile with high tissue levels (16,17). The correlation between in-vitro activity, animal pharmacological efficacy and human therapeutical results appears to be good. The laboratory data obtained with itraconazole are predictive for therapeutic efficacy. The therapeutic efficacy of itraconazole, not only in various superficial mycoses, but also in invasive infections has been predicted from the results in animal models. The combination therapy of itraconazole with fluconazole in cryptococcosis suggests that there is no contraindication, but also no advantage to combine lipophilic and lipophobic compounds. The combination of itraconazole and flucytosine, or itraconazole and amphotericin B appeared to have at least additive efficacy in cryptococcosis (3,4,7). The same conclusion could be drawn from earlier experiments in aspergillosis of guinea-pigs with itraconazole or ketoconazole and amphotericin B. In predisposed or immunocompromised patients antifungal prophylaxis with itraconazole has been used with success. The results of this study justify the evaluation and the use of itraconazole in larger series of patients (18,19,20).

Prophylaxis with itraconazole in patients undergoing remission-induction therapy has indicated that the mortality induced by opportunistic fungi can be significantly reduced in this patient group (19). For treatment of systemic mycoses an oral pelleted formulation, an IV formulation and an oral solution based on cyclodextrins are currently available or under development. No major toxicity has been observed at therapeutic doses up to 40 mg/kg in animals as well as in over 150,000 patients treated.

REFERENCES

1. J. Van Cutsem, The in-vitro antifungal spectrum of itraconazole, Mycoses, 32, S1: 7-13 (1989).
2. A. Espinel-Ingroff, S. Shadomy and R. J. Gebhart, In-vitro studies with R 51211 (itraconazole), Antimicrob. Agents Chemother., 26: 5-9 (1984).
3. J. Van Cutsem, Oral, topical and parenteral antifungal treatment with itraconazole in normal and in immunocompromised animals, Mycoses, 32, S1: 14-34 (1989).
4. J. Van Cutsem, Oral and parenteral treatment with itraconazole in various superficial and systemic experimental fungal infections. Comparison with other antifungals and combination therapy, Br. J. Clin. Pract., Sympos. Suppl. London, 1989, in press 1990.
5. J. R. Graybill, Azole therapy of systemic fungal infections, Diagnosis and Therapy of systemic fungal Infections (K. Holmberg and R. Meyer, eds.) Raven Press, Ltd., New York, p 133-143 (1989).
6. R. M. Tucker, P. L. Williams, E. G. Arathoon and D. A. Stevens, Treatment of mycoses with itraconazole, Ann. N Y Acad Sci (V. S. Georgiev, ed.), 544: 451-470 (1988).
7. A. Polak, Combination therapy with antifungal drugs, Mycoses, 31: 45-53 (1988).
8. J.R. Perfect, D. V. Savani and D. T. Durack, Comparison of itraconazole and fluconazole in treatment of cryptococcal meningitis and Candida pyelonephritis in rabbits, Antimicrob. Agents Chemother, 29: 579-583 (1986).
9. D. W. Denning, R. M. Tucker, L. H. Hanson and D. A. Stevens, Treatment of invasive aspergillosis with itraconazole, Am. J. Med., 86: 791-800 (1989).
10. B. Dupont and E. Drouhet, The treatment of aspergillosis with azole derivatives. Aspergillus and Aspergillosis, (H. Vanden Bossche, D. W. R. MacKenzie and G. Cauwenbergh, eds.) Plenum Publ. Corp., New York, p 243-251 (1988).
11. R. J. Hay and Y. M. Clayton, Treatment of dermatophytosis and chronic oral candidosis with itraconazole, Rev. Infect. Dis., 9, S1: 114-118 (1987).
12. A. Restrepo, I. Gomez, J. Robledo, M. M. Patino, L. E. Carro, Itraconazole in the treatment of paracoccidioidomycosis, Rev. Infect. Dis., 9, S1: 51-56 (1987).
13. M. A. Viviani, A. M. Tortorano, M. Langer, M. Almaviva, C. Negri, S. Cristina, S. Scoccia, R. De Maria, R. Fiocchi, P. Ferrazzi, A. Goglio, G. Gavazzeni, G. Faggian, R. Rinaldi and P. Cadrobbi, Experience with itraconazole in cryptococcosis and aspergillosis, J. Infect., 18: 151-165 (1989).
14. P. A. Thomas, D. J. Abraham, G. M. Kalavathy and J.Rajasekaran, Oral itraconazole therapy for mycotic keratitis, Mycoses, 31: 271-279 (1989).
15. J. Van Cutsem, Fungal models in immunocompromised animals, Mycoses in AIDS Patients, (H. Vanden Bossche, D. W. R. MacKenzie, G. Cauwenbergh, E. Drouhet, B. Dupont and J. Van Cutsem, eds.)Plenum Publ. Co., New York, (in press 1990).
16. J. Heykants, A. Van Peer, V. Van de Velde, P. Van Rooy, W. Meuldermans, K. Lavrijsen, R. Woestenborghs, J. Van Cutsem and G. Cauwenbergh, The clinical pharmacokinetics of itraconazole : an overview, Mycoses, 32, S1, 67-87 (1989).
17. G. Cauwenbergh, Skin kinetics of antifungal drugs, Current Topics in medical Mycology, Vol. IV, (M. Borgers, R. J. Hay and M. J. Rinaldi, eds.),Springer Verlag, New York (in press 1991).
18. M. A. Boogaerts, G. E. Verhoef, P. Zachee, H. Demuynck, L. Verbist and K. De Beule, Antifungal Prophylaxis with itraconazole in prolonged neutropenia : correlation with plasma levels, Mycoses, 32, S1: 103-108 (1989).
19. G. Cauwenbergh, Antifungal prophylaxis, Antifungal Drug Therapy (P. H. Jacobs and L. Nall, eds.) Marcel Dekker Inc., New York, p 297-313 (1990).
20. A. G. Prentice and G. R. Bradford, Prophylaxis of fungal infections with itraconazole during remission-induction therapy, Mycoses, 32, S1: 96-102 (1989).

Table 1: Antifungal activity of itraconazole in vitro (BHI broth)

Fungi	Tested No. of		% of strains with absence of growth	
	Species	Strains	0.1 $\mu g.ml^{-1}$	1 $\mu g.ml^{-1}$
Dermatophytes	25	750	94	99.6
Candida spp.	18	3869	78	98
Cr. neoformans	1	62	100	100
Torulopsis spp.	5	344	87	97
Pityrosporum spp.*	2	115	97	100
A. fumigatus	1	243	75	99.2
Asperg. spp. & Penicil. spp.	37	225	44	93
Sp. schenckii	1	34	100	100
Dimorphic fungi (MP+YP)	8	51	98	100
Phaeohyphomycetes	13	33	97	100
Eumycetoma agents	10	13	77	85
Fusarium spp.	11	36	3	8
Zygomycetes	13	30	10	23
Entomophthorales	2	3	33	100

* Test medium for P. ovale : Dixon broth

Table 2: Oral therapeutic treatment of superficial mycoses with itraconazole

Animals				Man				
Infection	mg.kg^{-1}	Days	Cure (%)	Infection (No. cases)	mg/day	Days	Cure (%)*	
Microsporosis (guinea-pig)	1.25	14	83	T. corporis/cruris (646)	100	15	clinical	88
" "	2.5	14	100				mycological	82
Trichophytosis (guinea-pig)	1.25	14	83	T. pedis/manus (197)	100	30	clinical	85
" "	2.5	14	100				mycological	79
Vaginal candidosis (rat)	2.5	3	91	Vaginal candidosis (211)	200	3	clinical	89
" "	2.5	2	83				mycological	84
" "	20	1	75	Vaginal candidosis (174)	200	2	clinical	82
" "	40	1	90				mycological	78
				Vaginal candidosis (146)	2x200	1	clinical	83
							mycological	81
Pityrosporosis (guinea-pig)	1.25	7	84	Pityriasis versicolor (351)	1000 mg total dose		clin. & myc.	80
" "	5	7	100					

* Two weeks after treatment for dermatophytosis and one month for candidosis and pityriasis versicolor

Table 3: Oral prophylaxis with itraconazole of systemic candidosis in guinea-pigs (groups of 10)

Oral treatment		Infection	No. of animals with					
mg.kg^{-1} b.i.d.	On days	CFU.g^{-1} B.W.	Skin folliculitis score				Negative cultures	
			o	+	++	+++	Skin	Kidneys
Excipient*	-3, -2, -1	1000		2	8		0	0
Itra 5	-1	1000	8	2			9	10
Itra 5	-2, -1	1000	10				8	10
Itra 5	-3, -2, -1	1000	10				9	9
Excipient	-3, -2, -1	2000		2	7	1	0	0
Itra 5	-1	2000	10				9	9
Itra 5	-2, -1	2000	10				10	7
Itra 5	-3, -2, -1	2000	10				10	10

* excipient: PEG200

Table 4: Treatment of candidosis in guinea-pigs and in man

Systemic candidosis in guinea-pigs								Candidosis in man treated with itraconazole					
Treatment for 14 days o.d.					Results (%)								
Drug*	mg.kg^{-1}	Route	Neutropenia	Start on day	Cured of folliculitis	Negative organs		Pathology	No.	Median		Global response rate (%)	Negative mycology (%)
						Skin	Kidneys			Daily dose (mg)	Treatment duration (days)		
Itra	2.5	oral	o	o	100	98	52	Invasive	21	400	48	35	30
Itra	5	oral	o	o	100	100	97	Non-invasive					
Fluco	2.5	oral	o	o	67	67	67	systemic	58	100	21	76	62
Fluco	5	oral	o	o	84	75	83	Oral/					
Itra	2.5	oral	+	o	100	100	67	oesophageal	14	200	79	86	57
Itra	5	oral	+	o	100	100	100	CMC	9	100	224	78	78
Itra	2.5	oral	o	+2	66	67	17	Cutaneous	4	175	69	100	100
Itra	5	oral	o	+2	83	83	50						
Itra	2.5	oral**	o	+2	100	100	83						
Itra	5	oral**	o	+2	100	100	100	Total	106				
Itra	2.5	IP	o	o	100	100	78						
Itra	5	IP	o	o	100	100	100						
Ampho B	2.5	IP	o	o	42	50	33						
Ampho B	5	IP	o	o	42	42	42						

* drug: itraconazole, fluconazole, amphotericin B
** oral: for 21 days

Table 5: Treatment of aspergillosis in guinea-pigs and in man

Systemic aspergillosis in guinea-pigs						
Treatment for 14 days o.d.					Results (%)	
Drug*	mg.kg^{-1}	Route	Neutropenia	Start on day	Survivors	Negative organs
Itra	2.5	oral	o	o	46	69
Itra	5	oral	o	o	83	94
Fluco	20	oral	o	o	0	3
Fluco	40	oral	o	o	33	17
Itra	2.5	oral	+	o	44	64
Itra	5	oral	+	o	93	93
Itra	2.5	oral	+	+1	33	23
Itra	5	oral	+	+1	83	92
Itra	2.5	IP	+	o	67	74
Itra	5	IP	+	o	83	94
Itra	2.5	IP	+	+1	67	76
Itra	5	IP	+	+1	83	96
Ampho B	2.5	IP	+	o	50	46
Ampho B	5	IP	+	o	83	72
Ampho B	2.5	IP	+	+1	33	43
Ampho B	5	IP	+	+1	50	69

Aspergillosis in man : median daily dose : 200 mg of itraconazole				
Aspergillosis	No.	Median treatment duration (days)	Global response rate (%)	Negative mycology (%)
Allergic	21	131	74	67
Aspergilloma	69	150	60	56
Pulmonary	72	104	62	76
Invasive pulmonary	63	97	54	74
Disseminated	14	60	46	25
Other types	12	40	83	90
Total	251			

* Drug: itraconazole, fluconazole, amphotericin B

Table 6: Therapeutic treatment of cryptococcosis in guinea-pigs and in man

Meningeal and disseminated cryptococcosis in guinea-pigs						
Treatment for 35 days o.d.				Results (%)		
Drug*	mg.kg^{-1}	Route	Neutropenia	Cure of skin cryptococcomas	Negative organs: Meningi	Negative organs: Others
Itra	5	oral	o	100	40	85
Itra	10	oral	o	95	55	96
Itra	5	oral	+	100	50	82
Itra	10	oral	+	100	33	95
Fluco	5	oral	o	50	13	86
Fluco	10	oral	o	88	0	84
Itra	10	IP	o	100	63	98
Fluco	10	IP	o	88	38	87
Itra+Fluco	5+5	oral/IP	o	100	50	99
Itra+Fluco	5+5	IP/oral	o	100	50	97

Cryptococcosis in man : oral treatment with itraconazole								
	International study (200 mg/day)				US study (400 mg/day)**			
Pathology	No.	Median treatment duration (days)	Global response (%)	Neg. mycology (%)	No.	Median treatment duration (days)	Global response (%)	Neg. mycology (%)
Meningitis	37	88	57	51	36	160-216***	86	64
Pulmonary	6	139	83	50	9	160	89	-
Others	4	349	75	50	-	-	-	-
Maintenance therapy	13	192	92	-	-	-	-	-

* Drug: itraconazole, fluconazole, amphotericin B
** Denning, Tucker, Hostetler, Gill, Stevens
*** Negative mycology in 160-216 days; partial response in 72-81 days

Table 7: Therapeutic treatment of meningeal and disseminated cryptococcosis in neutropenic guinea-pigs : combination therapy

Treatment for 35 days o.d.			Results (%)		
Drug	$mg.kg^{-1}$	Route	Cure of crypto-coccomas	Negative organs	
				Meninges	Others
Itra	5	oral	67	33	69
5FC	10	IP	0	0	25
5FC	40	IP	17	0	43
Itra+5FC	5/10	oral/IP	100	33	96
Itra+5FC	5/40	oral/IP	100	50	100
Ampho B	1.25	IP	33	0	44
Ampho B	2.5	IP	100	50	81
Itra+ampho B	5/1.25	oral/IP	100	33	88
Itra+ampho B	5/2.5	oral/IP	100	67	100

Table 8: Oral treatment of sporotrichosis in guinea-pigs and in man

Sporotrichosis in guinea-pigs (I.V. infection)					Sporotrichosis in man : median daily dose : 100 mg of itraconazole				
Treatment starts on day +3			Results %						
Drug*	$mg.kg^{-1}$	Duration	Cured	Improved	Pathology	No.	Median treatment duration (days)	Global response (%)	Negative mycology (%)
Itra	2.5	14	67	33	Cutaneous	32	100	100	93
Itra	5	14	83	17	Lymphatic	38	93	90	82
Itra	2.5	28	100	0	Disseminated	2	-	50	50
Fluco	5	28	0	17					
					Total	72			

* Drug: itraconazole, fluconazole

Table 9: Oral treatment of histoplasmosis in guinea-pigs and in man with itraconazole

Histoplasmosis in guinea-pigs (I. test)			Histoplasmosis: clinical studies in man				
Treatment for 14 days o.d. mg.kg-1	Results (%)		Parameters	Dismukes et al.*	Graybill, Stevens et al.*	Dupont et al.*	
	Cured	Improved				H. capsulatum	H. duboisii
10	63	37	No. of patients	31	26 (13 AIDS)	9 (2 AIDS)	3
40	100	-	Median treatment duration (days)	263 (151-557)	391 (35-829)	180 (30-300)	365 (180-600)
			Median dose (mg)	239 (100-400)	50-400	100-400	100-200
			Responders	97%	96%	89%	100%
			Relapse during therapy	3%	4% (AIDS)	11% (AIDS)	0%
			Relapse during follow up (months)	8% (14)	0% (28)	0 % (5)	0 % (11.5)**

* Unpublished results
** One patient still under therapy

Table 10: Oral treatment of human blastomycosis with itraconazole

Parameters	Dismukes et al.*	Graybill, Stevens et al.*
No. of patients	44	33
Median treatment duration (days)	183 (31-368)	222 (32-439)
Median dose (mg)	230 (100-400)	50-400
Responders	98%	100%
Relapse during therapy	2%	0%
Relapse during follow up (months)	0% (18)	11%

* Unpublished results

Table 11: Oral treatment of human chromomycosis with itraconazole

Fungi and No. of patients		Median		Global response	Negative mycology
		Daily dose (mg)	Treatment duration (days)	(%)	(%)
Fonsecaea pedrosoi	35	200	336	59	39
Cladosporium carrionii	10	100	73	89	70
Others*	13	200	180	70	46

* Others: Phialophora parasitica: 1; Ph. verrucosa: 1; Wangiella dermatitidis: 1; Fonsecaea and Cladosporium spp.: 10

Table 12: Oral treatment of various systemic mycoses in man with itraconazole

Fungi (mycosis) and No. of patients		Infection site	Median		Global result	
			Daily dose (mg)	Treatment duration (days)	Cured and improved	Failed
Pseudallescheria boydii	1	pulmonary	200-400	79	1	-
Dermatophytes	1	generalized	200	100	2	-
Trichosporon beigelii	1	generalized	200-400	7	-	1
Mucor sp.	1	generalized	100	545	1	-
Rhizopus sp.	1	pulmonary	200	86	1	-
Loboa loboi	3	subcutaneous	100-200	113	1	2
Fungal mycetoma	11	various	50-400 (200)	148	4	7
Actinomycotic mycetoma	1	foot	200	85	-	1
Prototheca sp.	1	bone, skin	200	52	1	-

PART IV

PROBLEMS IN THE TREATMENT OF FUNGAL INFECTIONS IN IMMUNOCOMPROMISED HOSTS

19

Historical Perspectives and State-of-the-Art Treatment of Systemic Mycoses Compared to Newer Problems in Management of Fungal Infections in Debilitated and Immunosuppressed Hosts

David A. Stevens, M.D.

Division of Infectious Diseases, Department of Medicine
Santa Clara Valley Medical Center
751 So. Bascom Avenue
San Jose, CA 95128 USA

Stanford University Medical School
Stanford, California

California Institute for Medical Research
San Jose, California

The breadth of my assigned topic permits me only an overview of the past (1), present and future of antifungal chemotherapy. Much of the State of the Art will be covered in more detail by other participants. The field of antifungal chemotherapy is presently rapidly moving. It began in 1903, with the successful use of KI in therapy of lymphocutaneous sporotrichosis. Then there was little progress for 50 years, when in 1951 Brown and Hazen introduced nystatin, the first of the useful polyenes. Four years later, amphotericin B was introduced, which is still the historical standard against which new systemic antifungals are commonly compared. Except for the development of flucytosine, which is still a useful drug for agents within its spectrum (essentially Candida, Cryptococcus and Torulopsis), there was little further progress until the early 1970's and the development of the azole drugs. Miconazole was the first useful drug in this series of broad-spectrum agents for systemic use(2). Although response rates with miconazole in deep mycoses such as coccidioidomycosis were satisfying, the need to give the drug intravenously and its short half life, requiring multiple administrations per day, made it logistically difficult to give long courses of therapy. The inability to eradicate or suppress residual disease undoubtedly contributed to the unsatisfactory relapse rate. Ketoconazole followed, and began the present era, which is characterized largely by the modification of azole drugs, bringing agents which can be given orally and have increasing potency, decreasing toxicity, and broader spectrum of activity (3).

The rapid expansion of our antifungal armamentarium is timely, because fungal infections are on the rise in the 1990's. This is related to the use of more powerful and broad spectrum antibacterials for prophylaxis and therapy, the increased use of prosthetics (from heart valves to joints), the increased use of invasive procedures and monitoring and of parenteral nutrition, more aggressive immunosuppression for a variety of conditions, more intensive chemotherapy of cancer and enhanced survival of patients in the immunosuppressed state, increased use of transplantation (parenchymal organs, bone marrow) as a means of therapy of organ dysfunction, the modern plague of AIDS, the rise in drug addiction, increased survival of premature infants in neonatal intensive care units, population growth in the U.S. "sunbelt" and in Latin America (zones for endemic mycoses) and increased travel and tourism to these areas.

Amphotericin B will continue to have an important role for many patients. Recent studies have examined ways to ameliorate its well-known toxicities, so as to utilize best its demonstrated efficacy. More rapid methods of infusion (e.g., for 1 hour) may decrease infusion-related side effects. However, in anuric patients, hyperkalemia may be associated with high drug concentrations, and as the patients cannot excrete the potassium load, ventricular fibrillation has been a problem (4). In these patients the drug can be given slowly, or during dialysis. Meperidine has been shown to decrease the frequency of shaking chills, but increases that of nausea and vomiting (5). Dantrolene may have a role in reducing infusion-related rigors (6). Salt repletion appears a possible method of reducing nephrotoxicity (7). The mechanism appears to involve tubuloglomerular feedback, where low sodium concentrations in the distal tubule results in vasoconstriction in the renal arterial vasculature. The source of the salt load in most studies has been concomitant ticarcillin; concurrent flucytosine may also have a role in reducing amphotericin nephrotoxicity.

A new approach to reducing amphotericin's toxicity has been complexing the drug with lipids or encasing it in liposomes (8). Liposomes are generally concentric bilayers (multilamellar) of lipid material with aqueous phase material between; however unilamellar vesicles are also included with this term. The interest generated related to the findings that lipid delivery systems for amphotericin are less toxic for mammalian cells, whereas activity against fungi is retained. However, some lipid formulations have been found less efficacious _in vitro_ than conventional amphotericin complexed with desoxycholate (so-called "free amphotericin"). Also of note is that *in vivo* lipid preparations are less toxic than conventional amphotericin. Moreover, much of the *in vivo* experimental toxicologic studies have been based on acute cardiotoxicity, and it is unclear how this lessened toxicity will relate to the usual amphotericin toxicities noted in man. The toxicology and pharmacokinetics of the lipid preparations reflect the types of lipid used, size of delivery vehicle, and surface charge. With most lipid preparations the pharmacokinetics of amphotericin is markedly altered, particularly in organ distribution. Generally, more is delivered to the liver and spleen, and less found in the kidney or serum, and distribution to the lung varies. The lower serum concentrations/dose administered with the lipid formulations may be compensated for by an ability to give more of the drug systemically by the latter method, and by increased tissue binding. The lower kidney concentrations could result in lowered amphotericin nephrotoxicity. With respect to the enhanced concentrations distributed to various organs, it is of concern that liposomes (and their amphotericin content) may not traverse capillaries. This may explain drug accumulation in the liver, where there are gaps between capillary cells. It is possible that liposomes may cross capillaries inside macrophages, as a result of phagocytosis by these cells, and that they may cross capillaries damaged by local disease. Of note, brain concentrations of lipid-complexed materials are greater than with free amphotericin and this may reflect passage through capillaries with damaged endothelium. However, it is not clear that increased amphotericin concentrations reported in some organs, detectable after extraction with lipophilic solvents, are truly available for therapy of local infection in those organs.

A likely mechanism for the decreased toxicity is binding of amphotericin to the lipids and delay in its transfer to the sites of its toxic actions. It is also possible that lipid complexing affects dispersion and orientation of the amphotericin molecules, and thus their relative affinity for fungal ergosterol versus mammalian cholesterol. A possible mechanism for its antifungal activity _in vivo_ is penetration of the lipid complex into phagocytes, and fusion of lysosomes containing degraded lipid material (with amphotericin) with parasitized phagosomes. Lipid-complexed amphotericin has been compared to conventional amphotericin in a variety of animal models. Almost without exception these studies have shown the conventional drug is more effective on a mg/kg basis (though this appears less so after chronic administration), but more lipid-complexed drug can be given. Some studies have thus concluded that more lipid complex preparation is more effective than less free amphotericin, but have not shown that doses used of the latter are the most they can give. (Moreover, most studies have compared intravenous lipid complex vs. intravenous free amphotericin, whereas intraperitoneal amphotericin in animals may more closely mimic pharmacokinetics after intravenous administration in man than does intravenous drug in animals, necessarily given by a rapid intravenous pulse.) Definite demonstration of lipid complexed drug superiority thus has generally required an effective dose that is greater than that which can be given as free drug in order to show a difference.

Flucytosine (9) is largely used at present to potentiate the activity of therapeutic regimens containing amphotericin. This has been most intensively exploited in the therapy of cryptococcosis. However, used alone for pathogens within its spectrum, it undoubtedly has the best record of success in treatment of infections of the urinary tract. This relates to its excretion in the active form in high concentrations. There has also been experience with it in therapy of neonatal candidosis, where demonstration of its lack of toxicity and efficacy and knowledge of its pharmacokinetics compares favorably with amphotericin and the imidazoles. There is much fear of its toxicity in patients with limited marrow reserve (e.g., AIDS patients), but frequent monitoring of serum levels would most likely make such fear ill-founded. However, our own studies have indicated nearly 20% of random C. albicans isolates in the US are resistant to it (10), and in vitro susceptibility has been shown by us to correlate with in vivo efficacy (in an animal model)(11).

Most current energies are related to the triazoles, which are replacing the imidazoles for reasons stated previously (3). The two most extensively studied drugs are itraconazole and fluconazole, though SCH 39304 appears very promising in early clinical trials, and superior to fluconazole in several animal models (12).

Itraconazole is a broad-spectrum antifungal whose largest advantages over the imidazoles are in its activity against cryptococcosis (13) and aspergillosis (14). It is highly lipophilic, penetrates well into tissues and accumulates in some key target tissue for fungal infections on chronic therapy. It has an active circulating hydroxylated metabolite (15). Absorption increases with food, and serum concentrations have been unpredictable. We have associated low serum concentrations with failure to respond in some opportunistic mycoses. Rifampin, phenytoin and carbamazepine all markedly depress its serum concentrations. The most efficacy data in the deep mycoses with triazoles have been accumulated with this drug. In addition to the endemic mycoses (e.g., coccidioidomycosis), over 75% of patients reported in the literature with invasive aspergillosis have responded (14). In 36 evaluable cryptococcal meningitis patients with AIDS, 23 (64%) achieved a complete response (complete resolution of all signs and symptoms, and negative cultures), 8 (22%) a partial response (symptomatic response without CSF sterilization), and 5 (14%) failed (13). Patients who failed prior therapy did as well. Sterilization of cultures was also seen in cryptococcemia (89%), cryptococcuria (40%), and pulmonary disease (89%). The median time to CSF sterilization was <30 days, which is slower than with amphotericin. That disease was largely suppressed but not cured is reflected in a 42% recrudescence rate on therapy. Our patients' survival at 8 weeks (77%) was equal to or better than that reported in AIDS with amphotericin with or without flucytosine, and the minimum mean survival of 12.1 months from the diagnosis of AIDS exceeded that in all previously published cryptococcosis series.

Fluconazole has low protein binding, appears in CSF and urine in the active form in high concentrations, and penetrates key tissues. Its in vitro activity is unimpressive compared to its activity in animal models. It has been shown to be efficacious in various forms of superficial candidosis and in coccidioidal meningitis (16). Ongoing dose escalating studies suggest the optimal dose for treating deep mycoses may not yet have been thoroughly studied. Results in cryptococcal meningitis very similar to ours with itraconazole have been attained in France by Bertrand Dupont and colleagues, and early American data appears similar or not as good (17). Late recrudescences in patients on therapy, and slower CSF sterilization than with amphotericin, are also a problem. We have shown that fluconazole maintenance therapy can completely prevent thrush in AIDS patients with recurrent thrush, in a randomized, double blind, placebo-controlled study, and possibly all deep and superficial mycoses (18).

Despite our increased weapons, we are faced with many therapeutic problems in compromised and debilitated hosts. We will have to do better diagnostically. Too often fungal infection is not considered in the differential diagnosis of the febrile compromised host, and appropriate diagnostic tests not utilized (19). Since a tissue diagnosis is often impossible because invasive techniques cannot be used in these precarious patients, we need improved rapid methods for diagnosis, detecting fungal antigen or antibody in body fluids with tests that will distinguish patients with disease and those with colonization.

Our literature is a confounding map in attempting to define our future directions. Patient disease is poorly characterized, and terminology of outcome is lax. Uniform scoring systems would alleviate many problems (20). More randomized studies are needed (21,22).

In vitro susceptibility testing will need to be standardized, and correlations made with in vivo results (23).

Our results in deep candida infections presently are difficult to interpret and there are too many failures. We have no good regimens for the zygomycoses, and the new azoles seem to offer nothing. As the best results have been achieved with aggressive surgical debridement plus local and systemic amphotericin therapy, perhaps the new amphotericin delivery systems may hold some promise. Aspergillus infections are also an area where therapeutic results are poor (8), though clinical results with itraconazole (14), animal model data in aspergillosis with lipid-amphotericin delivery systems (24) and results with saperconazole (25) hold promise for the future. Measures that appear useful in therapy of aspergillosis are valve replacement in endocarditis, local chemotherapy in ocular, pleural or renal disease, and surgical excision in disease of bone, burn wounds, and the vitreous, in epidural abscesses and in recurrent significant hemoptysis in aspergillomas, and removal of catheters for peritonitis and of silk sutures in bronchial stump (post-pneumonectomy) aspergillosis. Rifampin almost always, and flucytosine sometimes, will potentiate the activity of amphotericin in vitro against aspergilli, and if synergy can be demonstrated in vitro, combination therapy appears a logical avenue to explore. Fusarium infections, common in keratomycosis, and now also being reported more frequently in systemic infections in compromised hosts, are generally resistant to presently available drugs.

A whole area as yet neglected in our current approach to fungal diseases is the host response to infection. Responses may be defective due to pre-existing immune impairment, or anergy may occur in normal hosts in the course of progressive disease. It is in the area of immunomodulating therapy that we may find new concepts for clinical applications. Many years of work on host defenses against infection have illustrated the central role of cell-mediated immunity in determining outcome in deep mycotic infection. Therefore, possible future targets for our therapy are the T cells and phagocytes (and their interactions) (26) that are critical in immunity.

An unanswered clinical question (one that can be generally applied to all antimicrobial therapy) is when to stop therapy in a patient apparently responding to treatment. Answers to such questions should properly come from the kind of clinical trials to which I previously referred.

Although development of resistance to antifungal therapy has fortunately been rare, we must be vigilant about this possibility with increasing polyenes and azoles use.

Even better than more efficacious treatment of fungal infection in the compromised host would be prevention. Azoles offer the greatest promise in this area, and examples in AIDS and neutropenic patients have already been reported.

In the development of new agents, there are several possible avenues of attack on fungi (that will also be sparing of the host). These include the cell wall, the membrane (interrupting the many steps in sterol synthesis with fungal enzyme-specific agents or agents active against pre-formed sites, which have specificity for fungal vs. mammalian membranes), metabolic inhibition, nuclear function, and nucleic acid synthesis, assembly and function.

We are working toward the ideal agent, which would have these properties: broad spectrum, fungicidal, no development of resistance during therapy, available for oral and intravenous administration, penetrate key target tissues and fluids, have no drug interactions or toxicity, and have a low cost.

References

1. D.A. Stevens. Drugs for systemic fungal infections. Rational Drug Therapy (Amer. Soc. for Pharmacology and Experimental Therapeutics, ed.), W.B. Saunders Co., Philadelphia, (1979).
2. D.A. Stevens. An update on miconazole therapy for coccidioidomycosis. Drugs 26:347 (1983).
3. D.A. Stevens. The new generation of antifungal drugs. Eur. J. Clin. Micro. 7:732 (1988).
4. P.C. Craven and D.H. Gremillion. Risk factors of ventricular fibrillation during rapid amphotericin B infusion. Antimicrob. Agents Chemother. 27:868 (1985).
5. L.C. Burks, J. Aisner, C.L. Forner, and P.H. Wiernik. Meperidine for the treatment of shaking chills and fever. Arch. Intern. Med. 140:483 (1980).
6. M.H. Gross, W.J. Fulkerson, and J.O. Moore. Prevention of amphotericin B-induced rigors by dantrolene. Arch. Intern. Med. 146:1587 (1986).
7. R.A. Branch. Prevention of amphotericin B-induced renal impairment. Arch. Intern. Med. 148:2389 (1988).
8. D.W. Denning and D.A. Stevens. The treatment of invasive aspergillosis. Rev. Infect. Dis., in press.
9. H.J. Scholer. Flucytosine. Antifungal Chemotherapy (D.C.E. Spiller, ed.), John Wiley, Toronto, p.35 (1980).
10. R.L. Stiller, J.E. Bennett, H.J. Scholer, M. Wall, A. Polak, and D.A. Stevens. Susceptibility to 5-fluorocytosine and prevalence of serotype in 402 Candida albicans isolates from the United States. Antimicrob. Agents Chemother. 22:482 (1982).
11. R.L. Stiller, J.E. Bennett, H.J. Scholer, M. Wall, A. Polak, and D.A. Stevens. Correlation of in vitro susceptibility test results with in vivo response: flucytosine therapy in a systemic candidosis model. J. Infect. Dis. 147:1070 (1983).
12. K.V. Clemons, L.H. Hanson, A.M. Perlman, and D.A. Stevens. Efficacy of SCH 39304 and fluconazole in a murine model of disseminated coccidioidomycosis. Antimicrob. Agents Chemother. 34:928 (1990).
13. D.W. Denning, R.M. Tucker, J.S. Hostetler, S. Gill, and D.A. Stevens. Itraconazole therapy of cryptococcal meningitis and cryptococcosis in patients with AIDS. Mycoses in AIDS patients (H. Vanden Bossche, D.W.R. Mackenzie, G. Cauwenbergh, E. Drouhet, B. Dupont, J. Van Cutsem, eds.), Plenum Press, in press.

14. D.W. Denning, R.M. Tucker, L.H. Hanson, and D.A. Stevens. Treatment of invasive aspergillosis with itraconazole. Amer. J. Med. 86:791 (1989).
15. J. Heykants, A. Van Peer, V. Van de Velde, P. Van Rooy, W. Meuldermans, K. Lavrijsen, R. Woestenborghs, J. Van Cutsem, and G. Cauwenbergh. The clinical pharmacokinetics of itraconazole: an overview. Mycoses 32 (Suppl. 1): 67 (1989).
16. R.M. Tucker, J.N. Galgiani, D.W. Denning, L.H. Hanson, J.R. Graybill, K. Sharkey, M.R. Eckman, C. Salemi, and D.A. Stevens. Treatment of coccidioidal meningitis with fluconazole. Rev. Infect. Dis. 12:S380 (1990).
17. D.A. Stevens. Fungal infections in AIDS patients. Brit J. Clin. Pract., in press.
18. O.S. Lang, S.I. Greene, and D.A. Stevens. Thrush can be prevented in AIDS/ARC patients: randomized double-blind placebo-controlled study of 100 mg fluconazole daily. 6th International Conference on AIDS, Abstracts, no. 2163, 2165
19. S.C. Deresinski and D.A. Stevens. Coccidioidomycosis in compromised hosts. Medicine 54:377 (1975).
20. W.E. Dismukes, J.E. Bennett, D.J. Drutz, J.R. Graybill, J.S. Remington, and D.A. Stevens. Criteria for evaluating therapeutic response to antifungal drugs. Rev. Infect. Dis. 2:535 (1980).
21. W.E. Dismukes, G. Cloud, H.A. Gallis, T.M. Kerkering, G. Medoff, P.C. Craven, L.G. Kaplowitz, J.F. Fisher, C.R. Gregg, C.A. Bowles, S. Shadomy, A.M. Stamm, R.B. Diasio, L. Kaufman, S-J. Soong, W.C. Blackwelder and the NIAID Mycoses Study Group. Treatment of cryptococcal meningitis with combination amphotericin B and flucytosine for four as compared with six weeks. New Eng. J. Med. 317:334 (1987).
22. J.N. Galgiani, D.A. Stevens, J.R. Graybill, W.E. Dismukes, and G.A. Cloud. Ketoconazole therapy of progressive coccidioidomycosis. Comparison of 400 and 800 mg doses, and observations at higher doses. Amer. J. Med. 84:603 (1988).
23. D.A. Stevens. Antifungal drug susceptibility testing. Mycopathol. 87:135 (1984).
24. T.F. Patterson, P. Miniter, J. Dijkstra, F.C. Szoka, J.L. Ryan and V.T. Andriole. Treatment of experimental invasive aspergillosis with novel amphotericin B/cholesterol-sulfate complexes. J. Infect. Dis 159:717 (1989).
25. D.W. Denning, L.H. Hanson, and D.A. Stevens. In vitro activity of saperconazole against aspergillus species compared with amphotericin B and itraconazole. Eur. J. Clin. Micro. Inf. Dis., in press.
26. D.A. Stevens. Interferon gamma and fungal infections. The Anti-Infective Applications of Interferon-Gamma (H.S. Jaffe, S.A. Sherwin, eds.), Marcel Dekker, in press.

20

Treatment of Systemic Fungal Diseases in Patients with AIDS

William E. Dismukes, M.D.*

Division of Infectious Diseases
Department of Medicine
University of Alabama at Birmingham School of Medicine
Birmingham, Alabama, U.S.A., 35294

Systemic mycoses are increasingly encountered opportunistic infectious diseases in HIV infected persons, and, in many patients, may be the initial AIDS defining illness. Among the systemic fungal diseases, cryptococcosis is the most common, occurring in 6-10% of AIDS patients(1,2). Histoplasmosis and coccidioidomycosis are the next most common; blastomycosis, sporotrichosis, and invasive or disseminated candidiasis and aspergillosis occur less frequently. The immunologic hallmark of AIDS is a reduction in the T-helper lymphocyte cell population, resulting in a virtual elimination of cell-mediated host defenses. Thus, it is not surprising that AIDS patients should fall prey to fungi which require a functional lymphocyte/macrophage system for containment and eradication. Because of the relentless decline

*Supported in part by U.S. Public Health Service contract NO1 A1 52562 with Microbiology and Infectious Diseases Program, National Institute of Allergy and Infectious Diseases.

in T-cell function over time in these patients, persistent or progressive disease while on antifungal therapy or relapse shortly after discontinuation of therapy is the rule. The therapy of cryptococcosis, compared with other mycoses, has been more thoroughly evaluated; hence, the primary focus of discussion here will be on this disease. The therapy of histoplasmosis, coccidioidomycosis, and blastomycosis will be only briefly addressed.

CRYPTOCOCCOSIS

The findings of two retrospective analyses of therapy of cryptococcosis, primarily cryptoccocal meningitis (CM), in AIDS patients indicated poorer outcomes compared with cure rates of 60 to 75 percent in non-AIDS patients(3). In 1985, Kovacs and colleagues reported treatment results in 24 patients with AIDS and first-episode cryptococcosis, including 18 with CM(4). This small group of patients received either amphotericin B (AMB) alone or AMB plus flucytosine. Success as defined by survival for four weeks after discontinuation of therapy, absence of symptoms, and negative cerebrospinal fluid (CSF) cultures was observed in only 10 patients (42%). Four of these 10 relapsed within six months of stopping therapy. There was no difference in outcomes by treatment regimen. In 1986, Zuger et al reported similarly poor outcomes.(5)

In 1989, investigators in San Francisco summarized their six-year experience with 106 patients with cryptococcosis and AIDS(2). Among 40 CM patients treated with AMB, the survival rate was 52%, compared with a survival rate of 37% among 49 CM patients who received both AMB and flucytosine. Flucytosine was discontinued prematurely in over half the patients because of cytopenia. However, in these patients no standardized approach to flucytosine therapy was used, and flucytosine serum levels were not monitored. These investigators also assessed the efficacy of long-term suppressive therapy in those patients who survived the primary episode. Among the 63 survivors, 37 received some form of suppressive treatment. Survival in the 22 patients who received ketoconazole (median, 238 days) or the 15 who received AMB (median, 280 days) was significantly longer than in the patients who did not receive any suppressive regimen (median, 141 days; $p < 0.004$), leading the authors to conclude that suppressive therapy is beneficial.

The development of new triazoles, such as fluconazole (FLU) and SCH 39304, with favorable pharmacologic properties including good to excellent penetration into CSF(1,6), has prompted several clinical trials with these antifungal agents in AIDS patients with CM. Itraconazole, another investigational triazole, also shows promise on the basis of results in in vivo animal models of cryptococcosis, although measurable concentrations in CSF are less than 10 percent of serum concentrations(7). To date, most trials have utilized FLU, which is available as either an oral or intravenous formulation.

Studies of FLU as primary therapy of CM in patients with AIDS have provided somewhat conflicting results. Larsen et al conducted a small prospective comparison of oral FLU (400 mg p.o. daily for 10 weeks) versus combination AMB (0.7 mg/kg/d x 1 wk, then 3 times/week x 9 weeks) and flucytosine (150 mg/kg/d x 10 weeks)(8). Among 14 patients randomized to FLU, 8 failed (57%); by contrast, none of the 6 assigned to combination therapy failed ($p = 0.04$). In addition, 4 of the 8 FLU failures died, whereas none of the AMB/flucytosine treated patients died. These findings in this small clinical trial led the authors to conclude that combination therapy has superior mycologic and clinical efficacy over FLU in AIDS patients with acute CM. Pietroski and coworkers, using a regimen of initial intravenous FLU followed by oral FLU, noted a failure rate of 62% (8 of 13 patients) (9), whereas Squires et al, using an all oral FLU regimen for 10 weeks reported a failure rate of only 30% (5 of 17) (10). Itraconazole has also been evaluated in AIDS patients with CM(7). Among 18 patients who received itraconazole as primary therapy in a small uncontrolled study, 10 failed (55%). Three of these initially responded to itraconazole, but had a recrudescence of disease while on therapy. One other failure relapsed after itraconazole was stopped.

The only large prospective randomized clinical trial to evaluate efficacy of primary therapy in CM in AIDS was conducted by the National Institute of Allergy and Infectious Diseases (NIAID) Mycoses Study Group and the AIDS Clinical Trials Group, together with a group of independent investigators(11). Eligible patients were assigned to either FLU, 200 mg p.o. daily, or AMB, minimum dose 0.3 mg/kg/d, with or without flucytosine. Among 194 evaluable patients, 131 received FLU, and 63 received AMB (the majority of patients in this regimen did not receive concomitant flucytosine). Preliminary analysis indicates that the failure rates in the two treatment groups were similar, FLU (66%) and AMB (60%), $p = 0.40$. Other analyses are also of interest. First, among AMB treated patients, there was no difference in the median total dose of AMB in the two outcome categories: cured/improved versus failure. Second, among patients who died during therapy, there were more deaths within the initial two weeks of therapy in the FLU treated patients (19 of 131) than in the AMB treated patients, (5 of 63) $p = 0.25$. Finally, the median time to conversion of CSF culture from positive to negative was shorter in cured or improved patients receiving the AMB regimen, 16 days versus 30 days, p = 0.02. Larsen and colleagues also observed that AMB plus flucytosine sterilized the CSF more rapidly than FLU(8).

Because of the high rate of relapse of CM in AIDS patients after primary therapy is stopped, investigators have sought to determine the optimum regimen for chronic, life-time maintenance or suppressive therapy. Results of two earlier noncontrolled studies suggested moderate efficacy of long-term oral FLU once the CSF had been sterilized by primary therapy, usually with AMB, with or without flucytosine(12,13). At least two prospective randomized clinical trials have been recently conducted to further evaluate suppressive therapy. The first, performed by the California Collaborative Treatment Group, compared FLU, 100 or 200 mg p.o. daily, to placebo(14). Among 36 FLU treated patients, there was one relapse (urinary); in contrast, among 27 placebo recipients, there were 10 relapses (4 CNS and 6 urinary), p = 0.0005. Based on the superior efficacy of FLU, the trial was terminated after 36 months by an independent data safety and monitoring board. The suppressive efficacy of FLU has been confirmed by the findings of a second larger trial, performed by the NIAID Mycoses Study Group, the NIAID Clinical Trials Group, and a group of independent investigators(15). Two suppressive regimens were compared: FLU, 200 mg p.o. daily, and AMB, 1 mg/kg/week. One-hundred eighty-nine patients met eligibility criteria for enrollment; 78 (41%) received AMB and 111 (59%) received FLU. Patients were classified as failures if they relapsed on therapy or study drug was discontinued because of a toxic event. The failure rate was significantly higher among those who received AMB, 26 of 78 (33%), versus FLU, 9 of 111 (8%), p = 0.00001. Because of the marked differences in efficacy of the two treatment regimens, this study was also halted by an independent data safety and monitoring board.

Based on the results of the multiple studies cited above, several conclusions can be drawn about the therapy of cryptococcosis, especially CM, in patients with AIDS. First, primary therapy, regardless of the regimen, is ineffective in about half of the patients. Second, antifungal azoles, such as FLU and itraconazole, while better tolerated than AMB and flucytosine, appear to be less effective in rapidly sterilizing CSF and in reversing disease in patients with severe neurologic impairment at time of initiation of therapy (data not shown). Third, chronic suppressive therapy, especially FLU, is effective in preventing relapse.

HISTOPLASMOSIS

Histoplasmosis in AIDS, like cryptococcosis, is moderately to highly refractory to therapy(16,17). Disseminated histoplasmosis (DH), involving multiple organs such as lungs, liver, spleen, bone marrow, lymph nodes, skin, gastrointestinal tract, and CNS, is the most common form of disease in HIV infected persons. Information about outcomes by treatment regimen has, for the most part, been based on retrospective analyses(18,19,20). To date, the three antifungal drugs which have been most utilized in DH in AIDS patients are AMB, ketoconazole, and itraconazole. Data from early in the AIDS epidemic indicated that the mortality rate during primary therapy was high, in the 40 to 50% range, and relapses were frequent, even in patients on some form of suppressive therapy. Ketoconazole alone, as either primary or suppressive therapy, was ineffective(17,20).

One potential explanation relates to reduced absorption of ketoconazole in patients with AIDS, largely as a result of gastric hypochlorhydria. Other problems with ketoconazole include its association with significant gastrointestinal intolerance, such as nausea and vomiting, symptoms already common in AIDS patients, and its potential at high doses to suppress steroid synthesis by the adrenal glands, with resulting adrenal insufficiency.

Amphotericin B is currently regarded as the most effective primary therapy of histoplasmosis in AIDS. Wheat and coworkers have noted an 80 percent response rate in 81 episodes of DH in 69 patients (L.J. Wheat, unpublished observation). While other earlier and smaller series have documented only moderate efficacy of AMB as primary therapy, especially when total doses >2.0 gm were employed(18,19,20), recent data confirm the encouraging results observed by Wheat et al. In an open pilot study, McKinsey and coworkers evaluated 22 AIDS patients with DH and employed two different AMB regimens(21). Only 16 of the 22 patients were evaluable for efficacy. Treatment group one consisted of 7 patients who received an initial intensive course of AMB, 1000 mg total dose, followed by weekly doses of 50-80 mg until a cumulative dose of 2.0 gm was reached; thereafter, 50-80 mg was given biweekly. Treatment group two consisted of 9 patients who received AMB, 2000 mg total dose, followed by long-term AMB, 80 mg weekly. Both regimens were effective in preventing relapse over a median period of follow-up of 14 months. Biweekly maintenance AMB was as effective as weekly maintenance AMB. Sixty-three percent of patients developed infection or other intravascular device-related complications, emphasizing the hazard of long-term vascular access which is necessary for the administration of AMB.

The NIAID Mycoses Study Group and the AIDS Clinical Trials Group are currently evaluating itraconazole as suppressive therapy in a pilot study of AIDS patients with DH. All patients receive itraconazole, 400 mg daily. Over 40 patients have been enrolled. Thus far, itraconzole has been well tolerated; it is also well absorbed in these patients. Although complete data on outcomes are not yet available, no relapses have been observed. Soon, the NIAID AIDS Clinical Trials Group will begin a second study to evaluate itraconazole as both primary and suppressive therapy. Until the results of these two studies with itraconazole are available, AMB should remain the drug of choice for AIDS patients with DH. An AMB regimen similar to the regimens described by McKinsey et al(21), is advocated.

COCCIDIOIDOMYCOSIS

Although considerably less common than cryptococcosis and histoplasmosis in HIV infected persons, coccidioidomycosis is being recognized with increased frequency, especially among individuals living in the coccidioidal endemic area(16,22). Coccidioidomycosis in the HIV population is associated with a wide range of manifestations, including both focal and diffuse pulmomary disease, extrathoracic lymph node or liver involvement, meningitis, brain abscess, peritonitis, and cutaneous disease. The treatment of coccidioidomycosis in AIDS patients has been generally unsatisfactory. As with most other fungal diseases in these patients, therapy is rarely curative, and relapse is common if treatment is discontinued.

Fish and coworkers have summarized the largest experience yet reported(22). Among 77 AIDS patients with coccidioidomycosis, 32 (42%) died. Diffuse pulmonary disease and low CD4 lymphocyte counts were predictors of death, $p < 0.001$ and $p < 0.01$, respectively. Ninety-nine courses of therapy were given to 68 of the 77 patients; 9 patients received no treatment. The treatments included 53 courses of AMB, 34 courses of ketoconazole, and 10 courses of FLU (including 5 to patients with coccidioidal meningitis). There were no differences in efficacy among the different antifungal drugs. Importantly, 3 patients developed coccidioidomycosis while receiving ketoconazole for other conditions.

To date, the optimum therapy of coccidioidomycosis in AIDS patients remains undefined in regard to specific antifungal drug, dose, or length of therapy. Extrapolation from the experiences in cryptococcosis and histoplasmosis suggests that some form of chronic maintenance therapy should be given indefinitely. Fluconazole may prove useful, especially in patients with meningitis(6).

BLASTOMYCOSIS

Among the so-called endemic mycoses, including blastomycosis, histoplasmosis, and coccidioidomycosis, blastomycosis occurs least commonly in HIV-infected persons(16). In a recent survey of 23 U.S. medical centers, only 12 cases of blastomycosis in AIDS were identified(23). The 12 cases were severely immunocompromised as evidenced by CD4 counts $< 200/mm^3$ at time of diagnosis and prior AIDS defining conditions in 11 of the 12. The most common site of blastomycotic involvement was lung (10 patients); 4 had CNS disease. No standardized treatment regimen was employed. Nine patients received AMB, median dose 1.0 gm; 1 patient received ketoconazole, and 2 patients were not treated. The outcomes were unsatisfactory. Six patients died secondary to active blastomycosis, including one patient who had received 3.0 gm AMB. Five of the deaths occurred within 21 days of diagnosis. Four patients died of unrelated causes. Two patients are alive and receiving AMB maintenance therapy. As with coccidioidomycosis, the optimum treatment regimen for blastomycosis in AIDS remains undefined. Amphotericin B should probably be used as primary therapy in all patients; FLU and itraconazole are promising agents for chronic maintenance therapy.

REFERENCES

1. Dismukes WE. Cryptococcal meningitis in patients with AIDS. J Inf Dis 1988; 157:624-628.
2. Chuck SL, Sande MA. Infections with Cryptococcus neoformans in the acquired immunodeficiency syndrome. N Engl J Med 1989; 321:794-799.
3. Dismukes WE, Cloud G, Gallis HA, et al. Treatment of cryptococcal meningitis with combination amphotericin B and flucytosine for four as compared with six weeks. N Engl J Med 1987:; 317:344-341.
4. Kovacs JA, Kovacs AA, Polis M, et al. Cryptococcosis in the acquired immunodeficiency syndrome. Ann Intern Med 1985; 103:533-538.
5. Zuger A, Louie E, Holzman RS, et al. Cryptococcal disease in patients with the acquired immunodeficiency syndrome. Ann Intern Med 1986; 104:234-240.
6. Galgiani JN. Fluconazole, a new antifungal agent. Ann Int Med 1990; 113:177-179.
7. Denning DW,Tucker RM, Hanson LH, et al. Itraconazole therapy for cryptococcal meningitis and cryptococcosis. Arch Intern Med 1989; 149:2301-2308.
8. Larsen RA, Leal MAE, Chan LS. Fluconazole compared with amphotericin B plus flucytosine for crypto-

coccal meningitis in AIDS. Ann Intern Med 1990; 113:183-187.

9. Pietroski N, Buckley RM, Braffman MN, Stern JJ. Intravenous and oral fluconazole in treatment of acute cryptococcal meningitis in AIDS. In: Program and Abstracts, 30th Interscience Conference on Antimicrobial Agents and Chemotherapy, 1990, #576.

10. Squires K, Rowland V, Gassyuk E, et al. Fluconazole as therapy for acute cryptococcal meningitis. In: Program and Abstracts, 30th Interscience Conference on Antimicrobial Agents and Chemotherapy, 1990, # 573.

11. Dismukes W, Cloud G, Thompson S, et al. Fluconazole versus amphotericin B therapy of acute cryptococcal meningitis. In: Program and Abstracts, 29th Interscience Conference on Antimicrobial Agents and Chemotherapy, 1989, # 1065.

12. Stern JJ, Hartman BJ, Sharkey P, et al. Oral fluconazole therapy for patients with acquired immunodeficiency syndrome and cryptococcosis: experience with 22 patients. Am J Med 1988; 85:477-480.

13. Sugar AM, Saunders C. Oral fluconazole as suppressive therapy of disseminated cryptococcosis in patients with acquired immunodeficiency syndrome. Am J Med 1988; 85:481-489.

14. Bozzette SA, Larsen R, Chiu J, et al. Successful secondary prophylaxis of cryptococcal meningitis with fluconazole: a placebo-controlled trial. In: Program and Abstracts, 30th Interscience Conference on Antimicrobial Agents and Chemotherapy, 1990, # 1161.

15. Powderly W, Saag M, Cloud G, et al. Fluconazole versus amphotericin B as maintenance therapy for

prevention of relapse of AIDS-associated cryptococcal meningitis. In: Program and Abstracts, 30th Interscience Conference on Antimicrobial Agents and Chemotherapy, 1990, # 1162.

16. Threlkeld MG, Dismukes WE. Endemic mycoses. In: Leoung G, Mills J, eds. Opportunistic Infections in Patients with the Acquired Immunodeficiency Syndrome. New York: Marcel Dekker, Inc, 1989:285-314.

17. Graybill JR. Histoplasmosis and AIDS. J Inf Dis 1988; 158:623-626.

18. Bonner JR, Alexander WJ, Dismukes WE, et al. Disseminated histoplasmosis in patients with the acquired immune deficiency syndrome. Arch Intern Med 1984; 144:2178-2181.

19. Mandell W, Goldberg DM, Neu HC. Histoplasmosis in patients with the acquired immune deficiency syndrome. Am J Med 1986; 81:974-978.

20. Johnson PC, Hamill RJ, Sarosi GA. Clinical review: progressive disseminated histoplasmosis in the AIDS patient. Sem Resp Inf 1989; 4:139-146.

21. McKinsey DS, Gupta MR, Riddler SA, et al. Long-term amphotericin B therapy for disseminated histoplasmosis in patients with the acquired immunodeficiency syndrome (AIDS). Ann Inter Med 1989; 111:655-659.

22. Fish DG, Ampel NM, Galgiani JN, et al. Coccidioidomycosis during human immunodeficiency virus infection: a review of 77 patients. Med (Baltimore) 1990:In press.

23. Pappas PG, Pottage JC, Tapper ML, et al. Blastomycosis in AIDS patients. In: Program and Abstracts, 30th Interscience Conference on Antimicrobial Agents and Chemotherapy, 1990, # 1166.

21

Problems in the Treatment of Fungal Infections After Renal Transplantation in Japan

S. Oka, H. Sugimoto, and K. Shimada

Institute of Medical Science, University of Tokyo
4-6-1, Shirokanedai, Minato-ku, Tokyo, 108, Japan

I. INTRODUCTION

In Japan, renal transplantations were performed on 4,736 cases from 1970 through 1987, 735 of whom (15.5%) have died so far. Among them, 396 cases (53.8%) died of bacterial, viral, and fungal infections. Cyclosporine, which raised the survival rate of patients after renal transplantation remarkably, has been available

Grant Support: In part by the Ministry of Education, Science, and Culture and by the Ministry of Health and Welfare of Japan.

in Japan since 1984. However, the incidence of death by infection per total deaths remained 37.5 % during this period. This fact indicates that infections are still the major factors which limit the prognosis of a recipient as well as the graft survival.

There are various problems in infections in renal transplant patients (1). First, they are receiving immunosuppressive therapy. Second, in some cases, it is difficult to discriminate the infection from the rejection of the graft (i.e., psuedo-rejection). For instance, urinary tract infection elevates the level of serum creatinine. Finally, when we start therapy for infection, we have to consider the interactions between antimicrobial drugs and cyclosporine (2). Among opportunistic infections, fungi are one of the major pathogenic agents (1). Therefore, it is very important to investigate fungal infections in renal transplant patients. In this study, clinical features of fungal infections in renal transplant patients in the Hospital of the Institute of Medical Science, the University of Tokyo were reviewed.

II. MATERIALS AND METHODS

A. *PATIENTS*

Two hundred and sixty cases of renal transplantations were performed in our hospital from 1970 through 1990. Among them, 18 cases (6.9 %) of fungal infections were observed and were studied retrospectively. The patients, 14 men and 4 women, ranged in age from 22 to 43 years, with a mean of 32 years. To make characteristics of the infections in renal transplantion clear, 17 consecutive cases of AIDS were also studied.

B. *THE CRITERIA FOR DIAGNOSIS OF FUNGAL INFECTIONS*

The criteria for a diagnosis of candida infection are as follows; 1. Candida is repeatedly isolated from the clinical specimens obtained from the infectious focus. 2. The patient has a clinical focus associated with the symptoms. 3. Candida antigen in serum is positive. 4. Infections by other pathogenic agents are excluded. If a case met three of these, it was diagnosed as a candida infection.

In case of cryptococcal, aspergillus, and mucor infections, we diagnosed each infection if the fungus was isolated.

C. *SEROLOGICAL TESTS*

CANDI-TEC (Ramco Lab. Inc., Houston, TX, USA) and CRYPTO-LA TEST (International Biological Lab. Inc., Crambury, NJ, USA) were used for both the diagnosis and the clinical marker to evaluate drug effects according to the manufacturer's instructions.

III. RESULTS AND DISCUSSION

A. *INCIDENCE OF OPPORTUNISTIC INFECTIONS*

The incidences of opportunistic infections in renal transplant patients from 1981 to 1987 are presented in Table 1. There were 135 cases of renal transplantations during this period. Among these, 94 cases received the conventional immunosuppressive therapy consisting of steroid and azathioprine, and 41 cases received the combination immunosuppressive therapy in which cyclosporine was added to the conventional therapy. Cyclosporine has improved the graft survival.

Table 1

Incidences of Opportunistic Infections from 1981 to 1987 in Hospital of Inst. Med. Sci., Univ. Tokyo

	C.I. (%)	CYA (%)
No.of patients	94	41
Pneumocystis carinii	9 (9.6%)	5 (11.9%)
Virus	7 (7.4%)	17 (40.5%)
Bacteria	16 (17.0%)	6 (14.3%)
Fungus	**7 (7.4%)**	**3 (7.1%)**

C.I. : Patients treated with conventional immunotherapy consisting of steroid and azathioprine.
CYA : Patients treated with combination immunotherapy consisting of cyclosporine, steroid, and azathioprine.

However, it has not affected the incidence of opportunistic infections. Particularly, the incidence of fungal infections has not been affected at all.

B. *FUNGAL INFECTIONS IN RENAL TRANSPLANT OR AIDS PATIENTS*

Table 2 shows the number of fungal infections occurring in renal transplant or AIDS patients. Nine of 18 cases with fungal infections observed in renal transplant patients had candida infections, six cryptococcal, one aspergillus, and two mucor infections. In contrast, of 17 AIDS cases, all had candida infections, one cryptococcal, and one aspergillus infection. This result suggests that patients in the renal transplant group had more diverse fungal infections than those in the AIDS group. Infections by histoplasma, blastomyces, and coccidioides were not found; the distribution of these fungi is limited geographically.

Table 2

Fungal Infections in Renal Transplant or AIDS Patients

	Renal Trans.*1)	AIDS *2)
Candida	9	17
Cryptococcus	6	1
Aspergillus	1	1
Mucor	2	0

*1) : 18 cases of renal transplantation
*2) : 17 cases of AIDS

Table 3 shows kinds of candida infections occurring in the two groups. In the renal transplant group, candida caused five kinds of infections: two oropharyngeal candidiasis, three pneumonia, three sepsis, two meningitis, and one urinary tract infection. In contrast, in the AIDS group, candida caused only oropharyngeal candidiasis including two esophagitis.

Table 3

Candida Infections in Renal Transplant or AIDS Patients

	Renal Trans.	AIDS
Candida	9	17
oropharyngeal	2 (1)*	17 (2)*
pneumonia	3	0
sepsis	3	0
meningitis	2	0
urinary tract	1	0

* no. of esophageal candidiasis

Table 4

Fungal Infections Other Than Candida in Renal Transplant or AIDS Patients

	Renal Trans.		AIDS	
Cryptococcus	6		1	
meningitis		4		1
sepsis		2		0
pneumonia		2		0
disseminated		1		0
Aspergillus	1		1	
pneumonia		1		1
Mucor	2		0	
pnuemonia		1		0
sepsis		1		0

Table 4 represents fungal infections other than by candida. Six patients with renal transplant had cryptococcal infection; four had meningitis, two sepsis, two pneumonia, and one disseminated infection including meningitis, pneumonia, phlegmone, and urinary tract infections. Therefore, five out of six cases had meningitis.

C. *ANTI-FUNGAL THERAPY AND OUTCOME*

Anti-fungal therapies and their outcome in patients with renal transplantation and candida infections are summarized in Table 5. Of nine candida infections, six were cured and three died. In the six cured patients, three were treated with miconazole, one with fluconazole, one with intrathecal administration of amphotericin B combined with flucytosine, and one with nystatin combined with flucytosine. In the three who died, in contrast, no treatment was conducted because all cases were diagnosed at autopsy. In other words, candida infections could be cured if found and treated.

Table 5

Therapy and Outcome in Patients with Renal Transplantation and Candida Infection

Outcome	No. of Pt.	Therapy
Cure	6	Miconazole 3; Fluconazole 1 Amp B (IT)* + Flucytosine 1 Nystatin + Flucytosine 1
Death	3	none 3

* intrathecal administration of amphotericin B

Outcome of anti-fungal therapies for cryptococcal infections in renal transplant patients are given in Table 6. Among six cases of cryptococcal infections, only one patient who recovered from the infection following the graft survived. Although amphotericin B is the first drug of choice for cryptococcal infections, the nephrotoxicity always becomes a subject of the graft survival. One patient died while amphotericin B was being administered. Cryptococcal infections are more serious than candida infection and affect the patient survival as well as the graft survival.

Table 6

Therapy and Outcome in Patients with Renal Transplantation and Cryptococcal Infection

Outcome	No. of Pt.	Therapy
Cure	1	Miconazole + Flucytosine 1
Return to HD	3	Amphotericin B + Flucytosine 1 Amphotericin B + Fluconazole 1 Amp (IT)* + Flucytosine 1
Death	2	Amphotericin B + Flucytosine 1 no therapy 1

* intrathecal administration of amphotericin B
HD: hemodialysis

Table 7

Outcome of Fungal Infections in Renal Transplant Patients

	Cure	Return to HD	Death	Total
before 1984	4	2	7	13
after 1985	4	1	0	5

HD: hemodialysis

Table 7 shows outcome of fungal infections in renal transplant patients before 1984 and after 1985. There have been no cases of death due to fungal infections after 1985. Two reasons may account for this: an early diagnosis and new anti-fungal drugs. Azole compounds which have been available in Japan since 1985 appear to be generally well tolerated with minimal toxic side effects. Therefore, they may play an important role in the treatment and prevention of fungal infections suffered by patients with renal transplantation (3).

IV. CASE REPORTS

A. *CANDIDA PNEUMONIA (FIGURE 1)*

A 32 year-old female was admitted to our hospital with chief complaints of fever and cough on June 20th, 1987. She received renal transplantation in 1982. She has been controlled with immunosuppressive therapy of 15 mg per day of prednisolone and 100 mg per day of azathioprine. The chest x-p and the tomography on admission revealed multiple nodular shadows in the right upper and the left middle lung fields. Candida albicans was isolated from sputa and the candida antigen was detected in serum. We diagnosed this case as a candida pneumonia using our criteria for candida infections described above. 600 mg per day of miconazole was started on June 20th. Four days after the initiation of the therapy, temperature had decreased to normal, candida in sputa was not isolated on the 24th, clinical symptoms of cough and sputa were improved and the candida antigen in serum had disappeared by June 30th. Administration of miconazole was continued until July 12th, and the patient was discharged from our hospital as cured.

Figure 1

J.S.; 32 year-old, female, Candida pneumonia

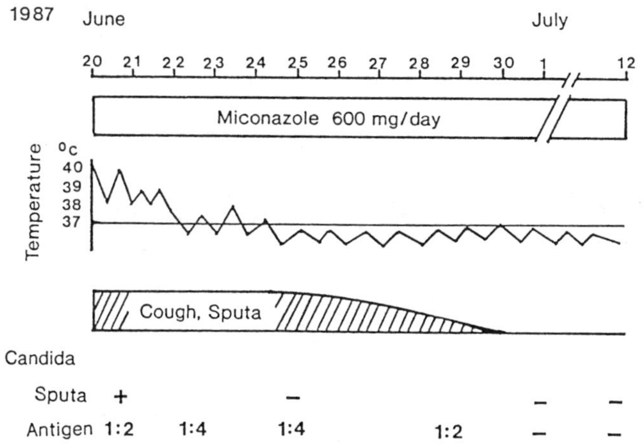

B. *DISSEMINATED CRYPTOCOCCOSIS (FIGURE 2)*

Figure 2

Clinical course of disseminated cryptococcosis

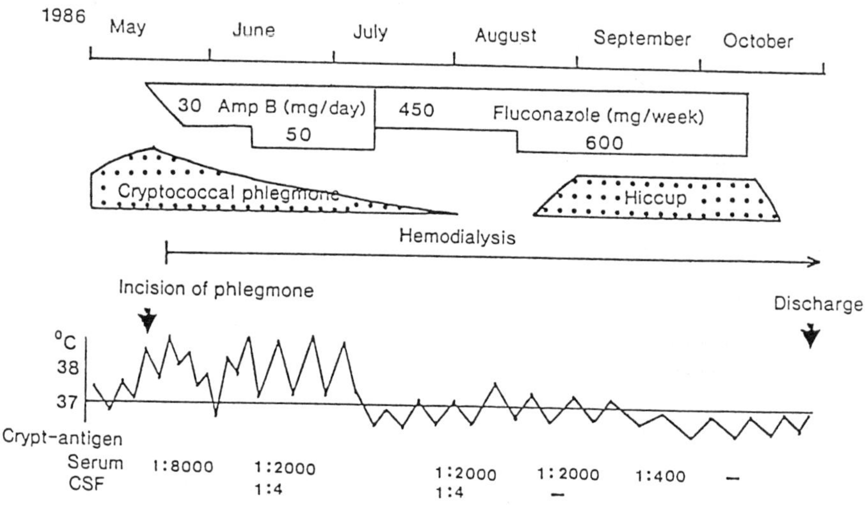

A 37 year old man was admitted to our hospital on May 2nd, 1986 because of redness, swelling, and pain in both lower extremities where many craters and pyorrhea were noted. Cryptococcus neoformans was isolated from skin, sputa, and urine. He received renal transplantation in 1981 and was administered 15 mg per day of prednisolone and 100 mg per day of azathioprine. He had a past history of cryptococcal meningitis in June, 1985. At that time, he had been treated with miconazole and flucytosine for 3 months and had shown clinical improvement. However, the antigen for cryptococcus in serum was still detected in the order of 1 : 1024; therefore, ketoconazole and flucytosine had continued to be administered orally after this discharge from the hospital.

From May 20th, 1986 intravenous administration of amphotericin B was started, and on May 24th, an incision was made of the phlegmone. As renal function has deteriorated after the procedure, he has returned to hemodialysis. Although the phlegmone was improved with a total dose of 2g of the drug, it has been difficult to continue the drug because of side effects: vasculitis and fever associated with intravenous administration of the drug. At that time, the antigen for cryptococcus in serum and the cerebrospinal fluid (CSF) were still positive with high titer. Therefore, we used fluconazole as a suppressive drug from July 10th. Clinical symptoms have improved and the antigen in CSF converted to negative on August 20th and in serum on October 3rd. He was discharged from our hospital as cured and has lived well without any drugs until now. He has had a unique side effect of severe hiccups which were probably related to fluconazole. Twenty hours after the administration of 200 mg of the drug, levels of the drug in serum and in CSF were 11.6 μg/ml and 9.2 μg/ml, respectively. These levels are not too high and are consistent with previously published levels (4). However, the hiccups could not be controlled despite a blocking of the phrenic nerve, whereas they disappeared after stopping the drug. Furthermore, we had another case of the hiccups associated with fluconazole therapy in a patient with AIDS and cryptococcal meningitis. Further investigations are needed to determine whether or not this unique side effect is related to the drug.

V. CONCLUSION

Fungal infections in renal transplant patients were more varied than those in AIDS cases in our hospital. Although the incidences of infections have not changed for 20 years, they have been well treated using azole compounds such as miconazole and fluconazole since 1985. However, in accordance with the widespread use of azole compounds, the safety of the drugs remains to be determined.

VI. REFERENCES

1. Sugimoto H., et al. Severe infections in renal transplant patients. Transplantation 21, 515 - 524, 1986. (In Japanese)
2. Kim JH. and Perfect JR. Infection and cyclosporine. Rev. Infect. Dis. 11, 677 - 690, 1989.
3. Saag MS. and Dismukes WE. Azole antifungal agents: Emphasis on new triazoles. Antimicrob. Agent. Chemother. 32, 1 - 8, 1988.
4. Larsen RA., et al. Fluconazole compared with amphotericin B plus flucytosine for cryptococcal meningitis in AIDS. Ann. Intern. Med. 113, 183 - 187, 1990.

22

Treatment of Fungal Infections in the Immunocompromised Host

Donald Armstrong

Infectious Disease Service, Department of Medicine
Memorial Sloan-Kettering Cancer Center
New York, New York, USA, 10021

Department of Medicine
Cornell University Medical College
New York, New York, USA, 10021

The first step in treating opportunistic fungal infection should be to attempt to correct the immune defect which predisposed the person to the infection. The immune defects are listed in Table 1 along with environmental factors which contribute to the infection.[1] Knowledge of these factors can help in preventing such infections. An example of correcting immune defects include removing intravenous catheters infected with a Candida species or infusing antifungal agents through the catheter, including the specific port of the catheter if it is documented that one port is infected. Another example is decreasing the doses of immunosuppressive agents such as prednisone in a patient with cryptococcosis. An example of prevention is to protect neutropenic patients from exposure, during

Supported in part by a grant from National Institutes of Allergy and Infectious Diseases, National Institutes of Health, # N01 A162533, AIDS Treatment and Evaluation Unit.

Table 1

FACTORS ASSOCIATED WITH OPPORTUNISTIC FUNGAL INFECTIONS

	Associated Environmental factors		Altered host factors*			
Fungi	External	Internal	Integument	Neutrophil	Mononuclear phagocyte	Humoral
Candida species	Intravenous and bladder catheters	Altered normal flora by antibiotics	+ + +	+ + +	+ + +	+ ?
Aspergillus species	Dust, soil	Altered normal flora (?)	+	+ + +	+ +	+ ?
Mucorales	Dust, soil	Altered normal flora (?)	+	+ + +	?	?
Cryptococcus neoformans	Pigeon feces, soil	Dissemination to CNS (?) by reactivation	+	- ?	+ + +	+ ?
Histoplasma capsulatum	River valleys, (especially Mississippi), in United States	Dissemination often by reactivation	±	-	+ + +	+ ?
Coccidioides immitis	Southwest North America, Central America, northern South America	Dissemination often by reactivation	±	-	+ + +	+ ?

NOTE: Table is adapted from Armstrong D and Gold J, Treatment of Opportunistic Mycoses in the Immunosuppressed Patient. In: Antifungal Chemotherapy, Speller DCE (Editor), John Wiley & Sons, 1980:333-364.
*Graded from - (absent) to + + + (most prominent)

hospital construction, to inhalation of aspergillus spores by using masks, re-routing through different hallways, or special air filters. Another example is to advise chronically T cell immunocompromised patients, such as HIV infected individuals, to avoid areas where they would be exposed to high concentrations of Histoplasma capsulatum (e.g., chicken coops), Coccidioides immitis (e.g., new world deserts, especially after rains), or Cryptococcus neoformans (e.g., pigeon coops).

If prevention fails and an infection occurs, there are adjunctive measures that can be used, such as removal of intravenous catheters for candidemia, although I would not always advise doing this alone without administering an antifungal agent; or surgical extirpation of some mucormycosis lesions (again, with concomitant antifungal agents). The choice of the antifungal agent will vary with the organism and the type of infection, but for most opportunistic fungal infections that are acute and invasive with possible dissemination, amphotericin B remains the treatment of choice.[2]

The approach to the six most common invasive fungal infections in the immunocompromised host will be discussed first and then the indications for the newer antifungal agents.

I. THE PATIENT WITH A NEUTROPHILE DEFECT

The most common neutrophile defect is neutropenia caused by cytotoxic chemotherapy for neoplastic disease. Others, such as chronic granulomatous disease or myeloperoxidase deficiency, are rare. The neutropenic patient is susceptible to infection with a number of bacteria and a few fungi. Candida species and the Aspergillus species are the fungi most commonly causing invasive diseases in the neutropenic patient. Less often, the mucorales cause invasive disease. There are scattered reports, but in slowly increasing numbers, of molds such as Pseudallescheria boydii, Fusarium species and others (Table 2) being documented as causing invasive disease in neutropenic patients.[3]

Table 2

OTHER FUNGAL ISOLATES IN IMMUNOCOMPROMISED HOSTS

1. Acremonium spp.
2. Alternaria spp.
3. Aureobasidium pullulans
4. Blastomyces dermatitidis
5. Cladosporium spp.
6. Cunninghamella spp.
7. Curvularia spp.
8. Drechslera spp.
9. Fonsecaea spp.
10. Fusarium spp.
11. Geotrichum spp.
12. Malassezia furfur
13. Paracoccidioides brasiliensis
14. Paecilomyces spp.
15. Penicillium marneffei
16. Pichia farinosa
17. Prototheca wickerhamii
18. Pseudoallescheria boydii
19. Rhodotorula rubra
20. Saccharomyces cerevisiae
21. Sporothrix schenckii
22. Torulopsis pintolopesii
23. Trichosporon beigelii

II. INVASIVE CANDIDIASIS (TABLES 3 AND 4)

Candida species are the fungi most often responsible for invasive disease. Candida albicans, followed by Candida tropicalis, and uncommonly Candida krusei, are those yeasts responsible for life-threatening and disseminated disease either via transmission through the g.i. tract or via IV catheters. Candida parapsilosis and Torulopsis glabrata usually invade via catheters and less often disseminate to and invade organs such as the kidney or lung.[4,5]

The diagnosis (Table 3) of invasive candidiasis is confounded by false positive clinical specimens and false negative or late positive blood cultures. Tests for antibody are inaccurate, both false negative and false positive results occur. Tests for circulating antigen are also similarly troubled, but some hold some promise. Tests for antigen in the urine also seen promising as do tests for specific metabolites in the serum such as d-arabinitol.[7-9]

Problems in diagnosis not only present daily dilemmas for clinicians, but make the evaluation of therapy most difficult. Specific diagnoses may rest on demonstrating organisms morphologically and on culture in normally sterile tissues. This is often not possible in thrombocytopenic patients. Blood cultures are positive in only about 50% of patients with invasive disease and may, in rare cases, represent transient catheter associated fungemia. Since more than 80% of neutropenic patients fungemic with C. albicans

Table 3

INVASIVE CANDIDIASIS - DIAGNOSIS

Hidden source
(IV catheters, g.i. tract)

Prevalent in body secretions
(false positives frequent, false negatives occur)

Blood culture yield poor
(about 50% and late)

Serology not standardized
(Tests for antigen experimental, for antibody unreliable)

Metabolite or Cell constituent detection under investigation

Table 4

INVASIVE CANDIDIASIS - THERAPY

Only amphotericin B reliable

Combined therapy appears promising
(e.g., flucytosine)

Newer azoles under evaluation

Susceptibility studies necessary

Prophylaxis does not prevent

or C. tropicalis have disseminated disease at autopsy, this is an acceptable setting to evaluate anti-candida therapy.[5,6] The only proven effective treatment for invasive candidiasis in this setting is amphotericin B with a response rate of about 50%.10 Any new agent must be compared to amphotericin B in controlled trials. Until this is done, amphotericin B at doses of 0.7 to 1 mgm/kgm/day remains the only proven effective therapy (Table 4). The addition of flucytosine appears to improve the response rate for C. tropicalis which is regularly more resistant by one double dilution than C. albicans to amphotericin B.[6] Relative resistance has been associated with poor outcome.[11] This clearly needs further documentation.

III. INVASIVE ASPERGILLOSIS (TABLES 5 AND 6)

Invasive aspergillosis usually starts in the lungs, but the clinical picture, including the x-ray, is not diagnostic and the sputum is positive in only about 1/3 of the cases[12] (Table 4). False positive sputum cultures do occur even in the neutropenic patient. Clinicians used to do open lung biopsies to document the diagnosis, but recently empiric therapy with amphotericin B, in a neutropenic patient with pulmonary infiltrates, has become commonplace. Thus, evaluation of antifungal therapy is difficult. Tests for antibody are positive in about one-half or more of the cases, if prospectively and persistently followed by testing at least weekly and then any time when the diagnosis is considered. Whether these positive antibody tests or tests for circulating antigen or antigen excreted in the urine will be positive in time to allow for effective therapy remains to be proven.[1]

Amphotericin B is the only treatment of proven efficacy (Table 5). The dose is 0.7 to 1 mgm/kgm/day and even up to 1.25 mgm/kgm/day in rapidly progressive cases. Because of *in vitro* and animal model synergy with rifampin, we often add rifampin at 600 mgm per day for an adult. There is no controlled clinical study to support this. Others have suggested adding flucytosine to amphotericin B, but there is neither *in vitro* nor animal model studies to support this. The duration of therapy is uncertain, but we recommend therapy until the patients bone marrow function returns and then 10 to 14 days more. Reports of responses to itraconazole[13] need to be substantiated by

Table 5

INVASIVE ASPERGILLOSIS - DIAGNOSIS

Specimen usually negative
(False negative common, false positives occur)
(positive sputum in neutropenic patient indication for therapy)

Blood cultures negative
(rare positive, contaminant ?)

Serology not standardized
(Tests for antigen experimental, but promising)
(Tests for antibody done regularly may help)

Metabolite and cell constituent detection under study

controlled comparative trials with amphotericin B. Other azoles have shown efficacy in animal models and are presently undergoing clinical trials.

In some instances extirpation of a persistent lung lesion on x-ray has been recommended, especially when a patient is to undergo further cytotoxic chemotherapy and neutropenia. These do tend to recur. An alternative is to treat with amphotericin B prior to and during the period of chemotherapy induced neutropenia.

IV. INVASIVE MUCORMYCOSIS (TABLES 7 AND 8)

The rhinocerebral form of invasive mucormycosis, first described in diabetics in ketoacidosis, is seen less often now. Pulmonary or brain lesions are the most common type of presentations in three-quarters of patients with neutropenia which is presently the most common predisposing immune defect[14] (Table 6). The ketoacidosis in diabetics appears to cause the neutrophile defect. In the rhinocerebral form, the diagnosis can usually be made rapidly by smear, scraping or biopsy, but the clinician should not wait for

Table 6

INVASIVE ASPERGILLOSIS - THERAPY

Inexact indications for initiation of therapy

Serologic tests promising but not established

Only amphotericin B proven effective

Combined therapy under evaluation (e.g., rifampin)

Newer azoles under evaluation

Susceptibility studies necessary

Prophylaxis poor or impractical (laminar flow)

Table 7

INVASIVE MUCORMYCOSIS - DIAGNOSIS

Rhinocerebral form positive on smear, scrape or biopsy

Lung or brain abscess require biopsy

Serology under study

results. Empiric, early therapy is important and should not await the microbiologic diagnosis. Patients rarely have a mucorales in the sputum with pulmonary lesions, which almost always requires biopsy, and brain abscess always requires biopsy. Serological tests are not reliable. Treatment is amphotericin B with surgical extirpation necessary in some cases (Table 7). Control of the immune defect is all important in mucormycosis and can be readily achieved in the face of ketoacidosis, but often takes longer in the face of neutropenia. In vitro tests have shown synergism between amphotericin B and rifampin against Rhizopus oryzae and in one instance this appears to have been supported by a clinical response (Armstrong and Edwards, unpublished data). This seems an important lead to follow since the response to amphotericin B alone is so unreliable. In some instances we are able to suppress, but not eradicate, the infection until the immune response returns. Duration of therapy or total dose is uncertain and must be decided on a case-by-case basis. As with all opportunistic fungal infections, return of the immune function is critical and treatment should continue through and beyond this time.

V. THE PATIENT WITH A T CELL MONONUCLEAR PHAGOCYTE DEFECT

Worldwide, the most commonly occurring opportunistic fungal infection in this setting is Cryptococcosis. Regionally, other fungi such as C. immitis, or H. capsulatum may surpass C. neoformans. The role as opportunistic fungi - or incidence of Paracoccidioides brasiliensis in South America or Penicillium marneffei in Southeast Asia or even Blastomyces dermatitidis in North America remains to be defined so that this discussion will concentrate on the first 3 fungi plus the local luxuriant growth of C. albicans in patients with T cell defects. The appearance of cases of invasive aspergillosis in HIV infected patients without other evident risk factors also requires further delineation. In our experience there have been other risk factors.[15]

VI. INVASIVE CRYPTOCOCCOSIS (TABLES 9 AND 10)

The diagnosis of invasive cryptococcosis is facilitated by the use of tests to detect antigen (Table 8). The latex agglutination tests are straightforward, inexpensive and technically readily adapted in diagnostic microbiology laboratories. In CSF it is specific above titers of 1:4. In serum it should be the same except that rheumatoid factor will non-specifically agglutinate latex particles. This should be apparent if appropriate controls are used (uncoated and non-immune serum coated particles), but makes unspecific reactive serum nonusable. Trichosporon beigelii cross reacts with anti-cryptococcal serum coated latex particles but the clinical setting is so different that this should not be a problem in practice. In patients with very high titer latex agglutination reactions either in CSF or serum the specimen may show a prozone phenomena at low

Table 8

INVASIVE MUCORMYCOSIS - THERAPY

Amphotericin B (± rifampin)

Duration varies with degree of immunocompromise

Adjunctive surgery may be necessary

dilutions so that screening should be done at 1:2 and 1:10 at a minimum.

The mainstay of treatment remains high dose amphotericin B and we use flucytosine in addition, including in patients with AIDS (Table 9). The amphotericin B should be given at doses of 0.7 to 1 mgm/kgm IV and the flucytosine at 100 mgm/kgm/day po in 4 divided doses. The dose of amphotericin B of 0.7 to 1 mgm/kgm/day should be achieved the first day and not slowly escalated over a number of days. A practical way to achieve early high levels is to give the 1 mgm test dose over 1 hour and if tolerated give the remaining 49 mgms over the next 4 to 6 hours. Thereafter, a 1 mgm/kgm/day dose can be administered. If the creatinine increases above 2.0 - then the dose should be decreased by 25% and if it increases to > 3.0 - by 50%. The flucytosine levels must be followed closely and maintained between 25 and 50 ugm/ml. If levels are not available the dose should be decreased to 75 to 50 mgm/kgm/day and the platelet and leucocyte count followed daily. The duration of initial or induction therapy should vary with the response of the individual patient. There is no set duration to be followed, nor is there a set amount of amphotericin B to be given. Response depends on a complex

Table 9

INVASIVE CRYPTOCOCCOSIS - DIAGNOSIS

Antigen detection accurate with few exceptions

Small capsule cryptococcus rarely yields false negative

Prozone phenomenon may yield false negative

Trichosporosis rarely yields false positive

Serum factors may yield false positive

Prostate may be haven for organisms

interaction of host factors and severity of infection at the time therapy is initiated. Four weeks of therapy and a total dose of 15 mgm/kgm may be adequate for some - but not for most, especially immunocompromised hosts. A total dose of 1.5 to 2 grams over 6 to 8 weeks is often necessary with the frequency of administration decreasing over the last 2 to 3 weeks to every other day or three times weekly. Parameters to follow include the usual clearing of signs and symptoms plus return of CSF to normal and disappearance of culturable organisms and antigen, or fall of antigen to low and stable levels. Since the relapse rate is high in immunocompromised hosts, suppressive or maintenance therapy should be given. A prospective controlled trial has shown that fluconazole at 200 mgm daily is equal to amphotericin B at 1 mgm/kgm/week and maintenance should be given for as long as the immunocompromised state continues, e.g., HIV infection where it should be given indefinitely.

In the final analysis, the treatment of cryptococcosis should be individualized, it should include amphotericin B in doses of close to 1 mgm/kgm/day and flucytosine at 100 mgm/kgm/day for a duration or total dose to be decided by the patients' response. If the patients' immunocompromised state does not change, then maintenance or suppressive therapy should be continued indefinitely using fluconazole at a dose of 200 mgm per day. Resistance to amphotericin B has recently been described and susceptibility studies should be done on all isolates.

VII. INVASIVE HISTOPLASMOSIS (TABLES 11 AND 12)

The diagnosis of invasive histoplasmosis can be difficult (Table 10). Respiratory secretions may contain the organism, skin lesions usually do, but the bone marrow most consistently affords the clinician a rapid diagnosis. The organism may even be seen in peripheral smears within leukocytes. Serological tests for antibody are not consistently positive in the immunocompromised host and often take time to obtain while being sent to reference laboratories. Experimental tests for antigen in serum and urines are very promising, but are so far only available from one laboratory. These

Table 10

INVASIVE CRYPTOCOCCOSIS - THERAPY

Antigen detection indication for therapy

Antigen clearance helps determine duration

Amphotericin B (1 mgm/Kgm/day) plus
Flucytosine (100 mgms/Kgm/day) treatment of choice

Consider maintenance for all consistently immunocompromised

Fluconazole treatment of choice for maintainence

Susceptibility studies necessary

are not only promising in early diagnosis, but in following therapy. Therapy should be started with amphotericin B and a course of induction therapy given at 1 mgm/kgm/day, following the patients' response and making decisions about when to stop according to each patients' response (Table 11). Maintenance therapy is under investigation but can probably be achieved with an azole. Failures

Table 11

INVASIVE HISTOPLASMOSIS - DIAGNOSIS

Skin or mucous membrane lesions require biopsy

Bone marrow requires smear and biopsy

(peripheral smears may be diagnostic in severe cases)

Serology for Antibody often negative in immunocompromised

Serology for Antigen promising (urine as well as serum)

with ketoconazole have prompted investigation with fluconazole, itraconazole and other azole trials are under development. At this time fluconazole at a dose of 200 mgm per day seems reasonable.

VIII. INVASIVE COCCIDIOIDOMYCOSIS (TABLES 13 AND 14)

The diagnosis of invasive coccidioidomycosis depends greatly on the proper history of exposure by travel or residence in an endemic area (Table 12). This includes Central and South America as well as Southwestern North America. Just as with histoplasmosis, cases can be due to reactivation of an old latent infection. The spherules are usually found in the sputum or other respiratory specimens including lung biopsies, but also may be found in skin or other tissue biopsies (bone) or aspirations (CSF or joint fluid). Serology for antibody may be falsely negative and dose not rule out coccidioidomycosis.

The treatment of the acute infection should be amphotericin B at doses of 1 mgm/kgm/day (Table 13). In patients with meningitis, some clinicians add intracisternal amphotericin B at a dose of 0.1 to 0.5 mgms to the regime. After induction with amphotericin B, when maintenance therapy is indicated, ketoconazole, fluconazole, and itraconazole have been tried. There have been failures with ketoconazole and insufficient experience with the other two azoles to make recommendations.

Table 12

INVASIVE HISTOPLASMOSIS - THERAPY

Amphotericin B initially (Induction) at 0.7 to 1 mgm/Kgm /day

An azole subsequently (Maintenance)

-fluconazole; itraconazole under study. Ketaconazole inadequate

-Duration - varies with degree of immunocompromise

(can follow urine antigen excretion for efficacy)

Table 13

INVASIVE COCCIDIOIDOMYCOSIS - DIAGNOSIS

Respiratory secretions often positive

Skin or mucous membrane lesions require biopsy

Serology for Antibody may be negative in immunocompromised

IX. OTHER OPPORTUNISTIC FUNGAL INFECTIONS (TABLE 2)

There are a number of other fungi which cause invasive infection less often, but are definitely associated with the immunocompromised host. Some, such as *Penicillium marneffei*, clearly take advantage of T cell defects, while others are less obvious but suspected of doing so, such as *Paracoccidioides brasiliensis*. Others, such as *Trichosporon beigelii* or *Fusarium* species take advantage of neutrophile defects as well as intravenous catheters, while fungi such as *Rhodotorula rubra* and the dematiaceous fungi are associated with intravenous catheters alone. Experience with amphotericin B as well as other antifungal agents needs to be expanded. *In vitro* resistance has been noted, particularly with molds, but some patients have, nevertheless, responded.

X. OLD AND NEW ANTIFUNGAL AGENTS

A. OLD

1. AMPHOTERICIN B. Amphotericin B remains the gold standard for the treatment of most opportunistic fungal infections. It is toxic but effective *in vivo* and fungicidal *in vitro*. Once the decision to give amphotericin B is made, the dose should be achieved within the first 24 to 48 hours of therapy unless a relatively benign condition, such

Table 14

INVASIVE COCCIDIOIDOMYCOSIS - THERAPY

Amphotericin B initially (Induction) at 0.7 to 1 mgm/kgm/day
An azole subsequently (Maintenance)
-fluconazole, itraconazole under study. Ketaconazole inadquate
-Duration - varies with degree of immunocompromise

as persistent Candida esophagitis, is the indication. For life-threatening fungal infections, one approach is to give a 1 mgm test dose over 1 hour and, if tolerated, give the remaining 49 mgms in the vial over 4 to 6 hours and thereafter 1 mgm/kgm/day. Some clinicians suspend the 50 mgms in 500 ml of 5% D/W and infuse the first 10 ml slowly. If this is tolerated then the remainder of the dose is infused over 4 hours. This obviates the need for a test dose.

An infusion of 500 ml to 1 liter of saline before the amphotericin B appears to ameliorate renal toxicity.

Amphotericin B can be given regionally such as by bladder instillation with minimal toxicity. Recent studies in animals[16] show that aerosol amphotericin B is effective in ameliorating pulmonary aspergillosis with greatly reduced potential toxicity. Amphotericin B in liposome solutions is less toxic and studies are underway to evaluate comparative efficacy with amphotericin B desoxycholate.

2. FLUCYTOSINE. As mentioned above, 100 mgm/kgm/day po in 4 divided doses should be the maximum dose and this should be decreased in the face of renal failure or leucopenia or thrombocytopenia. Blood levels are very helpful and should be maintained in the 25 to 50 µgm/ml range.

3. RIFAMPIN. By itself, rifampin has no effect on fungi <u>in vitro</u>. In combination with amphotericin B it decreases the amount necessary

to inhibit many fungi. This effect has been demonstrated in animal models, but not by controlled trials in humans. The usual dose is 10 mgm/kgm/day po with a maximum dose of 600 mgms/day for adults.

B. NEW DRUGS

1. AZOLES. Systemic miconazole was the first of the azoles used and reports of its efficacy in treating cryptococcosis or candidiasis have varied. Because of toxicity and questions about its efficacy, it is seldom used. It must be given intravenously. In contrast, ketoconazole must be given orally and is irregularly absorbed. In the absence of gastric acid it is not absorbed. When absorbed it is usually, but not always, effective against oropharyngeal candidiasis or esophagitis, but efficacy against invasive candidiasis has not been documented. It can cause endocrine hypoplasias and hepatotoxicity. It will be replaced by a new triazole.

2. FLUCONAZOLE. The fist of the new triazoles to reach widespread clinical use is well absorbed, widely distributed in body fluids including the CSF and excreted in the urine. Rare reversible hepatotoxicity has been noted. It is effective against oropharyngeal and esophageal candidiasis.

Efficacy in invasive candidiasis remains unproven. It does show effect in invasive cryptococcosis, but comparative tests versus adequate doses of amphotericin B have not been done. Since it is so relatively non-toxic, some clinicians prefer to use it in mild cryptococcosis, others prefer to use it only in early maintenance after induction with amphotericin B. The optimal dose of fluconazole is not certain, most studies have used 200 to 400 mgms in life-threatening diseases including histoplasmosis and coccidioidomycosis, but higher doses may well be tolerated and more effective. At present we recommend it for maintenance of these two diseases after induction with amphotericin B. An intravenous preparation is available as well as oral.

Itraconazole is an experimental triazole which is given orally and reported effective in invasive cryptococcosis and aspergillosis.

We need further experience to confirm this. Studies are also underway evaluating this drug in histoplasmosis and coccidioidomycosis.

One new triazole which was active in an animal model of aspergillosis was recently withdrawn from clinical trials because of hepatic carcinomas seen in rats on long term (2 years) of therapy.

XI. CONCLUSIONS

There are old antifungal agents with predictable toxicities which we have learned to manage. There are variations on the formulations of amphotericin B which reduce toxicity as well as regional therapy which achieves similar or greater reduction in toxicity. Combination therapy is under study to evaluate reduction of amphotericin B and thus toxicity or just increased efficacy.

New drugs are under intense study including new azoles, polysaccharides, echinocandins and nikkomycins. With new drug development and combination chemotherapy we can expect further improvement in the treatment of opportunistic fungal infection.

XII. REFERENCES

1. Armstrong, D. Problems in management of opportunistic fungal diseases. Rev Infect Dis 1989; 11(Suppl):1591-1599.
2. Schmitt, H.J., and Armstrong D. Antifungal chemotherapy. In: Current Therapy in Infectious Disease - 3, Kass, E.H., and Platt, R. (Eds)., 1990, pp. 12-17.
3. Anaissie, E., Bodey, G.P., Kantarjian, H., Ro, J., Vartivarian, S.E., Hopfer, R., Hoy, J., and Rolston, K. New spectrum of fungal infections in patients with cancer. Rev Infect Dis 1989; 11(3):369-378.
4. Kiehn, T.E., Edwards, F.F., and Armstrong D. The prevalence of yeasts in clinical specimens from cancer patients. Amer J Clin Pathol 1980; 73:518-1521.
5. Meunier-Carpentier, F., Kiehn, T.E., and Armstrong D. Fungemia

in the immunocompromised host: Changing patterns, antigenemia, high mortality. Amer J Med 1981; 71:363-370.

6. Horn, R., Wong, B., Kiehn, T.E., and Armstrong D. Fungemia in a cancer hospital: Changing frequency, earlier onset and results of therapy. Rev Infect Dis 1985; 7:646-655.

7. Ferreira, R.P., Yu, B., Niki, Y., and Armstrong D. Detection of candida antigenuria in disseminated candidiasis by immunoblotting. J Clin Microbiol 1990; 28(5):1075-1078.

8. Kiehn, T.E., Bernard, E.M., Gold, J.W.M., and Armstrong, D. Candidiasis: Detection by gas-liquid chromatography of D-arabinitol, a fungal metabolite, in human sera. Science 1979; 206:577-580.

9. Wong, B., Baughman, R.P., and Brauer, K.L. Levels of the Candida metabolite D-arabinitol in sera of steroid-treated and untreated patients with sarcoidosis. J Clin Microbiol 1989; 27(8):1859-1862.

10. Whimbey, E., Kiehn, T.E., Brannon, P., Blevins, A., and Armstrong D. Bacteremia and fungemia in patients with neoplastic disease. Amer J Med 1987; 82:723-730.

11. Powderly, W., Kobayashi, G., Herzig, G., and Medoff, G. Amphotericin B resistant yeast infection in severely immunocompromised patients. Amer J Med 1988; 84:826-831.

12. Fisher, B., Armstrong D., Yu, B., and Gold, J.W.M. Invasive aspergillosis: Progress in early diagnosis and treatment. Amer J Med 1981; 71:571-577.

13. Denning, D.W., and Stevens, D.A. Antifungal and surgical treatment of invasive aspergillosis: Review of 2,121 published cases. Rev Infect Dis 1990; 12(6):1147-1201.

14. Skahan, K., Wong, B., and Armstrong, D. Clinical manifestation and management of mucormycosis in the compromised patient. In Fungal Infections in the Compromised Patient, Warnock, D.W., and Richardson, M. (Eds.)., Second edition, John Wiley & Sons, Ltd., Sussex, England (in press).

15. Pursell, K.J., Telzak, E.E., and Armstrong D. Invasive aspergillosis in AIDS patients: Report of four cases and review. Rev Infect Dis (submitted).

16. Schmitt, H.J., Bernard, E.M., Hauser, M., and Armstrong, D. Aerosol amphotericin B is effective for prophylaxis and therapy in a rat model of pulmonary aspergillosis. Antimicrob Agents Chemo 1988; 32(11):1676-1679.

PART V

BIOLOGICAL RESPONSE MODIFIERS AND CYTOKINES POTENTIALLY USEFUL FOR IMMUNOTHERAPY OF FUNGAL INFECTIONS

23

Stimulation of Nonspecific Resistance to Infection by MDP-Lys (L18) (Romurtide)

T. Otani

Research Institute, Daiichi Pharmaceutical Co., Ltd.
Tokyo 134, Japan

1. INTRODUCTION

The minimum essential structure in the bacterial cell wall required for adjuvant activity has been defined as an N-acyl-muramic acid, linked to the dipeptide of L-alanyl-D-isoglutamine (1). N-acetylmuramoyl-L-alanyl-D-isoglutamine(MDP for muramoyl dipeptide) was synthesized and was shown to be fully active for increasing humoral and cellular immunity (2, 3). In the past decade, Chedid and his colleagues have found that MDP and certain of its analogs are also capable of enhancing host resistance to microbial infections (4). This finding opened a new field for the clinical application of MDP analogs, especially in immunosuppressed or immunodeficient patients in whom difficulties were encountered in the treatment and control of infectious diseases. We found a synthetic MDP analog, N^2-[(N-acetylmuramoyl)-L-alanyl-D-isoglutaminyl]-N^6-stearoyl-L-lysine (MDP-Lys(L18), romurtide), exhibiting higher protective activity but less pyrogenicity than MDP (5, 6).

This paper deals with the profile of the stimulating effect of MDP-Lys(L18) on host resistance to microbial infections.

2. THE PROTECTIVE ACTIVITY OF MDP-LYS(L18)

2.1. ANTI-INFECTIVE SPECTRUM OF MDP-LYS(L18)

The protective activity of MDP-Lys(L18) against bacterial and fungal infections was examined in systemic infection models in mice; MDP-Lys(L18) was administered at a dose of 100 μg/mouse 1 day before infection with *Escherichia coli*, *Pseudomonas aeruginosa*, *Staphylococcus aureus*, and *Candida albicans* (Table 1). The protective activity was estimated in terms of survival percentage on day 7 after infection, since control mice injected with saline all died by the 7th day. By subcutaneous treatment with MDP-Lys(L18), the survival rates were increased significantly in all organisms tested.

2.2. FACTORS INFLUENCING PROTECTIVE ACTIVITY

The factors influencing the protective activity of MDP-Lys(L18) and MDP were examined using the systemic infection model with *E. coli* in mice. A good dose dependency was observed at doses between 1 and

Table 1: Protective effect of MDP-Lys(L18) against systemic infection in mice.

Organism	Inoc. size (CFU/mouse)	% Survival in MDP-Lys(L18) treated mice	
P. aeruginosa PI-III	6.0×10^6	60	$P<0.01$
S. aureus E46	1.6×10^9	65	$P<0.01$
C. albicans D12	5.0×10^6	40	$P<0.05$

a) Expressed as the difference in the percentage of survival between the treated group and control group on day 7. Source: Ref. 6

Table 2: Effect of treatment timing of MDPs on protective activity against E. coli infection in mice.

Intervals before infection in hour (day)	% Survival MDP	MDP-Lys(L18)
112 (5)	ND	35*
72 (3)	60***	45**
24 (1)	65***	85***
0	5	0

ND: Not done. * P<0.05; ** P<0.01; *** P<0.001. Source: Ref. 6

100 μg of MDP-Lys(L18) and from 10 to 100 μg of MDP . The peak activity was shown at doses of 100 μg of MDP-Lys(L18) and of 300 μg of MDP. There was no difference in activity dependent on the parenteral routes of administration, such as subcutaneous, intraperitoneal, or intravenous routes. Oral application of 1 mg/mouse of MDP-Lys(L18) also provided significant protection.

Bacterial inoculum sizes significantly influenced the protective activity of these compounds; MDPs could not afford protection when the inoculum size was four times as much as the minimal lethal dose. The activity of MDP-Lys(L18) was less affected, and that of MDP was greatly affected.

The administration timing of MDPs largely affected the protective activity (Table 2). It was found that the optimal treatment timing for inducing protective activity was 1 day before infection. The activity decreased when treatment was made more than 1 day before infection. Treatment simultaneous with infection had no protective effect at all.

3. RESTORATION BY MDP-LYS(L18) OF THE RESISTANCE TO INFECTION IN IMMUNOSUPPRESSED ANIMALS

3.1. PROTECTIVE EFFECT OF MDP-LYS(L18) ON E. COLI INFECTION IN IMMUNOSUPPRESSED MICE

When mice were injected intraperitoneally with cyclophosphamide (CY) at a dose of 100 mg/kg one day before infection, their resistance to E. coli infection was significantly suppressed in comparison with that of untreated normal mice; the minimal lethal dose of E. coli in CY-treated mice was one third of that of normal mice. All of the CY-treated mice died of infection with minimal lethal dose of E. coli for CY-treated mice, whereas 70% of normal mice survived the infection. Treatment of mice with 100 μg/mouse of MDP-Lys(L18) simultaneously with CY administration afforded some protection against death from infection: the percent survival of mice with CY plus MDP-Lys(L18) was 65%. Thus, the depressed resistance of CY-treated mice to E. coli infection was restored to the normal level by treatment with MDP-Lys(L18), indicating a countering of the immunosuppressive action of CY.

3.2. PROTECTIVE EFFECT OF MDP-LYS(L18) AGAINST PSEUDOMONAS PNEUMONIA IN IMMUNOSUPPRESSED GUINEA PIGS

Experimental pseudomonas pneumonia was induced in guinea pigs immunosuppressed by subcutaneous treatment with cortisone acetate (CA) at a dose of 100 mg/kg a day for 5 consecutive days. The animals were treated subcutaneously with MDP-Lys(L18) (100 μg/animal) simultaneously with the last CA treatment, and were challenged with an aerosol of P. aeruginosa one day later. The survival study showed that all animals treated with CA alone died within 4 days of infection, while five out of six normal controls treated with saline instead of CA survived the infection. Treatment of CA-injected animals with MDP-Lys(L18) protected the animals to such a degree that the survival rate was equal to that of the normal controls.

The organisms were recovered not only from the lung but also from the liver, spleen, and blood in CA-treated animals, indicating that all the animals were infected systemically whereas the organisms were recovered only from the lung in saline-treated normal controls. From almost all the [CA + MDP-Lys(L18)]-treated animals (5/6), the organisms were recovered only from the lung, suggesting that MDP-Lys(L18) prevented systemic bacterial dissemination from the lung. The logarithmic mean population of organisms in the lungs on day 3 of infection of the [CA + MDP-Lys(L18)]-treated animals (mean ± S.D., 8.36 ± 1.04) was significantly less than that of the CA-treated controls (9.57 ± 0.85) ($P<0.05$ by Fisher's least significant difference test), but significantly higher than that of the normal controls (4.31 ± 0.10) ($P<0.01$).

The lesions in the lungs were classified histopathologically and are summarized in Table 3. In the [CA + MDP-Lys(L18)]-treated animals, the lesions of five out of six animals were characterized by purulogranulomatous changes around the grains which consisted of bacterial colonies surrounded by an eosinophilic shell (granulomatous pneumonia). The organisms appeared to be localized only in the grains around which neutrophils responded extensively. The lesions in one case were characterized by severe necrosis accompanied by massive hemorrhaging over all the lobes (necrotic pneumonia). Some grains were fused and disrupted, and the organisms were spread outside of the grains. In contrast, all CA-treated controls developed necrotic pneumonia. Most of the normal controls (4/6) were found to have quite mild catarrhal broncho-pneumonia characterized by intra-alveolar and -bronchiolar infiltrations of small numbers of neutrophils accompanied by serous exudation.

Table 3: Protective effect of MDP-Lys(L18) on pseudomonas pneumonia under immunosuppression assessed by type of pneumonia.

Type of pneumonia	Treatment with		
	Saline	CA	MDP-Lys(L18)
Mild catarrhal bronchopneumonia	4/6[a)]	0/6	0/6
Granulomatous pneumonia	1/6	0/6	5/6
Necrotic pneumonia	1/6	6/6	1/6

a) Expressed as the number of animals with the indicated type of pneumonia/number of animals tested. Source: Ref. 7

In the previous report (8), attention was focused on the course of grain formation in the lung. The grains developed near the centers of the multifocal accumulations of infiltrated neutrophils, and then granulomas were formed around the neutrophil accumulations, indicating that neutrophil-response in the early stage of infection might play an important role in grain formation. Furthermore, continuous response of neutrophils may be necessary for the development and consistency of grains because the neutrophil response was very poor around the disrupted grains, as seen in necrotic pneumonia. Depression of host resistance to pseudomonas pneumonia caused by CA and resulting in systemic infection is attributable to the suppressive effect of CA on neutrophil functions such as chemotaxis, mobilization and infiltration to the inflammation site, as has been reported for various corticosteroids (9, 10). In order to clarify the mechanism of the restorative effect of MDP-Lys(L18) on the resistance to pseudomonas pneumonia, we focused our interest on its effect on neutrophil functions.

The effect of MDP-Lys(L18) on the functions of neutrophils derived from guinea pigs with pseudomonas pneumonia were examined at 12 hours after infection. Chemotactic activity of peritoneal neutrophils induced by 0.1% glycogen was estimated according to the boyden chamber method. Comparing with the chemotactic activities of peritoneal neutrophils from normal guinea pigs, those of neutrophils from CA-treated ones were significantly depressed (Table 4). The treatment of the immunosuppressed animals with

Table 4: Effect of MDP-Lys(L18) on chemotactic activity of guinea pig peritoneal neutrophils.

Treated with	Migration (no. of cells/field)
Saline (normal control)	122.4 ± 19.0*
CA	94.6 ± 10.6
CA + MDP-Lys(L18)	111.2 ± 30.5*

* $P<0.05$ vs. CA

MDP-Lys(L18) one day before infection restored the depressed chemotactic activity to the normal level. On the other hand, phagocytic activity to P. aeruginosa of peritoneal neutrophils was slightly suppressed by treatment with CA, though the difference was not statistically significant. However, the phagocytic activity of neutrophils from MDP-Lys(L18) treated animals was significantly augmented over normal level. Furthermore, superoxide anion productivity of neutrophils was compared in each group. There was no significant change in NBT reduction potency of neutrophils between normal and immunosuppressed group. By additional treatment with MDP-Lys(L18), NBT reduction potency of neutrophils from the animals treated with CA was significantly augmented. Thus, it is supposed that the restorative effect of MDP-Lys(L18) on the depressed resistance of CA-treated animals to pseudomonas pneumonia might at least be responsible for the restoration of neutrophil response by the compound.

This study demonstrated that MDP-Lys(L18) saved the animals from death caused by bacteremic pneumonia in an immunosuppressed condition, but could not cure the pneumonia itself. Therefore, combined therapy using antibiotics and MDP-Lys(L18) was performed (See next section).

4. COMBINED EFFECT OF MDP-LYS(L18) AND ANTIBIOTICS

The ability of MDP-Lys(L18) to assist in experimental chemotherapy against infections with various species of pathogens in normal and immunosuppressed mice was studied. The mice were given 100 μg/mouse of MDP-Lys(L18) one day before infection, then treated with antibiotic 2h after infection. To confirm the combined effect of MDP-Lys(L18) with antibiotics, the 50% effective doses (ED_{50}s) of the combined agents were compared to those of the antibiotics alone.

In normal mice, the infections were produced by intraperitoneal inoculation with 4 or 8 times of minimal lethal dose of each pathogen except for C. albicans. With such severe infections, MDP-Lys(L18) did not offer effective protection against infection. In the case of C. albicans, mice were inoculated with minimal lethal

Table 5: Combined effect of MDP-Lys(L18) and antibiotics on microbial infections in normal mice.

Organism	Antibiotic	ED_{50}(mg/kg) of antibiotic with Saline	MDP-Lys(L18)
E. coli E77156	cefazolin	27.4	11.1
P. aeruginosa PI-III	gentamicin	4.0	1.4
S. aureus E46	ampicillin	5.6	1.1
C. albicans D12	amphotericin B	7.1	4.0

Source: Ref. 6

dose because the dose of amphotericin B could not be increased because of its toxicity. Combined therapy with MDP-Lys(L18) and with cefazolin or with gentamicin against *E. coli* and *P. aeruginosa*, respectively, reduced the ED_{50} values to approximately one-third of those of antibiotics alone. Likewise, against *S. aureus* or *C. albicans* infection, the ED_{50} values of ampicillin and amphotericin B fell to approximately one-fifth and almost to one-half, respectively (Table 5).

In the mice immunosuppressed with CY, infection was produced by subcutaneous inoculation with 4 times the minimal lethal dose of *E. coli*: the inoculum size was equivalent to minimal lethal dose for normal mice. The resistance of CY-treated mice to *E. coli* infection was markedly suppressed in comparison with that of normal mice, and the therapeutic effect of cefazolin on CY-treated mice was considerably less than that on normal mice(Table 6). The restoration of host defense by MDP-Lys(L18) was also demonstrated in

Table 6: Combined effect of MDP-Lys(L18) and cefazolin on *E. coli* infection in immunosuppressed mice.

Cyclophosphamide	Inoculum size (CFU/mouse)	Treatment	ED_{50} (mg/kg)
No (normal control)	6×10^6	cefazolin alone	21.9
Yes	6×10^6	cefazolin alone	98.9
Yes	6×10^6	cefazolin + MDP-Lys(L18)	13.5

the experimental chemotherapy of the CY-treated mice with cefazolin: the ED_{50} value of the antibiotic was reduced to the same range as that for normal mice.

The combined effect noted would be of advantage in the chemotherapy of infections which necessitate the use of highly toxic antibiotics, such as amphotericin B and gentamicin, in view of the reduction of the dosage of antibiotic, and may be important in the future therapy of opportunistic infections.

5. DISCUSSION

From the results presented in this paper, it is concluded that MDP-Lys(L18) can effectively prevent the establishment of a variety of infectious microorganisms in the normal and immunosuppressed host. In *E. coli* infection model, the greatest anti-infectious activity was attained by treatment 1 day before infection while treatment simultaneous with infection was not effective. It is supposed that activation of host cells is necessary to develop optimal resistance to infections, probably for the synthesis and secretion of mediating factors. In the *E. coli* infection model, the organisms disseminated rapidly from the injection site(6), so that it may not be possible by therapeutic regimens to stimulate the immune system soon enough to control the infection.

It is well known that the host defense for microbial infection depends mainly upon the presence of an adequate number of phagocytes plus serum opsonic activity as well as the function of phagocytes (11). Augmentation of these factors that organize the host defense mechanism is theoretically advantageous for enhancement of host resistance. The present study and another report(12) revealed that the neutrophil functions were augmented directly or indirectly by MDP-Lys(L18). Besides the augmenting effects of MDP-Lys(L18) on phagocytes functions, Ono et al. (13, 14) found that MDP-Lys(L18) increased the number of white blood cells in dogs and mice. Furthermore, Nakajima et al. (15) showed that MDP-Lys(L18) promoted recovery of mice from leukopenia induced by CY or X-ray irradiation.

These stimulating effects of MDP-Lys(L18) on myelopoiesis are thought to be attributable primarily to its augmenting effect on M-CSF production from macrophages(16).

Besides the effects of MDP-Lys(L18) on phagocytes, Endo (17) reported that the treatment of mice with the compound caused an increase either in the serum level of the third component of complement (C3), one of the potent serum opsonins (18), or in the plasma level of fibronectin (19), which is involved in the process of phagocytosis of microorganisms (20). Macrophages may also play an important role in augmentation of C3 production by MDP-Lys(L18), since mouse peritoneal macrophages incubated in vitro with the compound acquired an enhanced productivity of C3 (21).

Although further work is necessary in order to define the mechanism whereby MDP-Lys(L18) enhances nonspecific resistance to infection, the mechanism may at least involve neutrophils as effector cells for eliminating invading organisms, and macrophages as target cells for inducing factors which facilitate the functions of phagocytes and stimulate the proliferation and differentiation of stem cells. The enhancement of host resistance to infection by MDP-Lys(L18) may be beneficial if resistance mechanism in man is primarily mediated by the mechanism by which this compound has been shown to be active.

REFERENCES

1. F. Ellouz, A. Adam, R. Ciorbaru, E. Lederer, Minimal structural requirements for adjuvant activity of bacterial peptidoglycan derivatives, Biochem. Res. Commun., 59: 1317 (1974).
2. A. Adam, M. Devys, V. Souvannavong, P. Lefrancier, J. Choay, E. Lederer, Correlation of structure and adjuvant activity of N-acetylmuramyl-L-alanyl-D-isoglutamine (MDP), its derivatives and analogs. Antiadjuvant and competition properties of stereoisomers, Biochem. Biophys. Res. Commun., 72: 339 (1976).
3. S. Kotani, Y. Watanabe, T. Shimono, I. Morisaki, T. Shiba, S. Kusumoto, Y. Tarumi, K. Ikenaka, Immunoadjuvant activities of

synthetic N-acetylmuramyl-peptides or -amino acids, Biken J., 18: 105 (1975).

4. L. Chedid, M. Parant, P. Lefrancier, J. Choay, E. Lederer, Enhancement of nonspecific immunity to Klebsiella pneumoniae infection by a synthetic immunoadjuvant (N-acetylmuramyl-L-alanyl-D-isoglutamine) and several analogs, Proc. Natl. Acad. Sci. U.S.A., 74: 2089 (1977).
5. K. Matsumoto, T. Otani, T. Une, Y. Osada, H. Ogawa, I. Azuma, Stimulation of nonspecific resistance to infection induced by muramyl dipeptide analogs substituted in the -carboxyl group and evaluation of N-muramyl dipeptide-N-stearoyllysine, Infect. Immun., 39: 1029 (1983).
6. T. Otani, T. Une, Y. Osada, Stimulation of non-specific resistance to infection by muroctasin, Arzneim.-Forsch./Drug Res., 38: 969 (1988).
7. T. Otani, K. Katami, T. Une, Y. Osada, H. Ogawa, Restoration by MDP-Lys(L18) of resistance to pseudomonas pneumonia in immunosuppressed guinea pigs, Microbiol. Immunol., 28: 1077 (1984).
8. T. Otani, K. Katami, T. Une, Y. Osada, H. Ogawa, Nonbacteremic pseudomonas pneumonia in immunosuppressed guinea pigs, Microbiol. Immunol., 26: 67 (1982).
9. W. Peters, J. Holland, H. Senn, W. Rhomberg, T. Banerjee, Corticosteroid administration and localized leukocyte mobilization in man, N. Engl. J. Med., 282: 342 (1972).
10. P. Ward, The chemosuppression of chemotaxis, J. Exp. Med., 124: 209 (1966).
11. L. Young, D. Armstrong, Human immunity to Pseudomonas aeruginosa. I. In vitro interaction of bacteria, polymorphonuclear leukocytes, and serum factors, J. Infect. Dis., 126: 257 (1972)
12. Y. Osada, T. Otani, M. Sato, T. Une, K. Matsumoto, H. Ogawa, Polymorphonuclear leukocyte activation by synthetic muramyl dipeptide analog, Infect. Immun., 38: 848 (1982).
13. Y. Ono, T. Iwasaki, M. Sekiguchi, T. Onodera, Subacute toxicity

of muroctasin in mice and dogs, Arzneim.-Forsch./Drug Res., 38: 1024 (1988).

14. Y. Ono, M. Sekiguchi, K. Aihara, T. Onodera, Chronic toxicity of muroctasin in mice, Arzneim.-Forsch./Drug Res., 38: 1028 (1988).
15. R. Nakajima, Y. Ishida, F. Yamaguchi, T. Otani, Y. Ono, M. Nomura, T. Une, Y. Osada, Beneficial effect of muroctasin on experimental leukopenia induced by cyclophosphamide or irradiation in mice, Arzneim.-Forsch./Drug Res., 38: 986 (1988).
16. K. Akahane, F. Yamaguchi, Y. Kita, T. Une, Y. Osada, Stimulation of macrophages by muroctasin to produce colony-stimulating factors, Arzneim.-Forsch./Drug Res., 40: 179 (1990).
17. N. Endo, T. Okuda, Y. Osada, H. Zen-yoji, Stimulation of complement production in mice by N-(N-acetylmuramyl-L-alanyl-D-isoglutamine)-N-stearoyl-L-lysine, Infect. Immun., 42: 618 (1983).
18. J. Winkelstein, M. Smith, H. Shin, The role of C3 as an opsonin in the early stages of infection, Proc. Soc. Exp. Biol. Med., 149: 397 (1975).
19. N. Endo, T. Okuda, Y. Osada, H. Zen-yoji, Stimulation of plasma fibronectin production in mice, Arzneim.-Forsch./Drug Res., 38: 997 (1988).
20. S. Wright, L. Craigmyle, S. Silverstein, Fibronectin and serum amyloid p component stimulate C3b- and C3bi-mediated phagocytosis in cultured human monocytes, J. Exp. Med., 158: 1338 (1983).
21. N. Endo, In vitro and in vivo augmentation by muroctasin of the production of the third component of complement by murine macrophages, Arzneim.-Forsch./Drug Res., 38: 993 (1988).

24

Enhancement of Resistance to Experimental Candidiasis and Cryptococcosis in Mice by Dihydroheptaprenol, a Synthetic Polyprenol Derivative

Yoshimura Fukazawa, Keiko Kagaya, Toshihiko Yamada, Seiichi Araki[1], Makoto Kimura[1], Yoshiki Sugihara[1], and Kyosuke Kitoh[1]

Department of Microbiology
Yamanashi Medical College
Tamaho-cho, Yamanashi 409-38, Japan

Research and Development Division
Eisai Co., Ltd.
Bunkyo-ku, Tokyo 112, Japan[1]

I. INTRODUCTION

In recent years, opportunistic fungal infections in compromised hosts have become an increasing problem in chemotherapy. Especially, candidiasis and cryptococcosis are increasing in occurrence and severity because of advances in modern medicine with the use of antibiotic and immunosuppressive therapies (1), and more effective chemotherapies of such infections are urgently required. It is known that various microorganisms and their components enhance host defense mechanisms against microbial infections or against tumor cells in mice. On the other hand, chemically defined immunostimulants, such as muramyl dipeptide and its synthetic derivatives, also have been shown to enhance nonspecific resistance to infections (2).

Because vitamin E and ubiquinone (3), which contain a few isoprene units, have been shown to enhance nonspecific defense mechanisms in mice, we have attempted to find chemically defined terpenoid compounds which enhance host resistance. We have found that a chemically synthesized polyprenol derivative, dihydroheptaprenol (DHP), enhanced the nonspecific resistance of mice to infection with *Escherichia coli* (4). In this study, we attempted to explore the ability of DHP to enhance the resistance to experimental candidiasis and cryptococcosis in mice in relation to the number and function of peripheral blood neutrophils (NP) and elicitations of C3 component and cytokines.

II. MATERIALS AND METHODS

DHP. DHP (Fig. 1) was chemically synthesized and prepared as a microemulsion with lecithin at a 1% concentration in the Research Laboratories, Eisai Co. Ltd., Tokyo., Japan (4).

Mice. BALB/c male mice were obtained from Charles River Japan Inc., Kanagawa, Japan. Mice were used at 5 to 6 weeks of age and weighed from 24 to 26 g.

Strains used. *C. albicans* M1012 (serotype A) and *C. neoformans* MCY2002 (serotype A) were used. They were subcultured on Sabouraud glucose agar for 48 hr and cultured in Sabouraud glucose broth for 24 hr at 27°C under shaking. The yeast cells were washed, suspended in sterile physiological saline solution (PSS) and cell number was determined by a hemacytometer.

$$H(CH_2-\overset{CH_3}{\overset{|}{C}}=CH-CH_2)_6-CH_2-\overset{CH_3}{\overset{|}{C}H}-CH_2-CH_2OH$$

$$C_{35}H_{60}O \quad M.W.=496.86$$

Fig. 1. Chemical structure of dihydroheptaprenol (DHP)

Protection experiment. Mice were injected intramuscularly (i.m.) with DHP (100 mg/kg) at an appropriate time before infection. As a control, mice were injected i.m. with the same volume of lecithin solution (surfactant for DHP). Mice were inoculated with 2 x 10^5 CFU of *C. albicans* or *C. neoformans*, and the effect of the agent on the resistance of mice to candidiasis or cryptococcosis was expressed as the mean survival day after 5 and 7 weeks, respectively.

Leukocyte counts. Mice were bled from the retroorbital sinus with a heparinized tube, and leukocyte counts and their differential cell counts were made.

Candidacidal activity of leukocytes. Polymorphonuclear leukocyte (PMN)-rich cells were harvested from mouse peritoneal fluid after stimulation with 0.5% glycogen for 4 hr. Peritoneal resident macrophages (PMP) were harvested from normal mice as described for PMN. The monolayers of phagocytes (1 x 10^6 per well) in 24-well plates (Falcon No. 3047) were made by incubating the cells for 1 hr at 37°C in 5% CO_2-95% air. After being washed, the monolayers were infected with 1 x 10^5 yeast cells in the presence of 10% fresh mouse serum obtained from normal or DHP-treated mice (total volume, 1.0 ml). The infected monolayers were incubated at 37°C for 2 hr, lysed with water, and viable yeast cells in the wells were scored by colony counting.

Assay for C3 component in serum. C3 concentration in serum from DHP-treated or control mice was determined by enzyme immunoassay using plates coated with anti-mouse C3 serum and peroxidase conjugated anti-mouse C3 IgG antibody. Serially diluted sera were assayed and results were expressed as dilution which gave absorbancy of 1.0 at 490 nm.

Assay for colony stimulating activity in serum. The bone marrow cells (1 x 10^5) were prepared from the femora of untreated mice, and cultured in McCoy 5A medium containing 20% mouse serum (sample), 20% horse serum and 0.8% methylcellulose in a total volume of 1 ml. After 7 day-cultivation, number of colonies appearing in the medium was determined microscopically.

Statistical analysis. The statistical significance of the data was analyzed by the Student *t* test.

III. RESULTS

A. EFFECT OF DHP ADMINISTRATION ON THE NUMBER OF NP IN PERIPHERAL BLOOD

The number of NP in the bloodstream of mice which had been administered 100 mg of DHP per kg i.m. was determined. The mice administered DHP 2 days previously exhibited significant increase of NP, and the level returned to normal 4 days after treatment. When the mice were repeatedly administered DHP every 4 days, increase of NP in the blood was still observed at 2 days after the 14th administration (Fig. 2). Four days after the 14th treatment, the level of NP returned to that prior to the treatment.

When mice were administered DHP daily for 3 days, the number of NP increased the day after the first administration, maintaining this level for the next 3 days, and showed a peak 3 days after the

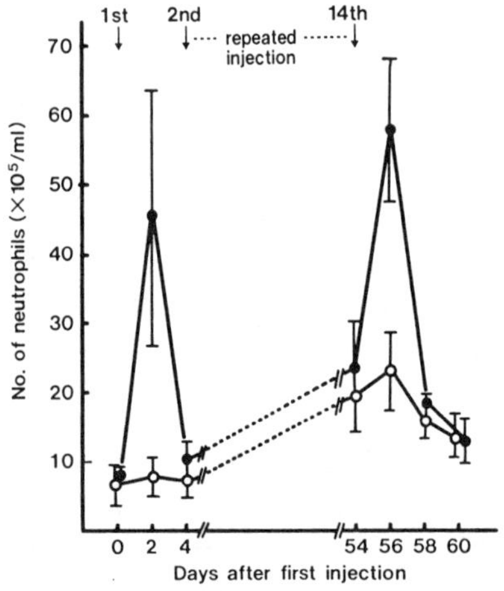

Fig. 2. Effect of repeated DHP administration on the number of neutrophils. ○, Control; ●, DHP (100 mg/kg, i.m.).

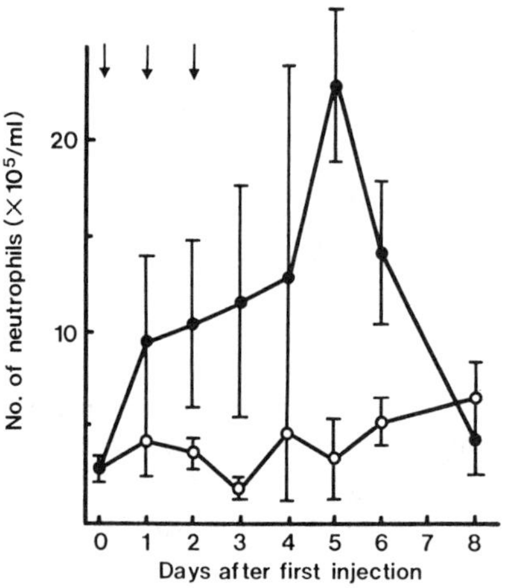

Fig. 3. Effect of consecutive DHP administration on the number of neutrophils. ○, Control; ●, DHP (100 mg/kg, i.m.).

last administration. The level of NP returned to normal 6 days after the last administration (Fig.3). These results indicate that mice respond to repeated DHP administration to generate NP, and that daily administration for 3 days induces prolonged increase in NP.

B. EFFECT OF DHP ON RESISTANCE OF MICE TO C. ALBICANS INFECTION

The effect of DHP administration on the resistance of mice to *C. albicans* infection was investigated. When mice were injected with DHP every 4 days from 2 days before infection for a 6 week period, they showed increased protection against *C. albicans* infection. In an observation period of 42 days, the mean survival day for the DHP-administered mice was longer than that for control mice ($P<0.05$) (Fig. 4A). On the other hand, mice which were daily administered DHP for 3 days before infection also showed increased protection against *C. albicans* infection. The mean survival day for the DHP-administered mice was longer than that for control mice ($P<0.05$) (Fig. 4B). Moreover, mice which were administered DHP once 2 days before infection showed apparent prolonged mean survival time, as compared with control mice, although the results were not statistically significant (data not shown). These results clearly indicate that protection of mice against *C. albicans* infection induced by DHP correlate well with increase in NP in blood at the time of infection.

C. EFFECT OF DHP ON CANDIDACIDAL ACTIVITY OF PHAGOCYTES

To determine whether DHP is able to activate phagocytes in addition to its ability to induce an increased number of NP in mice, candidacidal activity of glycogen-induced PMN and PMP from DHP-treated mice were examined. The monolayers of phagocytes were infected with *C. albicans* in the presence of autologous fresh serum (phagocytes: *C. albicans* =10:1), incubated for 2 hr and the number of viable cells was determined by colony counting. The effective candidacidal activity of NP was readily demonstrated in control mice, and further enhanced killing activity was not observed in NP of DHP-treated mice. Moreover, candidacidal activity of PMP either

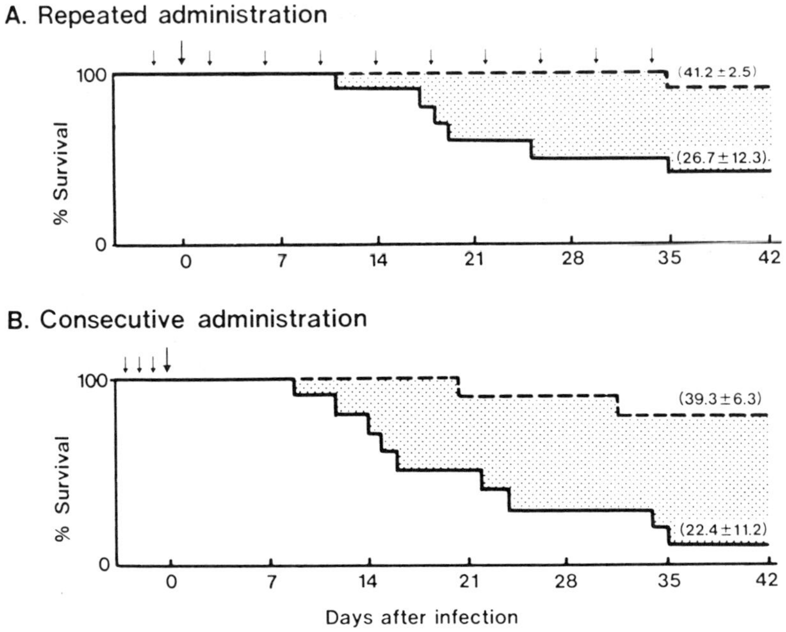

Fig. 4. Effect of DHP on protection against *C. albicans* infection. →, Placebo or DHP (100 mg/kg, i.m.); ➔, infection. —, Control; ---, DHP; ( ), mean survival day ± S.E..

from normal or from DHP-treated mice was not demonstrated (data not shown). These results suggest that resistance to infection with *C. albicans* in DHP-treated mice may be exclusively due to increase in NP.

D. EFFECT OF DHP ON RESISTANCE OF MICE TO C. NEOFORMANS INFECTION

The effect of DHP on the resistance of mice to *C. neoformans* infection was investigated by the same schedule of administration as used for *C. albicans* infection. Mice receiving repeated injections of DHP at 4 day intervals starting at 2 days before infection, exhibited a more prolonged survival time than did control mice ($P < 0.05$) (Fig. 5A). Moreover, when injected with DHP daily for 3 days before infection, they also exhibited increased protection against

C. neoformans infection. The mean survival day for DHP-treated mice was longer than that for control mice ($P<0.05$) (Fig. 5B). These results suggest that DHP induces enhanced resistance in mice against *C. neoformans* infection as well, and that resistance is induced when NP are increased at the time of infection in DHP-treated mice.

E. EFFECT OF DHP ON C3 LEVEL IN SERUM

Sera from mice injected with DHP or placebo were collected at 1 to 4 days after injection, and assayed for C3 concentration. In sera from mice injected with DHP (100 mg/kg) 1 or 2 days before assay, C3 levels were found to increase to double that in control sera. The C3 level returned to normal 4 days after injection. The results suggest that DHP enhances host defense, in part, by increasing the C3 component, in addition to stimulation of the generation of NP.

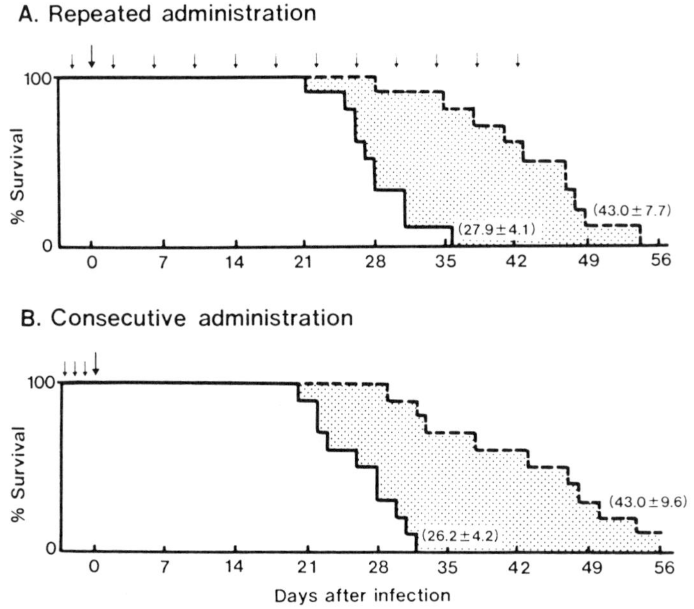

Fig. 5. Effect of DHP on protection against *C. neoformans* infection.
, Placebo or DHP (100 mg/kg); ⟶, infection.
—, Control; ---, DHP; ( ), mean survival day ± S.E.

F. EFFECT OF DHP ON INDUCTION OF COLONY STIMULATING FACTOR (CSF)

The colony stimulating activity of sera from DHP-injected mice was assayed to seek the primary action of DHP *in vivo*. The colony stimulating activity was detected in sera 6 hr after DHP injection, reached a peak at 18 hr and returned to normal 48hr after injection, suggesting that DHP induces CSF *in vivo* leading to increase in the number of NP, although the molecular species was not defined.

IV. DISCUSSION

In this study, we demonstrated the effect of DHP on protection of mice against subacute infections with *C. albicans* or *C.. neoformans* and suggested that the mechanism of resistance to both candidal and cryptococcal infections was mainly accountable for the increased population of NP induced by DHP.

To clarify kinetics of the protective effect of DHP on subacute fungal infections, we examined the effect of repeated DHP treatment on the generation of NP and found that mice responded to long term repeated injections at 4-day intervals. Furthermore, consecutive injections of DHP were shown to induce prolonged increase of NP as well. The important role of NP in protection against candidiasis is well known. Our data indicated the correlation between the increased number of NP and enhanced protection against candidiasis. Since the killing activity of DHP-induced NP against *C. albicans* was the same as that of control NP, the enhanced protection against candidiasis in DHP-injected mice is deemed to depend solely on the increased number of NP.

Our data suggest that CSF is induced by DHP treatment leading to increased generation of NP, although the CSF family is not characterized. It has been reported that both GM-CSF and G-CSF stimulate NP and macrophage function including enhancing the H_2O_2-generating capacity of NP and PMP in mice (5), and phagocytes obtained from DHP-treated mice exhibited enhanced H_2O_2 generation. However, the facts that *C. albicans* is relatively resistant to H_2O_2, and thereby the O_2-independent killing mechanism of NP is required, and that DHP did not enhance the killing activity of NP and PMP *per se*, suggest that DHP is not able to enhance O_2-independent microbicidal mechanism in phagocytes.

On the other hand, the factor(s) predisposing to cryptococcosis is not well defined. It has been generally considered that NP was not an essential defensive phagocyte against cryptococci (6). Nevertheless, we found that mice treated with DHP exhibited enhanced protection against *C. neoformans* infection. This evidence suggests that NP play a role in resistance to primary infection with *C. neoformans* infection to a certain degree. However, since DHP was also shown to stimulate RES (4), the possibility that enhanced protection against *C. neoformans* infection by DHP is based on such enhanced cellular events cannot be ruled out.

Opsonization of heavily encapsulated *C. neoformans* cells by normal fresh serum is low and C3 fragments were mostly bound in the sites beneath the capsule (7). Since the sera from DHP-treated mice showed higher C3 binding to *C. neoformans* cells than did sera from control mice (data not shown), it is suggested that increase in C3 in addition to phagocyte stimulation is attributable to enhanced protection against *C. neoformans* infection in DHP-treated mice.

Recently, it has been suggested that major factors in compromised patients leading to infection are leukopenia and depressed functions of phagocytes. In this respect, DHP might be applied as an agent to aid in prophylaxis or in chemotherapy for opportunistic bacterial and fungal infections in compromised patients.

V. SUMMARY

We demonstrated the enhancement of resistance to candidiasis and cryptococcosis in mice by DHP treatment in relation to the number and function of NP. The increased generation of NP was demonstrated at 2 days after single injection, 2-4 days after 3 consecutive injections, and also at 2 days after long-term injections of DHP at 4-day intervals. Increased generation of NP was shown to be mediated by colony stimulating factor(s) generated in the serum of DHP-treated mice. Mice injected with DHP 3 consecutive days before challenge, or given repeated injections for more than 35 days at 4-day intervals, which started at 2 days before challenge, showed longer survival time after infection with *C. albicans* or *C. neoformans* than did untreated controls. Evidence that killing activity of NP or PMP against *C. albicans* was not affected by DHP, and that concentration of the C3 component in the serum was increased, suggested that enhanced protection against candidiasis or cryptococcosis in mice by DHP is based mainly on the increased number of NP, and partly on an increase in C3, and that DHP can be applied as an agent to aid in prophylaxis or in chemotherapy for opportunistic fungal infections in compromised patients.

VI. REFERENCES

1. M. Amano, and H. Tanaka, Effect of antibiotics on phagocytosis and bactericidal activity of human leukocytes, *Chemotherapy (Tokyo)*, *34*: 157-164 (1986).
2. L. Chedid, M. Parant, F. Parant, P. Lefrancier, J. Choay, and E. Ledere, Enhancement of nonspecific immunity to *Klebsiella pneumoniae* infection by a synthetic immunoadjuvant (*N*-acetylmuramyl-L-alanyl-D-isoglutamine) and several analogs, *Proc. Natl. Acad. Sci. U.S.A.*, *74*: 2089-2093 (1977).
3. L. H. Block, A. Georgopoulos, P. Meyer, and J. Drews, Nonspecific resistance to bacterial infections: enhancement by ubiquinone-8. *J. Exp. Med.*, *146*: 1226-1240 (1978).
4. S. Araki, K. Kagaya, K. Kitoh, M. Kimura, and Y. Fukazawa, Enhancement of resistance to *Escherichia coli* infection in mice by dihydroheptaprenol, a synthetic polyprenol derivative, *Infect. Immun.*, *55*: 2164 (1987).
5. A. M. Cohen, D. K. Hines, E. S. Korach, and B. J. Ratzkin, In vivo activation of neutrophil function in hamsters by recombinant human granulocyte colony-stimulating factor, *Infect. Immun.*, *56*: 2861 (1988).
6. J. W. Murphy, Cryptococcosis. *In* Immunology of the Fungal Diseases (R. A. Cox, ed.), CRC Press, Boca Raton, Florida, U.S.A. (1990).
7. R. Ikeda, T. Shinoda, K. Kagaya, and Y. Fukazawa, Role of serum factors in the phagocytosis of weakly or heavily encapsulated *Cryptococcus neoformans* strains by guinea pig peripheral blood leukocytes, ..., *28*: 51 (1984).

25

Modulation of the Immune Defenses Against Fungi by Amphotericin B and Its Derivatives

Jacques Bolard

Laboratoire de Physique et Chimie Biomoléculaires (L.P.C.B.) - Université Pierre et Marie Curie - Tour 22, 4, place Jussieu 75252 Paris cedex 05, France

SUMMARY

The polyene antibiotic amphotericin B is the drug of choice for the treatment of fungal infections. It is toxic for fungi and to a lesser degree to host-cells. At sublethal doses it has stimulating properties, in particular for cells of the immune system. We shortly review the in vivo and in vitro characteristics of this immunomodulation. Then we describe the potent in vitro effects of amphotericin B derivatives (N-fructosyl and N-thiopropionyl) and the early events accompanying their activation of lymphocytes.

This work was supported in part by a grant from Institut Curie.

I. INTRODUCTION

Polyene antibiotics, in particular amphotericin B (AmB), are the most widely used antifungal drugs. Their activity is assumed to originate from the permeability changes induced in the membrane of fungi by pore formation or lipid peroxidation (see 1, 2). They exhibit also a non negligible, although weaker, toxicity for host-cells. Independently of these toxic effects, the polyene antibiotics at sublethal doses present in contrast stimulating effects for fungal cells as well as for mammalian cells. The action of these drugs is therefore complex and besides toxicity, stimulation of the cells of the immune system can be expected. We shall describe in this article the experimental evidence showing that it is indeed the case and shall recall then the studies performed on the mechanism of this stimulation.

II. IMMUNE DEFENSES AGAINST FUNGI.

The primary mechanism of host resistance to candidosis is centered around cellular immunity but there are contributions made by humoral systems. Fungi are not lysed directly by antibodies and complement, and the protective activity of Candida albicans antibodies, for instance, appears to be associated with optimizing complement-mediated phagocytosis by neutrophils, opsonization for monocyte phagocytosis and inhibition of attachment to host epithelium. Different immunocompetent cells may interfere depending on the nature of the fungal infection, namely in the presence of pathogenic fungi (Histoplasma, Coccidoides or Cryptococcus) or opportunistic fungi (Candida, Aspergillus). They are not always well specified and their interference is often subject to debate. In particular, the characteristics of the immune defenses can be totally modified by AIDS.

The role of macrophages is well established for Histoplasma capsulatum. It seems to be also the case for Cryptococcus neoformans but there is contest for Candida and Aspergillus. Polymorphonuclear leukocytes play an important role in resistance against Aspergillus, certainly also against Candida in its visceral infections and in a general manner against opportunistic fungi, which seem to be more sensitive to hydrogen peroxide toxicity than pathogenic fungi. Normal T-cell function is required for efficient host protection against superficial Candida albicans and also against pathogenic fungi as evidenced by the development of these infections in association with AIDS. Finally, it should be noted that cell wall of Candida albicans stimulates Natural Killer cell activity.

III. IN VIVO MODULATION BY AMPHOTERICIN B OF IMMUNE DEFENSES AGAINST FUNGI.

Numerous in vivo studies have shown that the cellular and/or humoral arms of the immune response may be affected by AmB or AmB methylester (AmE) (for reviews see 2-5). These drugs enhance the response in most of the common inbred mouse strains (6,7). AmB produces striking but reversible changes in murine thymus and splenic weights as well as histological modifications in lymphoid organs (6). Indeed, in our hands (N. Henry-Toulmé, M. Séman and J. Bolard, unpublished observations) in vivo treatment of DBA/2 mice with AmB appeared to have a severe but reversible toxic effect on lymphocytes. 90 % of the cells were eliminated from the thymus 5 days upon AmB injection. Splenic T and B lymphocyte populations were more resistant to AmB toxicity, both in vivo and in vitro. Fluorescence analysis of thymocytes from day 5 to 12 after treatment revealed that AmB is selectively toxic for cortical Lyt-2, L3T4 double positive cells. During the accute depletion phase, 46 % of the surviving thymocytes were $L3T4^{+}$, $Lyt\text{-}2^{-}$, 31 % were $L3T4^{-}$, $Lyt\text{-}2^{+}$ and 23 % were L3T4, Lyt-2 double negative cells. Double positive thymocytes reappeared by day 7 to 9 as the fraction of double negative cells decreased. This demonstrated that AmB has a similar effect on adult cortical thymocytes as corticosteroids. However, no modification of lymphocyte subpopulations was observed in the spleen although an important increase of the absolute number of cells was seen in this organ on day 10 after treatment. Moreover, a significant stimulation of spontaneous Ig secreting cells was detected from day 5 to day 12. Together, this demonstrated that

AmB, as an immunomodulator, is toxic for immature or non-mature cortical thymocytes and simultaneously behaves as a polyclonal B cell activator in vivo.

The possible enhancement of phagocytic activity of macrophages by AmB was first demonstrated on peritoneal macrophages of AKR mice (7). The clinical significance of this observation was demonstrated using the "skin window" test (8). It was applied for the study of the phagocytary capacity of mononuclear phagocytes in 6 patients with mucocutaneous candidiasis. The comparison with 9 control subjects showed the stimulating property of AmB for the ingestion and digestion capacity of mononuclear cells. On the other hand, mice receiving a single intraperitoneal injection of AmB showed resistance to subsequent challenge with Candida albicans (5, 9). This enhancement of resistance was obvious in terms of both survival criteria and clearance of the intravenously injected organism from different organs. The protective effect of AmB was conditioned by dose, time of drug administration, and size of yeast inoculum. A highly candicidal cell population appeared in the spleen and was characterized as macrophages (10). In another study (11) AmB - elicited macrophages from AKR mice exhibited enhanced superoxide release upon challenge with Histoplasma capsulatum and zymosan.

IV. IN VITRO MODULATION BY AMPHOTERICIN B AND ITS DERIVATIVES OF IMMUNOCOMPETENT CELLS.

A. The in vitro modulation of the macrophage activity could be demonstrated for the tumoricidal capability of activated macrophages (12,13). The in vitro activation against Candida albicans is now well documented (9, 10). AmB has been shown to induce secretion of TNF-α by murine macrophages in vitro (14, 15) and to induce serum levels of colony - stimulating factors in mice given AmB i.p. (7). However, another study (16) showed in contrast that AmB (but not liposomal AmB) was highly suppressive of macrophage differentiation and effector functions at doses of about 10^{-6}M. Similarly, we were not able to observe an increased tumoricidal capability of trehalose dimycolate activated macrophages with AmB concentrations ranging from 0.1 to 2×10^{-6}M (unpublished data). AmE and N-fructosyl AmB also were without effect.

B. Several experiments have suggested the critical central role of the neutrophil respiratory burst in the prevention and containment of disseminated candidiasis. Consequently, numerous in vitro studies have been performed on the influence of AmB on the activity of polymorphonuclear leukocytes. Conflicting data have been described. Phagocytosis was shown to be inhibited by clinically achievable concentration of 0.5 - 2×10^{-6}M in two cases (17,18) but only at very high concentrations (20×10^{-6}M) in another case (19). Phagocytosis could also be increased at 2×10^{-6}M (20). The role of the experimental conditions in these discrepancies has been discussed (21). Chemiluminescence and chemotaxis are generally shown to be decreased by AmB (17, 19, 22-24). However, there are two examples where it was either not modified (25) or even increased by Fungizone (26), although neither AmB nor deoxycholate did it. The toxic role of deoxycholate has been demonstrated for human PMN (27).

C. Consequently, based on the above results, positive as well as negative effects of AmB on the activation of macrophages and neutrophils can be deduced. These contradictions could be attributed to differences in the experimental protocol used. However, recent observations (5), indicating the strong correlation between the magnitude of the in vitro effects and the in vivo adjuvant effects of AmB or AmE in different mouse strains, has opened new perspectives for the comprehension of the variability in the results. Most of the common inbred mouse strains show AmB-induced immunostimulation (AmB-high responders) but mice of the C 57 BL strains are AmB-low responders. Lymphoid cells from AmB-high responder strains also exhibit greater resistance to H_2O_2 toxicity in vitro compared with cells from AmB-low responders. This result led to an evaluation of differences in the tissue catalase levels of AmB-high and -low responder strains. The C 57 BL mouse strains expressed low levels of tissue catalase activity while several AmB-high responder strains had high spleen cell, macrophage and liver catalase. It was therefore suggested that cellular peroxidation is a major determinant of the genetic regulation of AmB--induced immunostimulation.

D. AmB and nystatin stimulation of murine B cells in culture has been several times reported (28-31). However, one study indicated, in contrast, inhibition of the LPS-induced activation of BALB/c B lymphocytes (32). Proliferation assays scored by [^{3}H]T dR incorporation as well as plaque-forming cells (PFC) assays showing enhanced frequency of antibody-secreting spleen cells were used to demonstrate polyclonal activation. AmB treatment led, for instance, to an approximately fourfold stimulation of immunoglobulin G, PFC in AKR mice (33).

Very interesting results were obtained with soluble derivatives of AmB which appeared to be much more potent PBA than the parent compound : AmB methyl ester (AmE) (33), N-thiopropionyl AmB (AmBSH) (34), N-Fructosyl AmB (38) and to a lesser extent N-ornithyl AmE (32). The effects of AmE were strongly dependent on cell density and on the mouse strain studied (33). They were also modulated by lipoproteins (36). At the optimal doses (around 50 x 10^{-6}M) the polyenes were as active on AKR or DBA/2 cells as LPS at 100 μg/ml.

In contrast with these positive results on murine cells, mitogen and antigen induced stimulation of human lymphocytes has been found to be suppressed by AmB *in vitro* (37-39). Human peripheral blood lymphocytes showed a decreased "natural killer" activity in the presence of AmB (40). Incubation of murine peritoneal and spleen natural killer cells with AmB had little or no effect on spontaneous "natural killer" cell activity *in vitro* (39).

E. Murine T cells were not stimulated by AmB (27,31). With BALB/c T cells, that could be explained by their much higher sensitivity to

AmB-induced toxicity as compared to B lymphocytes (6) but this difference was not observed in DBA/2 cells (Henry-Toulmé, personal communication). Human T cells manifested decreased "natural killer" activity in the presence of AmB (40). In contrast, N-Fru AmB was shown to be mitogenic for murine peripheral T cells (35) although to a lesser extent than for B cells.

V. MECHANISMS BY WHICH AMPHOTERICIN B AND ITS DERIVATIVES MODULATE THE ACTIVITY OF LYMPHOCYTES.

We have seen that some derivatives of AmB (AmE, AmBSH, N-Fru AmB) are potent polyclonal activators. These drugs afford excellent tools to analyse the mechanism underlying lymphocyte activations because much information has been gained on their mechanism of action (see 2). In particular, they form trans membrane pores through which fluxes of ions can occur. As a matter of fact, changes in free cytosolic calcium concentration and in membrane voltage are thought to be important initiating events in lymphocyte activation. AmB derivatives may then exert their stimulating activity through the production of early ionic signals similar to those delivered by the classical activators lipopolysaccharide (LPS) and anti-immunoglobulin (anti-Ig). We addressed this question (41) in a B-cell line (WEHI 231) which has previously been shown to exhibit characteristic response to LPS and anti-Ig. AmBSH protected these cells against anti-Ig-induced cell growth inhibition, providing a LPS-like response. In contrast, the parental compound AmB did not. The two polyene antibiotics did not modify the resting $Ca^{2+}{}_i$ level of the cells, neither did LPS, whereas anti-Ig induced a rapid increase in the cytosolic calcium concentration. On the other hand, polyene antibiotics and LPS promoted membrane depolarization, whereas membrane voltage remained unchanged after anti-Ig treatment. Polyene antibiotics-induced depolarization originated from the increase of membrane permeability to Na^+ ions and occurred independently of Ca_i^{2+} changes.

The mitogen-induced rise in intracellular Ca^{2+} observed in activable cells is (at least in T-lymphocytes) accompanied by hyperpolarization. T line is assumed to be in relation with the existence of Ca^{2+}_{-} dependent K^{+} channels. Therefore, we concluded from the polyene-induced depolarization occurring independently of Ca^{2+}_{i} changes, the absence of these channels in the WEHI 231 cell line.

Finally, none of the early events observed after addition of AmBSH could specifically be related to WEHI 231 activation since they were observed, as well, with AmB which poorly activates this cell line. It should be added that neither protein kinase C nor phospholipase were significantly activated after addition of AmBSH (P. Sarthou personal communication).

It appears, therefore, that, at the present time, no good mechanistic explanation can be afforded to the lymphocyte stimulation obtained by AmBSH or N-Fructosyl AmB. We are currently investigating the modulation by these drugs of the membrane receptor internalization as a possible origin of this effect. On the other hand, up to now, AmB and its derivatives have always been assumed to act solely at the membrane level. It is quite possible that these drugs are internalized as we were able to show by fluorescence energy transfer from AmB to the probe DPH in T lymphocytes (42). They would act, therefore, by a totally different mechanism. It should be noted that the toxicity of AmBSH is smaller than that of AmB which, whatever is the activation mechanism, may allow greater amounts of drug to be added to lymphocytes and develop a type of activity impossible to obtain with AmB.

VI. CONCLUSIONS

The stimulation of immune defenses by AmB or AmE at sublethal doses is well established in mice. Some observations on patients go in the same direction. The origin of this effect is not clear, despite the numerous in vitro studies which have been performed but are often contradictory. Some AmB derivatives are potent activators of B lymphocytes in vitro. They deserve, therefore, further studies, the more as some of them have low toxicity for host-cells while keeping high activity against fungi. In vivo studies are currently being done.

BIBLIOGRAPHY

1. J. Brajtburg, W.G. Powderly, G.S. Kobayashi and G. Medoff, *Amphotericin B : Current understanding of mechanisms of action*, Antimicrob. Ag. Chemother., 34:183 (1990).
2. J. Bolard, *How do the polyene macrolide antibiotics affect the cellular membrane properties*, Biochim. Biophys. Acta, 864:257 (1986).
3. G. Medoff, J. Brajtburg, G.S. Kobayashi and J. Bolard, *Antifungal agents useful in therapy of systemic fungal infections*, Ann. Rev. Pharmacol. Toxicol., 232:303 (1983).
4. W.E. Hauser and J.S. Remington, *Effect of antibiotics on the immune response*, Am. J. Med., 72, 711 (1982).
5. S.H. Stein, J.R. Little and K.D. Little, *Parallel inheritance of tissue catalase activity and immunostimulatory action of amphotericin B in inbred mouse strains.* Cell. Immunol., 105:99 (1987).
6. T.J. Blanke, J.R. Little, S.F. Shirley and R.G. Lynch, *Augmentation of murine immune response by amphotericin B.* Cell. Immunol., 33:180 (1977).
7. H.S. Lin, G. Medoff and G.S. Kobayashi, *Effects of amphotericin B on macrophages and their precursor cells.* Antimicrob. Ag. Chemother., 11:154 (1977).
8. T. Dikeacou, E. Drouhet, B. Dupont et C. Romana, *Action de l'amphotéricine B sur la capacité phagocytaire des phagocytes mononucléaires, étudiée in vivo en employant le test fenêtre cutanée.* Bull. Soc. Mycol. Méd., 9:59 (1980).
9. F. Bistoni, A. Vecchiarelli, R. Mazzolla, P. Pucetti, P. Marconi and E. Garaci, *Immunoadjuvant activity of amphotericin B as displayed in mice infected with* Candida albicans. Antimicrob. Ag. Chemother., 27:625 (1985).
10. A. Vecchiarelli, G. Verducci, S. Perito, P. Pucetti, P. Marconi and F. Bistoni, *Involvment of host macrophages in the immunoadjuvant activity of amphotericin B in a mouse fungal infection model.* J. Antibiotics, 39:846 (1986)
11. J.E. Wolf and S.E. Masoff, *In vivo activation of macrophage oxidative burst activity by cytokines and amphotericin B.* Infect. Immunity, 58:1296 (1990).
12. H.A. Jr Chapman and J.B. Jr. Hibbs, *Modulation of macrophage tumoricidal capability by polyene antibiotics : support for membrane lipid as a regulatory determinant of macrophage function.* Proc. Natl. Acad. Sci. USA, 75:4349 (1978).

13. J.R. Perfect, D.L. Granger and D.T. Durack, *Effects of antifungal agents and gamma interferon on macrophage cytotoxicity for fungi and tumor cells.* J. Infect. Dis., 156:316 (1987).
14. J.A. Gelfand, K. Kimball, J.F. Burke and C.A. Dinarello, *Amphotericin B treatment of human mononuclear cells in vitro results in secretion of tumor necrosis factor and interleukin-1.* Clin. Res., 36:456 A (1988).
15. J.K.S. Chia and M. Pollack, *Amphotericin B induces tumor necrosis factor production by murine macrophages.* J. Infect. Dis., 159:113 (1989).
16. R.T. Mehta, K. Mehta, G. Lopez-Berestein and R.L. Juliano, *Effect of liposomal amphotericin B on murine macrophages and lymphocytes.* Infect. Immunity, 47:429 (1985).
17. D.J. Marmer, B.T. Fields, G.M. France and R.W. Steele, *Ketoconazole, amphotericin B and amphotericin B methyl ester : comparative in vitro and in vivo toxicological effects on neutrophil functions.* Antimicrob. Ag. Chemother., 20:660 (1981).
18. E.M. Johnson, D.W. Warnock, M.D. Richardson and C.J. Douglas, *In vitro effect of itraconazole, ketoconazole and amphotericin B on the phagocytic and candidacidal function of human neutrophils.* J. Antimicrob. Chemother, 18:83 (1986).
19. B. Bjorksten, C. Ray and P.G. Quie, *Inhibition of human neutrophil chemotaxis and chemiluminescence by amphotericin B.* Infect Immunity, 14:315 (1976).
20. H.D. Gresham, L.T. Clement, J.E. Volanakis and E.J. Brown, *Cholera toxin and pertussis toxin regulate the* F_c *receptor-mediated phagocytic response of human neutrophils in a manner analogous to regulation by monoclonal antibody IC2.* J. Immunology, 139:4159 (1987).
21. P. Van der Auvera and F. Meunier, *In vitro effects of cilofungin, amphotericin B and amphotericin B-deoxycholate on human polypor-phonuclear leukocytes.* J. Antimicrob. Chemother., 24:747 (1989).
22. K.M. Lohr and R. Snyderman, *Amphotericin B alters the affinity and functional activity of the oligopeptide chemotactic factor receptor on human polymorphonuclear leukocytes.* J. Immunology, 129:1594 (1982).
23. K. Yasui, M. Masuda, T. Matsuoka, M. Yamazaki, A. Komiyama, T. Akabane and K. Murata, *Miconazole and amphotericin B alter polymorphonuclear leukocytes functions.* Antimicrob. Ag. Chemother., 32:1864 (1988).
24. E. Roilides, J.W. Walsh, M. Rubin, D. Venzon and P.A Pizzo, *Effects of antifungal agents on the function of human neutrophils in vitro*, Antimicrob. Ag. Chemother., 34:196 (1990).

25. J.P. Siegel and J.S. Remington, *Effect of antimicrobial agents on chemiluminescence of human polymorphonuclear leukocytes in response to phagocytosis.* J. Antimicrob. Ag. Chemother., 19:284 (1982).
26. S.R. Supapidhayakui, L.R. Kizlaitis and B.R. Andersen, *Stimulation of human and canine neutrophil metabolism by amphotericin B.* Antimicrob. Ag. Chemother., 19:234 (1981).
27. E. Lingaas and T. Midtvedt, *Dissociated effect of amphotericin B and deoxycholate on phagocytosis of Escherichia Coli by human polymorphonuclear neutrophils.* Drugs Exptl. Clin. Res. XI:747 (1985).
28. L. Hammarström and E. Smith, *In vivo activating properties of polyene antibiotics for murine lymphocytes.* Acta Path. Microbiol. Scand., 85:277 (1977).
29. H. Ishikawa, H. Narimatsu and K. Saito, *Adjuvant effect of nystatin on in vitro antibody response of mouse spleen cells to heterologous erythrocytes.* Microbiol. Immunol., 21:137 (1977).
30. H. Ishikawa, H. Narimatsu and K. Saito, *Mechanisms of the adjuvant effect of nystatin on in vitro antibody response of mouse spleen cells : indication of nystatin as a B-cell mitogen and a stimulant for polyclonal antibody synthesis in B cells.* Cell. Immunol., 17:300 (1975).
31. E.V. Walls and J.E. Kay, *Inhibition of proliferation of a murine myeloma cell line and mitogen-stimulated B lymphocytes by the antibiotic amphotericin B (Fungizone).* Immunology, 47:115 (1982).
32. G.S. Kobayashi, J.R. Little and G. Medoff, *In vitro and in vivo comparisons of amphotericin B and N-D-ornythyl amphotericin B methyl ester.* Antimicrob. Ag. Chemother., 27:302 (1985).
33. J.R. Little, A. Abegg and E. Plut, *The relationship between adjuvant and mitogenic effects of amphotericin B methyl ester.* Cell. Immunol., 78:224 (1983).
34. P. Sarthou, D. Primi and P.A. Cazenave, *B cell triggering properties of a non toxic derivative of amphotericin B.* J. Immunol., 137:2156 (1986).
35. N. Henry-Toulmé, J. Bolard, B. Hermier and M. Seman, *Immunomodulating properties of the N-(1-deoxy-D-fructos-1-yl) derivative of amphotericin B, in mice.* Immunol. Lett., 20:63 (1989).
36. J.R. Little and V. Shore, *Modulation by lipoproteins of amphotericin B-induced immunostimulation.* Cell. Immunol., 93:212 (1985).
37. A. Tärnvik and S. Ansehn, *Effect of amphotericin B and clotrimazole on lymphocyte stimulation.* Antimicrob. Ag. Chemother., 6:529 (1974).

38. G.A. Roselle and C.A. Kauffman, *Amphotericin B and 5-fluorocytosine : in vitro effects on lymphocyte functions.* Antimicrob. Ag. Chemother., 14:398 (1978).
39. R.H. Alford and B.B. Cartwright, *Comparison of ketoconazole and amphotericin B in interference with thymidine uptake and blastogenesis of lymphocytes stimulated with histoplasma capsulatum antigens.* Antimicrob. Ag. Chemother., 24:575 (1983).
40. M.P.N. Nair and S.A. Schwartz, *Immunomodulatory effects of amphotericin B on cellular toxicity of normal human lymphocytes.* Cell. Immunol., 70:287 (1982).
41. N. Henry-Toulmé, P. Sarthou and J. Bolard, *Early membrane potential and cytoplasmic calcium changes during mitogenic stimulation of WEHI 231 cell line by polyene antibiotics, lipopolysaccharide and anti-immunoglobulin* . Biochim. Biophys. Acta, 1051:285 (1990).
42. N. Henry-Toulmé, M. Séman and J. Bolad, *Interaction of amphotericin B and its N-fructosil derivative with murine thymocytes : a comparative study using fluorescent membrane probes.* Biochim. Biophys. Acta, 982:245 (1989).

26

Granulocyte-Macrophage Colony Stimulating Factor with Amphotericin B for the Treatment of Disseminated Fungal Infections in Neutropenic Cancer Patients

E. Anaissie and G. P. Bodey

Section of Infectious Diseases
Department of Medical Specialties
The University of Texas, MD Anderson Cancer Center
Houston, Texas 77030, USA

Fungal infections remain one of the most frequent causes of morbidity and mortality in patients with hematological malignancies. When we recently looked at our experience at the University of Texas and the Anderson Cancer Center with causes of death in patients with acute leukemia, we realized that infection alone or infection plus hemorrhage constituted the majority of cases of death in this patient population. More specifically, fungal infections now constitute alone or with bacterial infection more than 50% of these causes of infectious death. This is a departure from previous experience which indicated that bacterial infections were much more frequent than mycotic ones. Several predisposing factors have been associated with these invasive, life-threatening fungal infections, including the use of broad spectrum antibacterial agents, the presence of indwelling central venous catheters, adrenocortical steroid therapy and other immunosuppressive drugs. However, the single most important factor remains what Bodey and others showed more than 25 years ago - that is, the presence of persistent and profound neutropenia: the neutrophil count decreases from normal to less than 100, the incidence of bacterial and fungal superinfection increases dramatically. The standard therapy for these fungal infections remains amphotericin B. However, while the drug is very active in patients with adequate neutrophil counts, its activity in a setting of profound persistent neutropenia is very poor.

Effect of Neutrophil Count on Response to Therapy of Systemic Candidiasis

	Treated		Untreated	
Neutrophil Count/mm^3	No.	% Response	No.	% Response
• > 1,000, Unchanges	2	50	14	0
• < 1,000, Increased	13	38	11	0
• < 1,000, Unchanged	25	0	68	0
• Total	40	15	93	0

The above figure shows the relationship of the neutrophil count to response in disseminated candidiasis, as collected from retrospective analysis of our cases of systemic Candida infection. You can see in the right-hand column that untreated patients, as expected, had a zero percent response rate. On the other hand, there was a 38% response rate in those patients who started with neutropenia and had subsequent increase in the neutrophil count. But please note the zero percent response rate, 0 out of 25 patients, in those who started with neutropenia and persisted with counts of less than 1000 throughout their episode. Similar results have been obtained from several other institutions and can be best explained by what was earlier referred to as the lack of availability of amphotericin B to the fungi.

Clearly, then, shortening the duration of neutropenia and improving the functional activity of neutrophils, macrophage and monocytes may perhaps be associated with better response rate in these patients. In order to address this question, we planned a pilot study using granulocyte macrophage colony-stimulating factor (GMCSF) together with the standard drug, amphotericin B. The treatment plan consisted of giving amphotericin B at 1mg/kg per day as a four-hour infusion for a minimum of 1 gram, until resolution of all signs and symptoms of infection. GMCSF was used as 400 ug/m^2 per day as a 24-hour continuous infusion, and was given from 2-6 weeks, depending on the response of the neutrophil count. Both drugs had dosage modification depending on response and toxicity. The eligibility criteria are shown in the figure above. We excluded patients with superficial infections and patients with positive blood cultures but without any clinical or radiologic evidence of invasive infection. In addition, a neutrophil count of less than 100 was required for patient inclusion, as well as a serum creatinine of less than 3 mg/dl.

Criteria for Patient Eligibility

- Documented Systemic Mycoses
  - Biopsy proven
  - Multiple positive blood cultures
  - Exclusions - superficial infection and catheter-associated fungemia without tissue invasion

- Other Requirements
  - Neutropenia < 100 μl
  - Renal function: Cr < 3 mg/dl

The response criteria were defined as follows: complete response meant total disappearance of all signs and symptoms of infection as well as laboratory and microbiologic evidence of eradication of infection. Partial response essentially addressed those patients with aspergillosis where there was clear evidence of clinical and radiologic improvement, but persistence of a pulmonary cavity that may not resolve with continuous therapy. Failure indicated the persistence or progression of any indicator of infection. We assessed all these patients at six weeks and, wherever possible, at six months after completion of therapy. The characteristics of the evaluable patients are shown at the top of the next page. We entered 11 patients, of which 8 were evaluable. Three were inevaluable: one pa-

Results of Therapy According to Infection

Infection	No Pts.	Outcome
Disseminated candidiasis	4	CR (3), F (1)
Disseminated aspergillosis	2	PR (1), F (1)
Disseminated candidiasis and aspergillosis	1	F
Disseminated trichosporinosis	1	CR
Pulmonary candidiasis	1	CR

CR: Complete Response. PR: Partial response. F: Failure

Drug-Related Side Effects

• Total patients	8
• No toxicity	4
• Hypotension	4
• Nephrotoxicity	4
• Capillary leak syndrome	3
• Hepatic	2

tient had an incorrect diagnosis, 2 received only one dose of granulocyte macrophage colony stimulating factor and died from other unrelated causes. We had 8 patients with a median age of 58; 7 patients had acute leukemia: myelogenous in 6 and lymphoblastic in one, while one patient had metastatic breast cancer and had undergone high dose chemotherapy with autologous bone marrow transplantation. The results of therapy showed response in 3 patients with disseminated candidiasis, one patient with disseminated trichosporiosis, and one patient with pulmonary candidiasis. As expected, the response was associated with the recovery of the neutrophils. All six patients whose neutrophil count recovered either spontaneously or because of GMCSF had some kind of a response: complete in 5 and partial in one, while both patients who remained profoundly neutropenic died of their fungal infection. This apparent improvement in response rate was, however, associated with substantial toxicities.

The final figure shows that we had 50% significant toxicity, including the capillary leak syndrome and severe hypotension. In fact, one of our patients may have died from GMCSF-induced toxicity. Other side effects included nephrotoxicity, but that was expected with amphotericin B, and in 2 patients significant hepatic dysfunction.

In conclusion, GMCSF plus amphotericin B appears to be associated with an improved response rate in invasive mycoses in the neutropenic cancer patient. A different dosage schedule may result in an improved therapeutic index. Additional prospective randomized studies can best address the issue of whether GMCSF does, indeed, improve the response rate in these infections.

27

Recombinant G-CSF Induces Anti-*Candida albicans* Activity in Neutrophil Cultures and Protection in Fungal Infected Mice

Y. Yamamoto, K. Uchida*, T. Hasegawa, H. Friedman, T.W. Klein, and H. Yamaguchi*

Department of Medical Microbiology and Immunology, University of South Florida College of Medicine, Tampa, FL U.S.A., 33612

**Research Center for Medical Mycology, Teikyo University School of Medicine, Tokyo, Japan*

INTRODUCTION

One of the most important host-defense mechanisms against invading microorganisms is phagocytosis, followed by intracellular killing and digestion of microorganisms by phagocytic cells. At the early phase of infection, neutrophils have a powerful defense ability against microorganisms. Recently it has been shown that the survival, growth, and differentiation of progenitor cells of these phagocytic cells are controlled by hemopoietic colony-stimulating factors (CSF)(1). Granulocyte colony-stimulating factor (G-CSF) is one of the hemopoietic factors which induces hemopoietic precursor cells to proliferate and differentiate to neutrophils (2). G-CSF administered to neutropenic animals causes the recovery to the normal level of neutrophils in the blood (3,4). Matsumoto, et al.(5) have recently reported the protective effect of natural G-CSF in microbial infection in neutropenic mice. These reports suggest that G-CSF might be a useful cytokine for treating neutropenic patients with secondary infections. However, there is little evidence that G-CSF activates the antimicrobial activity of neutrophils in culture against bacterial and fungal infections. The study reported here was designed to investigate the potential effects of G-CSF on the anti-*Candida albicans* activity of cultured human blood neutrophils. Furthermore, it was also studied whether G-CSF treatment of neutropenic mice can protect following infection with fungi such as *Candida, Cryptococcus* and *Aspergillus*. The results of this study suggest that G-CSF can readily activate neutrophils in culture to restrict the growth of yeast. And G-CSF was also able to protect significantly against systemic infections caused by either *C. albicans, C. neoformans* or *A. fumigatus*. These *in vitro* and *in vivo* data suggest that prophylactic therapy with G-CSF may be useful against fungal infections in immunocompromised patients.

MATERIALS AND METHODS

Animals: Female outbred mice, ICR, were obtained from Charles River Japan, Kanagawa, Japan. The mice were 6 to 8 weeks of age at the time of the experiments.

Neutrophils: Human neutrophils were isolated from leukocyte buffy coats obtained from healthy volunteers. The white cell layer lying on the surface of the red blood cell pellet after Ficoll-Hypaque (Pharmacia Fine Chemicals, Piscataway, NJ) centrifugation was collected and was treated with 10 vol of ACK solution (0.83% NH_4Cl, 0.1% $KHCO_3$, 0.1mM Na_2EDTA) to lyse red blood cells. The cells were washed twice in Hanks' balanced salt solution (HBSS) and then suspended in RPMI 1640 medium (Gibco Laboratories, Madison, WI) containing 1 % heat inactivated fetal calf serum (FCS, Hyclone Laboratories, Logan, UT). Cytocentrifuged preparations of neutrophil showed greater than 98 % pure and

99 % viable by the Giemsa staining method and the trypan blue dye exclusion method, respectively.

Microorganisms: *Candida albicans* TIMM 0239 and TIMM 1768, *Cryptococcus neoformans* TIMM 0362 and *Aspergillus fumigatus* F-48 were used in this study. The yeast were maintained on Sabouraud's dextrose agar and at the time of use were inoculated onto fresh Sabouraud's agar plates for 24 hrs at 37 C and harvested into pyrogen free saline. The suspension of *Aspergillus* conidia were prepared from 7 days old culture on Sabouraud's agar plates at 27 C. The number of yeast or conidia was measured by hemocytometer counts and adjusted to a working concentration with saline.

G-CSF: Recombinant human G-CSF was produced in an *E. coli* expression system and purified to homogeneity using HPLC as previously described (6). The CSF activity of the protein was 2.1×10^8 U/mg. Endotoxin was not detected by *Limulus* amoebocyte lysate assay (E-toxate, Sigma Chemical Co., St. Louis, MO) in this preparations.

Assay for growth inhibition of *Candida* in neutrophil cultures: Inhibition of *Candida* growth by neutrophils was accomplished by the following procedures. Briefly, 50 ul of the neutrophil suspension (1×10^6/ml) in 1 % FCS-RPMI 1640 medium was added to triplicate wells of a 96-well flat bottomed microplate. Then 20 ul of the appropriate concentrations of G-CSF and 50 ul of *C. albicans* at 1×10^4/ml were added to wells containing effector cells, yielding effector:target (E:T) ratio of 100:1. After the cell mixtures were incubated for 15 hrs at 37 C in 5 % CO2, 80 ul of 0.25 % saponin (Sigma) was added to lyse effector cells. The number of viable *Candida* in the wells was determined by the plate count method. The cell lysates were diluted with HBSS and plated on Sabouraud's dextrose agar plates. The plates were incubated at 37 C for 48 hrs and then counted for colony forming units (CFU). Saponin and G-CSF had no effect on *Candida* viability.

Phagocytosis assay: For phagocytosis assay of neutrophils, 1×10^6 neutrophils in 100 ul of 1 % FCS-RPMI 1640 medium, with and without appropriate concentrations of G-CSF, were placed in polypropylene tubes (10 x 75 mm, Falcon, Oxnard, CA) and incubated for 3 hrs at 37 C in 5 % CO2. The opsonized FITC labeled heat killed *Candida albicans*, 1 x 10^7/100 ul, were added to the tubes, incubated with shaking for 10 min at 37 C and phagocytosis measured by FACS (fluorescence activated cell sorter, Ortho Diagnostic System, Westwood) analysis using trypan blue quenching technique as previously described (7,8). Microscopic observation was also performed on these samples.

Animal study: The mice were injected intraperitoneally (i.p.) with 200 mg of cyclophosphamide (CY, Shionogi Pharmaceuticals, Osaka, Japan) per kg. Beginning on the day after CY injection, the mice were injected subcutaneously (s.c.) once a day with G-CSF (15, 60, 120 or 240 ug/kg/day) or vehicle for 3 days. Fungi were injected intravenously (i.v.) one day after the final injection of G-CSF or vehicle. In the case of *A. fumigatus* infection, G-CSF was injected twice (total of 5 injections) more following infection. The number of deaths was counted for 22 days after infection. The number of viable *Candida* in infected organs was detected by the following procedures. Mice were injected i.v. with 2 x 10^4 of *C. albicans* 4 days after CY injection. G-CSF or vehicle was given i.v. to mice once a day for 3 days starting one day after CY injection. At one to five days after infection, mice were sacrificed and the number of viable *Candida* in the homogenates of kidneys which were prepared in sterile saline was detected on Sabouraud's agar plates. Colonies were counted 2 days after incubation.

Statistical analysis: Variations are expressed as the standard error of the mean. *P* values were calculated with Student's *t* test.

RESULTS AND DISCUSSION

Activation of neutrophils in vitro.

Recently it has been reported that G-CSF regulates not only differentiation of hemopoietic progenitor cells but also the functions of mature neutrophils such as reactive oxygen production and membrane potential changes stimulated by

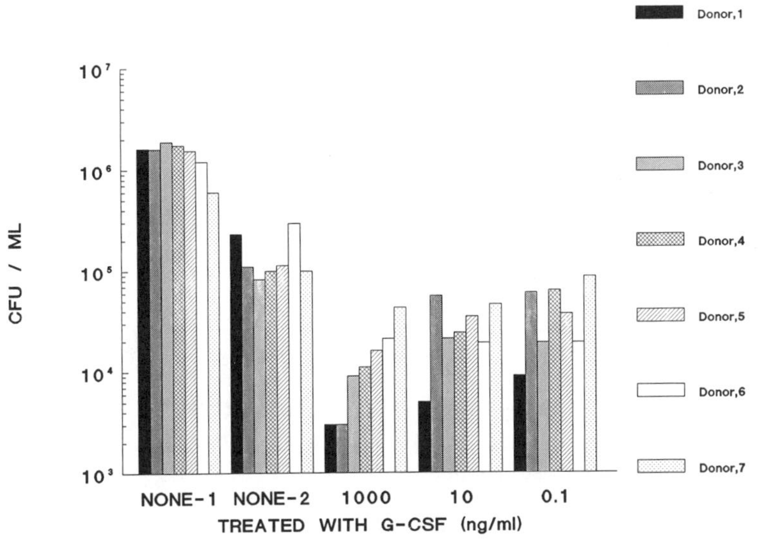

Fig.1 Effect of G-CSF on the anti-*C. albicans* activity of neutrophils. Isolated human neutrophils, 5 x 10^4 were cultured with or without G-CSF and infected with 5 x 10^2 of *C. albicans*. The cultures were incubated for 15 hrs at 37°C in 5% CO2 and the number of viable yeast per culture determined by culture lysis and dilution plating on Sabouraud's agar plates. Each column shows the mean of triplicate cultures of individual donor. None-1; yeast only, None-2; yeast cultured with normal neutrophils.

fMLP (N-formyl-methionyl-leucyl-phenylalanine)(9-11). More recently, Buckle and Hogg (12) reported that the treatment with G-CSF induced the up-regulation of expression of FcRIII receptor on neutrophils. These reports apparently suggest that G-CSF can modulate the functions of mature neutrophils directly. However, up to now, there is little information about whether G-CSF can boost the anti-microbial activity of neutrophils. Here, we report that G-CSF can enhance the anti-microbial activity of mature neutrophils in vitro.

Human peripheral neutrophils were isolated from buffy coats of healthy volunteers and 5 x 10^4cells were added to individual wells. Five hundred *Candida albicans* were added either to culture wells alone (none-1), wells containing untreated neutrophils (none-2), or wells containing neutrophils treated with G-CSF. The cultures were incubated for 15 hrs and then the number of viable *Candida* measured after lysis of neutrophils. It can be seen from Fig 1

Table 1. The effect of G-CSF on phagocytosis by neutrophils of *C. albicans*[a]

Treatment of G-CSF[b]	Neutrophils Phagocytizing (%)[c]	Fluorescent Intensity[d]	Phagocytic Index[e]
None	59.6	528.5	31499
10 ng/ml	86.8	653.0	56680

[a] Phagocytosis of neutrophils was measured by FACS using FITC labeled heat killed *C. albicans*.
[b] Neutrophils were incubated for 3 hrs with or without G-CSF.
[c] Neutrophils (3,000) were evaluated by FACS and the percentage of cells positive for internalized yeast calculated.
[d] Fluorescent intensity is indicator of the relative number of internalized yeast.
[e] Phagocytic index was calculated (neutrophils phagocytizing x fluorescent intensity). This value is an index of the total phagocytic capacity of the neutrophil population.

that G-CSF apparently boosted the anti-*Candida* activty of neutrophils. That is, 100 to 10 times fewer CFU's were found in neutrophil cultures treated with 1,000 ng/ml of G-CSF in comparison with non-treated neutrophil cultures. Even 0.1 ng/ml of G-CSF treatment induced significant restriction of *Candida* growth in neutrophil cultures (three of seven donors). The phagocytic activity of G-CSF treated neutrophils was measured by FACS analysis using FITC labeled *C. albicans*. Isolated neutrophils were incubated with or without 10 ng/ml of G-CSF for 3 hrs and then treated with FITC labeled *Candida*. The effector:target (E:T) ratio was 1:10. Following a 10 min incubation with shaking, neutrophils were fixed with paraformaldehyde and treated with trypan blue for quenching the extracellular yeast fluorescence. Trypan blue excludes extracellular yeast from counting process (8). Table 1 shows representative results from five donors. The treatment with G-CSF enhanced both the percent of cell phagocytizing and also the fluorescent intensity which is an indicator of the number of yeast particles internalized per neutrophil. The total phagocytic capacity of the G-CSF treated cells (i.e. phagocytic index) was almost double that of the non-treated cells. These findings were also confirmed microscopically by staining portions of the samples with Giemsa stain. Buckle and Hogg have recently shown that membrane expression of FcRIII was increased by G-CSF treatment (12). Yuo et al. have also reported the G-CSF increased the expression of C3bi receptors on human granulocytes and enhanced granulocyte adherence to nylon fiber (13). These previous reports support our findings, in that yeast uptake could be mediated by increased surface receptors such as FcR and CR3. From these in vitro studies, it is apparent that G-CSF can enhance the anti-*Candida* activity of mature neutrophils including enhancement of phagocytosis.

Protective activity against *Candida* infection.

It is widely accepted that neutrophils are protective against invading microorganisms such as pathogenic fungi. Neutrophils ingest and kill microorganisms and play a role as a first defense line in microbial infections. Therefore, leukopenia especially neutropenia carries a serious risk of infection in patients. Administration of G-CSF is known to restore the level of neutrophils in neutropenic animals (3, 4). So, it was expected that G-CSF treatment would protect against infections in immunocompromised patients. However, until now there is little information available concerning the protective activity of G-CSF against microbial infections, especially fungal infections in vivo. In this study, we used cyclophosphamide (CY) to induce neutropenia in mice. The number of blood neutrophils was reduced to approximately one fifth of normal levels by 3 to 4 days after injection of CY. Treatment with G-CSF, 30 ug to 240 ug/kg/day x 3 days, caused the number of peripheral neutrophils to increase at 24 hrs after the last injection of G-CSF (data not shown). Infection with a relatively low dose (2 x 10^4 yeast/mouse) of *C. albicans* in CY treated mice caused the death of all mice by 7 days after infection. As can be seen from Fig 2, all of the G-CSF treatments significantly prolonged the survival of *Candida* infected mice and this prolongation was cytokine dose dependent. The number of viable *Candida* in the kidney of infected mice was also investigated. Mice

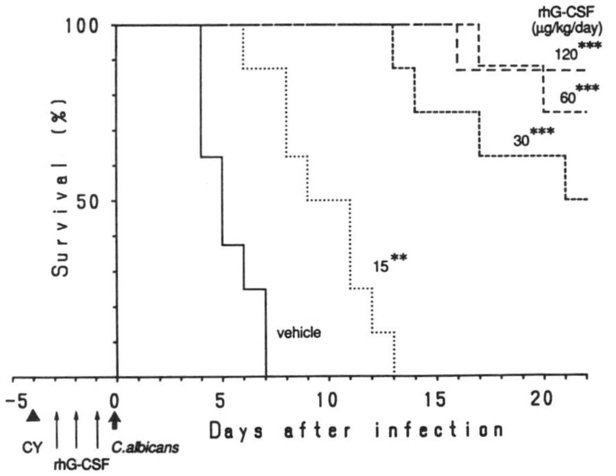

Fig. 2 Protective effect of rhG-CSF against *C. albicans* infection in CY-pretreated mice. Mice were inoculated intravenously with *C. albicans* ($2x10^4$/mouse) 4 days after CY injection. rhG-CSF (dashed line) or vehicle (solid line) was given subcutaneously to mice once a day for 3 days starting one day after CY injection. Each group consisted of 8 mice. **;p<0.01, ***;p<0.001: significantly different from the group of mice injected with vehicle.

were infected with 2 x 10^4 yeasts 4 days after CY injection. The G-CSF was given to mice once a day for 3 days starting one day after CY injection. The kidneys were taken from the mice at one to five days after infection and the number of CFU measured in the homogenates of kidneys. Fig 3 shows the results of this study. Vehicle treated mice (CY treated only, no G-CSF treatment) showed a high number of yeasts recovered from the kidney which is known to be a target organ of experimental *Candida* infection in mice. Treatment with G-CSF significantly reduced the number of yeasts in kidney (i.e. greater than 100 fold) compared with the number of yeasts in the kidney of non-treated control mice. Even the relatively low concentration of 15 ug/kg of G-CSF induced a significant inhibition of yeast growth in kidney. These data correlated well with the results of the mortality curves of G-CSF treated animals (Fig 2). That is, recovery of low numbers of viable yeast from the kidney in G-

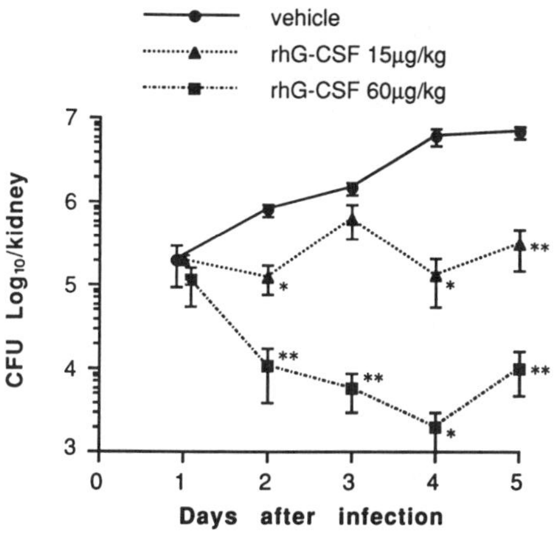

Fig. 3 Effect of rhG-CSF on the number of *C. albicans* cells in the kidney of CY-pretreated mice. Mice were inoculated intravenously with *C. albicans* ($2x10^4$/mouse) 4 days after CY injection. rhG-CSF or vehicle was given intravenously to mice once a day for 3 days starting one day after CY injection. The results are expressed as means of 3 mice ± SEM. *;$p<0.05$, **;$p<0.01$: significantly different from the group of mice injected with vehicle.

CSF treated mice coincided with relatively long survival times in these animals.

Protective activity against *Cryptococcus* and *Aspergillus* infections.

Cryptococcosis and aspergillosis are common fungal infections in immunocompromised hosts (14). From previous reports, it was suggested that the development of these infections correlates with the host immune conditions, especially defects of the certain immunological functions (15). Neutropenia and defective neutrophils also contribute to problems of resistance to these fungal infections (16). In this study, we investigated the immunotherapeutic efficacy of G-CSF for these fungal infections in neutropenic mice. In the case of *C. neoformans* infection, mice were injected with CY and treated with G-CSF as in the *Candida* infection studies. Fig 4 shows that all control mice which received

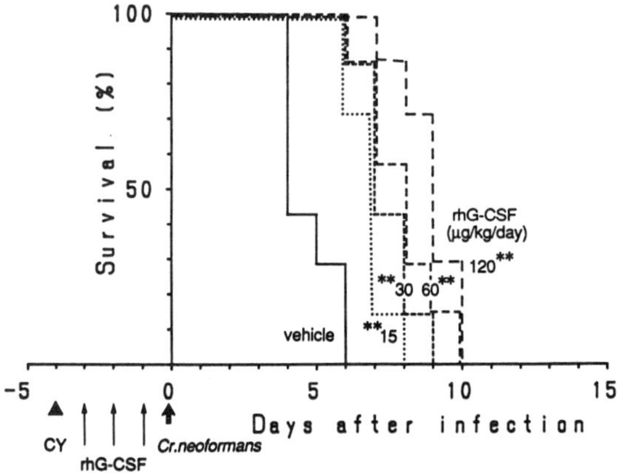

Fig. 4 Protective effect of rhG-CSF against *C. neoformans* infection in CY-pretreated mice. Mice were inoculated intravenously with *C. neoformans* ($1x10^6$/mouse) 4 days after CY injection. rhG-CSF (dashed line) or vehicle (solid line) was given subcutaneously to mice once a day for 3 days starting one day after CY injection. Each group consisted of 7 mice. **;p<0.01:significantly different from the group of mice injected with vehicle.

CY and were infected with *C. neoformans*, died within 6 days after infection. In contrast, G-CSF treated mice showed significantly prolonged survival. The effect of G-CSF on *Aspergillus* infection in mice was also investigated. Mice were given G-CSF a total of five times, that is, once a day with either 15, 30, 60 or 120 ug/kg of G-CSF for 3 days before infection, and 2 daily doses after infection. As can be seen in Fig 5, G-CSF treatment resulted in the prolongation of survival periods of *Aspergillus* infected mice.

When the effects of G-CSF on these fungal infections were compared with each other, the cytokine appeared to be the least effective against *C. neoformans* infection. It was well documented that infections caused by these encapsulated fungi are major causes of morbidity and mortality in patients with impaired cell-mediated immunity (17), and cell-mediated immunity is an important protective mechanism against *C. neoformans* (18-20). Moreover, the capsule of *C.*

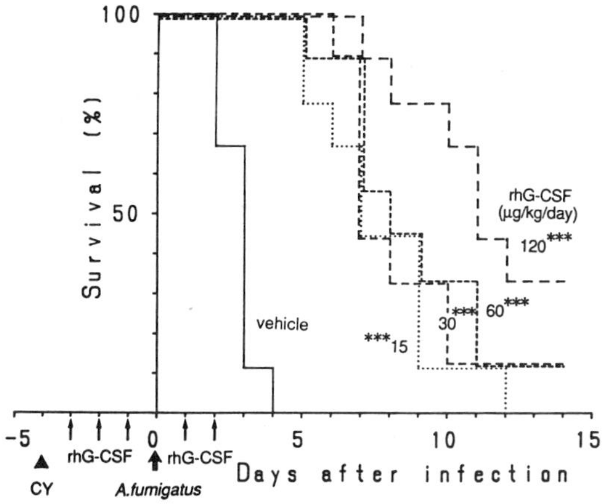

Fig. 5 Protective effect of rhG-CSF against *A. fumigatus* infection in CY-pretreated mice. Mice were inoculated intravenously with *A. fumigatus* ($1x10^6$/mouse) 4 days after CY injection. rhG-CSF (dashed line) or vehicle (solid line) was given subcutaneously to mice once a day for 3 days before inoculation and for 2 days after inoculation. Each group consisted of 9 mice. ***;$p<0.001$: significantly different from the group of mice injected with vehicle.

neoformans appears to inhibit phagocytosis by macrophages, monocytes, and neutrophils (21). From these results it is not surprising that *C. neoformans* was relatively virulent in our system. However, it is noteworthy that G-CSF treatment had some effect in neutropenic mice. Besides *Cryptococcus* infection, neutropenic mice were also significantly protected against *Candida* and *Aspergillus*. This protection may be related to enhancement of the neutrophil phagocytic capacity as suggested by our in vitro findings or to other mechanisms.

Recently Matsumoto et al. (5) have reported that treatment of neutropenic mice with natural human G-CSF protected against systemic infections caused by bacteria and yeasts. Cohen et al. (22) have also demonstrated the treatment with recombinant human G-CSF induced resistance to lethal injection with *S. aureus* in neutropenic hamsters. Our results confirm and extend these reports, and support the efficacy of G-CSF as an immunotherapeutic agent in fungal infection.

In summary, recombinant human G-CSF readily activated human peripheral neutrophils in culture to restrict the growth of *C. albicans* and also enhanced the phagocytosis of *Candida*. In in vivo studies, G-CSF was able to protect significantly against systemic infections caused by all fungi tested including *C. albicans, C. neoformans* and *A. fumigatus*. Moreover, G-CSF treatment caused a decrease in the number of viable yeast in the kidneys of *Candida* infected mice. These in vitro and in vivo data suggest that prophylactic therapy with G-CSF may be useful against fungal infections in immunocompromised patients.

ACKNOWLEDGMENT

This work was supported by grants-in aid from Kirin Brewery Co., Tokyo and Amgen Biologicals, Thousand Oaks, CA.

REFERENCES

1) Nicola,N.A., and Vadas,M. Hematopoietic colony-stimulating factors. *Immunol. Today*, **5**:76-80, 1984.

2) Metcalf,D. The molecular biology and functions of the granulocyte-macrophage colony-stimulating factors. *Blood*, **67**:257-267, 1986.

3) Welte,K., Bonilla,M.A., Gillion,A.P., Boone,T.C., Potter,G.K., Gabrilove,J.L., Moore,M.A.S., O'Reiely,R.J., and Souza,L.M. Recombinant human granulocyte colony-stimulating factor: Effects on hematopoiesis in normal and cyclophosphamide-treated primates. *J.Exp.Med.*, **165**:941-948, 1987.

4) Tamura,M., Hattori,K., Nomura,H., Oheda,M., Kubota,N., Imazeki,I., Ono,M., Ueyama,Y., Nagata,S., Shirafuji,N., and Asano,S. Induction of neutrophilic granulocytosis in mice by administration of purified human native granulocyte colony-stimulating factor (G-CSF). *Biochem.Biophys.Res.Commun.*, **142**:454-460, 1987.

5) Matsumoto,M., Matsubara,S., Matsuno,T., Tamura,M., Hattori,K., Nomura,H., Ono,M., and Yokota,T. Protective effect of human granulocyte colony-stimulating factor on microbial infection in neutropenic mice. *Infect.Immun.*,

55:2715-2720, 1987.

6) Souza,L.M., Boone,T.C., Gabrilove,J., Lai,P.H., Zesbo,K.M., Murdock,D.C., Chazin,V.R., Bruszewsk,J., Lu,H., Chen,K.K., Barendt,J., Platzer,E., Moore,M.A.S., Mertelsman,R., and Welte,K. Recombinant human granulocyte colony-stimulating factor: Effects on normal and leukemic myeloid cells. *Science*, **232**:61-65, 1986.

7) Ogle,J.D., Noel,J.G., Sramkoski,R.M., Ogle,C.K., and Alexander,J.W. Phagocytosis of opsonized fluorescent microspheres by human neutrophils. *J.Immunol.Methods*, **115**:17-29, 1988.

8) Hed,J., Hallden,G., Johansson,S.G.O., and Larsson,P. The use of fluorescence quenching in flow cytofluorometry to measure the attachment and ingestion phase in phagocytosis in peripheral blood without prior cell separation. *J.Immunol.Methods*, **101**:119-125, 1987.

9) Kitagawa,S., Yuo,A., Souza,L.M., Saito,M., Miura,Y., and Takaku,F. Recombinant human granulocyte colony-stimulating factor enhances superoxide release in human granulocytes stimulated by chemotactic peptide. *Biochem.Biophys.Res.Commun.*, **144**:1143-1146, 1987.

10) Yuo,A., Kitagawa,S., Okabe,T., Urabe,A., Komatsu,Y., Itoh,S., and Takaku,F. Recombinant human granulocyte colony-stimulating factor repaires the abnormalities of neutrophil in patients with myelodysplastic syndromes and chronic myelogenous leukemia. *Blood*, **70**:404-411, 1987.

11) Sullivan,R., Griffin,J.D., Simons,E.R., Schafer,A.I., Meshulan,T., Fredette,J.P., Mass,A.K., Gadenne,A-S., Leavitt,J.L., and Melnick,D.A. Effects of recombinant human granulocyte and macrophage colony-stimulating factors on signal transduction pathways in human granulocytes. *J.Immunol.*, **139**:3422-3430, 1987.

12) Buckle,A.N., and Hogg,N. The effect of IFN-gamma and colony-stimulating factors on the expression of neutrophil cell membrane receptors. *J.Immunol.*, **143**:2295-2301, 1989.

13) Yuo,A., Kitagawa,S., Ohsaka,A., Ohta,M., Miyazono,K., Okabe,T., Urabe,A.,

Saito,M., and Takaku,F. Recombinant human granulocyte colony-stimulating factor as an activator of human granulocytes: potentiation of responses triggered by receptor-mediated agonists and stimulation of C3bi receptor expression and adherence. *Blood*, **74**:2144-2149, 1989.

14) Frason,D.W., Ward,J.I., Ajello,L., and Plikaytis,B.D. Aspergillosis and other systemic mycoses: the growing problem. *J.A.M.A.*, **242**:1631-1635, 1979.

15) Warnock,D.W. Immunological and other defects predisposing to fungal infections in the compromised host. In: Fungal Infection in the Compromised Patient, Warnock,D.W., and Richardson,M.D.(ed.), John Wiley and Sons, Chichester, pp.29-47, 1982.

16) Cohen,M.S., Isturiz,R.E., Malech,H.L., Root,R.K., Wilbert,C.M., Gutman,L., and Buckley,R.H. Fungal infection in chronic granulomatous disease: the importance of the phagocyte in defense against fungi. *Am.J.Med.*, **71**:59-66, 1981.

17) Diamond,R.D. *Cryptococcus neoformans*, In: Principles and Practice of Infectious Diseases, 2nd ed., Mandell,G.L., Douglas,Jr.R.G., and Bennett,J.E.(ed.), John Wiley and Sons, New York, pp.1460-1468, 1985.

18) Graybill,J.R., and Drutz,D.J. Host defense in cryptococcosis II. Cryptococcoses in the nude mouse. *Cell.Immunol.*, **40**:263-274, 1978.

19) Lim,T.S., and Murphy,J.W. Transfer of immunity to cryptococcoses by T-enriched splenic lymphocytes from *Cryptococcus neoformans*-sensitized mice. *Infect.Immun.*, **30**:5-11, 1980.

20) Fung,P.Y.S., and Murphy,J.W. In vitro interactions of immune lymphocytes and *Cryptococcus neoformans*. *Infect.Immun.*, **36**:1128-1138, 1982.

21) Kozel,T.R., Pfrommer,G.S.T., Guerlain,A.S., Highison,B.A., and Hizhison,G.J. Role of capsule in phagocytosis of *Cryptococcus neoformans*. *Rev.Infec.Dis.*, **10**:S436-S439, 1988.

22) Cohen,A.M., Hines,D.K., Korach,E.S., and Ratzkin,B.J. In vivo activation of neutrophil function in hamsters by recombinant human granulocyte colony-stimulating factor. *Infect.Immun.*, **56**:2861-2865, 1988.

PART VI

DRUG DELIVERY SYSTEMS FOR ANTIFUNGAL AGENTS

28

Use of Ambisome, Liposomal Amphotericin B, in Systemic Fungal Infections: Preliminary Findings of a European Multicenter Study

Presented by R. J. Hay

Department of Dermatology, Guys Hospital
St. Thomas's Street, London SE1 9RT, U.K.

INVESTIGATORS: M. Abecassis, R. Alemeleh, S. Blanche, N. Clumeck, P. Fenaux, F. Fraschini, A. Goldstone, N. Gorin. A. Gouvia, R. Hay, J. Klastersky, E. Kuse, A. Lindemann, F. Meunier, P. Meusers, P. Pierce, G. Prentice, O. Ringden, S. Rodenhuis, W. Schroyens, C. Stoutenbeek, S. Tura, M. Viviani, R. Walner, R. Zirkulnig, R. Zittoun

SUMMARY

This preliminary analysis of the drug Ambisome, liposomal amphotericin B, in systemic fungal infections was based on a study of the drug in patients who have failed to respond to or tolerate alternatives or who were in acute renal failure. The clinical and mycological responses were better in candidosis than aspergillosis, but in both groups a significant number of patients achieved remission. Work is proceeding on more detailed studies of different subgroups of patients with fungal disease. One important finding so far has been the lack of serious toxicity and the ability of patients to tolerate doses of amphotericin B considerably in excess of those used for conventional formulations of the compound.

INTRODUCTION

In the management of systemic mycoses the commonest choice of treatment is amphotericin B given by intravenous injection [1]. Amphotericin B (AmB), a polyene antifungal, has a broad spectrum of activity against the main fungal pathogens, wider than the other drugs and has been used for a considerably longer period. There have been few objective comparative studies with alternatives and therefore much of the information on dosages and adverse reactions is based on open studies and clinical experience [2]. It has been the treatment of choice, though, for most serious fungal infections including systemic candidosis, aspergillosis and mucormycosis. It is also used for the treatment of cryptococcal meningitis in nonAIDS patients in combination with flucytosine [3]. The major disadvantage of amphotericin B is the high incidence of adverse reactions. These range from hyperpyrexia, severe malaise, hypotension, thrombophlebitis, azotaemia, renal tubular damage, hypokalaemia, anaemia and hepatitis [2,4]. These are commonly encountered and most patients receiving amphotericin will show at least one of these side effects. Renal tubular damage is a predictable response occurring when total doses of this formulation of amphotericin B exceed 4g. However, rising urea and creatinine will often occur early in treatment leading to interruption or abandonment of therapy [5]. This common problem often leads to reluctance on the part of the physician to use the drug. Because of its usefulness for the severely sick attempts have been made to avoid or diminish the adverse effects [6,7,8]. Although it is possible to reduce the frequency of early reactions such as pyrexia with a slow build up of dosage or by using drugs such as antihistamines, it has not been feasible to prevent the renal side effects. For this reason considerable effort has been expended to find alternative analogues of the drug such as the methyl esters or a different formulation with reduced toxicity. The liposomal amphotericin B formulations [9,10] are examples of such developmental work where an alternative to the conventional form of amphotericin has been produced. Liposomes are phospholipid vesicles with a single or multiple layered membrane (uni- or multi-lamellar). The drug reported in this study, Ambisome, is an example of a uni-lamellar lipsomal formulation.

PATIENTS AND METHODS

The assessment of the efficacy of liposome encapsulated amphotericin B (Ambisome) has been carried out in open fashion in 115 episodes of infection in 109 patients (41F, 68M,). These were recruited under three main criteria - failure of prior treatment including amphotericin B in 34 patients (30%), 43 patients who had AMB related toxicity (37%) and 38 patients with significant renal impairment (33%). Data for 80 of these patients was available for analysis. The underlying diseases are reported in Table 1. The infections treated were as follows: systemic candidosis (46), invasive aspergillosis (28), mucormycosis (1), cryptococcosis (3), mycetoma due to *Madurella grisea* (2). The identity and extent of the infection were assessed on the basis of the clinical appearances and laboratory findings. Where possible, patients selected for inclusion in the study were those in whom the diagnosis was supported by objective evidence of infection. In practice the laboratory diagnosis was established in the patients as follows: culture (37), culture and histology (12), culture and serology (10), histology alone (11), histology and serology (2), serology (8). With those infections whose diagnosis was confirmed by histology or blood culture or even the demonstration of circulating cryptococcal antigen there is a measure of agreement on the validity of such tests in supporting the diagnosis. In seven acutely ill patients the interpretation of the diagnostic tests was

Table 1

Predisposing factors in patients receiving Ambisome

Acute Leukaemia	30	
AIDS	4	
Solid organ transplant	15	(liver in 8)
Lymphoma	5	
Diabetes mellitus	5	
Others*	21	

* - sarcoidosis, chronic lymphatic leukaemia, neutropenia, bone marrow aplasia, renal failure, chronic granulomatous disease.

more difficult to assess - candidosis supported by serology or sputum cultures alone (5) and aspergillosis in non neutropenic patients diagnosed by positive sputum culture (2). In 10 patients the diagnosis was presumptive, it not being possible to establish, by any objective criteria, the nature of the infection.

Toxicity was assessed in all patients by monitoring blood parameters at least twice weekly. These included renal and liver function and full blood counts as well as urine chemistry. A full clinical assessment was recorded at least twice weekly and often more frequently.

Treatment was given daily and Ambisome was administered by intravenous infusion. Patients started therapy either at the same dose of AmB they had been receiving previously or the dose was increased rapidly daily to 3mg/kg or higher. In the later stages of this work doses of 1mg/kg were administered without a test dose and slow build up of daily dose levels.

RESULTS

Fifty four patients who survived completed at least 10 days therapy. Thirty seven patients died during therapy and in four cases treatment was stopped at the request of the patient. In addition, four patients developed severe intercurrent illnesses and the therapy was stopped, four ceased Ambisome because of suspected adverse reactions and data from two were not analysed because of protocol violations. Data from 80 patients are available for analysis because these were clinically evaluable.

The mean time on Ambisome was 21.1 days (SD 26.5). The mean dose administered was 2370 mg (SD 2639) or 40.7 mg/kg. The mean maximum daily dose was 2.13 mg/kg (range 0.45 - 4.0). In total 48 (60%) patients had resolution of signs and symptoms and were rated as "in remission" at the end of treatment by the investigator. A further 14 (18%) were said to be improved and 18 (22%) did not respond and were rated as failures. In contrast, 42 patients developed mycological recovery on the basis of the reversal of previous laboratory findings. A further 17 could not be evaluated, because samples were not obtained from the relevant site after therapy. Twenty one patients showed no mycological improvement.

When the results were analysed for different organisms the results are shown in Table 2. It is interesting to note that 35 or

Table 2

Clinical and mycological efficacy after therapy with Ambisome

Infection	Clinical efficacy (%)			Mycological efficacy (%)		
	Cure	Improved	Fail	Cure	Persistent	NE[1]
Aspergillosis	7(25)	7(25)	14(50)	7(25)	13(50)	6(25)
Candidosis	35(76)	4(9)	7(15)	32(68)	7(15)	9(17)
Mucormycosis	1			1		
Cryptococcosis	2	1		2	1	
Mycetoma		2				2

1 - Not evaluated (see text)

76 % of the patients with systemic candidosis recovered clinically, 32 of whom (69%) also attained mycological remission. By contrast, 7 of the patients with aspergillosis (25%) were rated as clinically in remission and 7 were also clear mycologically (25 %). Twelve of the *Aspergillus* patients had persistent cultures and 14 were rated as clinical failures. By contrast the one patient with mucormycosis cleared on therapy and two of three patients with cryptococcosis (all three had meningitis) achieved clinical and mycological remission. Where efficacy ratings took into account both complete clinical recovery and improvement the response rates are 84.8% and 50% for candidosis and aspergillosis, respectively.

Of the patients with a presumptive diagnosis of fungal infection there were five clinical "cures", 5 patients improved and one failed to respond.

ADVERSE REACTIONS

The results have been analysed using different baseline biochemical parameters. This was necessary because the underlying state of the patients and the fact that many already had evidence of renal dysfunction meant that some of the tests of renal or hepatic function were abnormal at the start of therapy and would be expected, even without antifungal therapy, to fluctuate or even deteriorate if the patient's condition worsened.

The results of monitoring renal function show a number of trends. Firstly, those patients with renal dysfunction at the outset of therapy generally normalised during treatment. There were only two cases where creatinine levels were reported to have risen during therapy and where this was ascribed by the investigator to Ambisome. It is difficult to interpret these results fully as both were receiving potentially nephrotoxic drugs - aminoglycosides or cyclosporin. A few patients had transient changes in creatinine which became normal during therapy. Changes in potassium levels, particularly hypokalaemia, bore no relation to changes in creatinine and urea although three patients developed hypokalaemia during therapy, one of of which was considered to be related to Ambisome.

Changes in liver function also occurred during therapy. In four cases patients with normal baseline values of tests of hepatic function had consistent rises during therapy. In no case was this ascribed to treatment; in one patient there was septic shock, two had border line values before therapy and the other had AIDS. The other changes seen were transient and reverted to normal with continued treatment.

Anaemia (normochromic, normocytic) has been reported with AmB therapy but no consistent changes were seen in these patients and none were reported to be drug related. Four patients developed evidence of anaemia during the study; three of these had haematological malignancies and the changes were thought to be due to the underlying disease. Other adverse effects reported included vomiting (1), pancreatitis (1), fever (1), injection site pain (1), confusion (1), neuropathy (1) and ventricular extrasystoles (2). The last two were not thought by the investigator to be drug related - the first occurred during an episode of secondary sepsis and one of the patients with extrasystoles had a prolonged episode of hypoxia.

CONCLUSION

Ambisome is a liposome encapsulated formulation of amphotericin B. The product is based on unilamellar liposomes containing phosphatidylcholine, cholesterol and distearoyl-phosphatidyl-glycerol. It is supplied in lyophilized form which has to be reconstituted with cool sterile water and allowed to equilibrate at 65° C for ten minutes before infusion in 5% dextrose. Like the conventional formulation of amphotericin it is not compatible with saline based infusions. The shelf life of the lyophilized form is at least six months. Data on the pharmacokinetics of Ambisome indicate that peak serum levels range from 6-14 mcg/ml after doses of 2mg/kg to 40-60 mcg/ml after 4mg/kg doses. These levels are considerably higher than those seen with AMB where maximum values after the usual maximum dose of 1mg/kg rarely exceed 5mcg/ml and are usually lower (Vestar Inc - data on file). In pharmacokinetic studies with Ambisome rats receiving high doses of the drug, 5.0mg/kg, showed no significant histopathological changes in potential target organs such as kidneys and liver, although in the latter there was some hypertrophy of Kupffer cells. Otherwise the only changes noted were interstitial lung infitrates in both control and treated groups of animals. The levels of drug in the kidney were significantly less in those receiving Ambisome than AMB. There was retention of drug particularly in the liver 28 days after the higher doses of Ambisome but this was not accompanied by tissue damage or biochemical changes. This work suggests that the distribution of drug in liposome form is different to that seen with AmB with some sparing of the kidney, but as with AmB accumulation not associated with damage in the liver.

The efficacy studies of Ambisome were carried out using an open design. Only those patients who had failed on or who could not tolerate AMB received the drug, i.e. those for whom there was no alternative therapy. A total of 115 episodes of fungal infection were treated at the time of analysis in which the remission rate (clinical and mycological) in those patients who were assessed was about 60%. This included a significant number of patients with continuing neutropenia. The results were better for patients with systemic candidosis than aspergillosis but once again the patients with invasive aspergillosis had well established infections. While in 17 cases (5 *Candida*, 2 *Aspergillus* and 10 treated empirically) the laboratory diagnosis may have been in doubt, the rest of the results suggest that Ambisome is effective in cases of systemic mycosis which have not responded to AmB.

It has not been necessary to use a low "test" dose with this preparation and the drug has been well tolerated at therapeutic levels without the conventional slow increase in dosage. Generally there was a low level of adverse reactions reported with Ambisome. It is very difficult to assign a cause to some of the changes observed as the patients were all acutely ill and many of the abnormalities could have been due to the underlying disease. However, there was no evidence of significant renal toxicity, anaemia or hepatic damage during this study. Further, there were no acute side effects such as hyperpyrexia or nausea and it appears that a slow build up of drug doses, the current practice with AmB, is not necessary with this compound.

Survival of cancer patients with aspergillosis is seldom achieved if therapy is delayed beyond 96 hours after the first appearance of lung infiltrates [11]. The results are better, but not optimal, if therapy is initiated earlier with survival of only 40-50% being seen. These results also appear to hold true for systemic candidosis in the neutropenic patient. One recent survey of systemic candidosis in cancer patients showed that the overall response rate to AmB was 26%, but no patients with continuing neutropenia survived [12]. Various reasons have been proposed for these observations. They include the finding that although tissue levels of the drug are comparatively high in infected organs the organisms appear to survive, presumably because the drug is not bioavailable [13]. Another reason for failed treatment responses in yeast infections is the finding that minimum inhibitory concentrations of AmB for yeasts are increased in severely immunocompromised patients [14], by not more than 6 fold, but sufficient to account for failure to eradicate organisms in some cases. It is not known why it also appears to be impossible to eradicate deep fungal infections permanently in AIDS patients but failure to achieve high enough concentrations of drug at the site of infection coupled with the absence of a host immune response, a major factor in determining the outcome of fungal invasion in the neutropenic patient, probably account for persistence of infection. It is hoped that by using preparations such as Ambisome it may be possible to overcome some of these problems.

Acknowledgement.
The drug Ambisome was kindly supplied by Vestar Inc, California who also helped to compile the data.

REFERENCES

1. Medoff G, Brajtburg J and Kobayashi GS (1983)
Antifungal agents useful in therapy of systemic fungal infections.
Ann.Rev.Pharmacol Toxicol. **2** 303-330.

2. Medoff G and Kobayashi GA (1980)
The polyenes.
In Antifungal Chemotherapy. Ed DCE Speller.
John Wiley and Sons, Chichester pp 3-34.

3. Bennett JE, Dismukes WE, Duma RJ et al (1979)
A comparison of amphotericin B alone and combined with flucytosine in the treatment of cryptococcal meningitis.
N.Eng J. Med **301** 126-131.

4. Butler WT, Bennett JE, Alling D and Wertlake PT (1964)
Nephrotoxicity of amphotericin B: early and late effects in 81 patients.
Ann.Intern.Med **61** 175-187.

5. Miller R and Bates JH (1969)
Amphotericin B toxicity. A follow up report of 53 patients.
Ann.Intern.Med **71** 1090-1095.

6. Stevens DA (1979)
Drugs for systemic fungal infections.
Pharmacology for Physicians **13** 1-7.

7. Warnock DW and Richardson MD Eds (1982)
Fungal infection in the compromised patient.
John Wiley and Sons Ltd, Chichester UK.

8. Herman PE and Keys TF (1983)
Antifungal agents used for deep seated mycotic infections.
Mayo.Clin.Proc. **58** 223-231.

9. Lopez-Berestein G, Fainstein V , Hopfer R et al (1985)
Liposomal amphotericin B for the treatment of systemic fungal infections in patients with cancer: a preliminary study.
J.Infect.Dis **151** 704-710.

10. Sculier J-P, Coune A, Meunier F et al (1988)

Pilot study of amphotericin B entrapped in sonicated liposomes in cancer patients with fungal infections.
Eur.J.Cancer.Clin.Oncol. **24** 527-538.

11. Aisner J, Schimpff SC and Wiernik PH (1977)
Treatment of invasive aspergillosis. Relationship of early diagnosis and treatment to response.
Ann.Intern.Med **90** 539-543.

12. Maksymiuk AW, Thonprasert S and Hopfer R (1984)
Systemic candidiasis in cancer patients.
Am.J.Med **77** 20-27.

13. Christiansen KJ, Bernard EM, Gold JWM and Armstrong D (1985)
Distribution and activity of amphotericin B in humans.
J.Infect Dis **152** 1037-1043.

14. Powderly WG, Kobayashi GS, Herzig GP and Medoff G (1988).
Amphotericin B resistant yeast infection in severely immunocompromised patients.
Am.J.Med **84** 826-832.

29

Amphotericin B Incorporated in Lipid Emulsion (lipid microsphere)

S. Kohno, K.Hara, N.Murahashi*, T.Watanabe*

Second Department of Internal Medicine, Nagasaki University School of Medicine, Nagasaki, Japan, 852

*Tsukuba Research Laboratories Eisai Co., 1-3 Tokodai 5-chome Toyosato-machi Tsukuba-gun Ibaragi, Japan, 300-26

I. INTRODUCTION

Amphotericin B has been the drug of choice for treating most systemic mycoses caused by opportunistic pathogen, however, its clinical utility is limited by its toxicity to host cells. Lipid vehicles are used to keep amphotericin B away from the host cells to reduce the toxicity. Several reports have shown that liposomes encapsulating amphotericin B have significantly reduced its systemic toxicity without a loss of efficacy against experimental fungal infection (1,2,3).

Lipid microspheres such as Intralipid®, which have been used for hyperalimentation, are good vehicles and they are already commercialized as steroids or prostaglandins incorporated in lipid emulsion (4). We describe amphotericin B incorporated in lipid emulsion that reduces the toxicity and shows therapeutic efficacy against murine candidiasis.

II. MATERIALS AND METHODS

A. Formulating the amphotericin B emulsion

The formulation method was reported by Kirsh et al.(5). Twenty mg of sodium deoxycholate was dissolved in 1 ml of dimethylacetamide. It was gently mixed with 45 mg of amphotericin B at 30 C. The amphotericin B solution was added to a vial containing Intralipid®-20%(Otsuka, Tokyo, Japan).

B. The size of the amphotericin B emulsion

Ten ul of amphotericin B (1.0 mg/ml) incorporated in emulsion, incubated at 4, 22, 45 °C for 2, 6, 24 hours, was diluted with distilled water. The change of size under each incubation condition was measured by dynamic light scattering (Otsukadenshi DLS 700) at 25 °C.

C. HPLC for measurement of amphotericin B

High-performance liquid chromatography (HPLC) was done using: a Jasco 851-A5 sampler, a Jasco 880-PU HPLC pump and a Jasco 875-UV UV/VIS detector operating at 405 nm. The column was Toso gel ODS-80TM CTR. The mobile phase was methanol - 4 m mole EDTA (8:2), delivered at 1.0 ml /min.

Amphotericin B emulsion was incubated at 4, 22 or 45 C for 1, 7 or 30 days, then the stability was measured by HPLC.

The concentrations of amphotericin B in sera from BALB/c mice injected with amphotericin B emulsion (1.25, 5 mg/kg) or amphotericin B (1.0 mg/kg) were measured by HPLC.

D. Stability of pH profile of the amphotericin B emulsion

Amphotericin B methanol solution (1.0 mg/ml) was mixed with citric acid Na_2HPO_4 buffer (pH 2.2, 3.0, 4.0, 5.0, 6.0, 7.0, 8.0) at the ratio of 1:9, then incubated at 22, 45, 55 °C for 1 week or 1 month. The concentrations were measured by HPLC in comparison with the solution kept at 4°C.

E. TOXICITY OF AMPHOTERICIN B & ITS EMULSION

Various concentrations (0.78, 1.56, 3.12, 6.25, 12.5 mg/kg) of Fungizone® (Squibb) were injected into ddY, ICR and BALB/c mice intravenously (ten mice in each group), and the number of animals that died and their pathology were observed.

Various concentrations (5, 7.5, 10, 12.5 mg/kg) of amphotericin B emulsion were injected into 5-week-old male BALB/c mice (ten in each group). Sonicated emulsion or incubated emulsion at 4, 22 or 45 C for various durations (1, 2, 4, 6, 18, 24 hours) was injected into 5-week-old BALB/c mice (ten in each group).

F. DIFFERENTIAL SCANNING CALORIMETRY

Twenty ul of amphotericin B(1.0 mg/ml) emulsion was put into an aluminum liquid container and thermal analysis was performed by the Perkin-Elmer model DSC 7. It was measured with rising temperature at 2 C/min and at fixed temperature of 45 C.

G. THE EFFICACY OF AMPHOTERICIN B INCORPORATED IN EMULSION AGAINST MURINE CRYPTOCOCCOSIS AND CANDIDIASIS

In the model of murine cryptococcosis, *Cryptococcus neoformans* C-28(1 x 10^6 cfu, a clinical isolate) was inoculated into the cranium of 5-week-old BALB/c mice. Shortly after inoculation, amphotericin B emulsion (5 mg/kg), amphotericin B (0.8 mg/kg) or lipid emulsion(20 % Intralipid®) was injected once intravenously. In the model of murine candidiasis, *Candida albicans* 7N (3.6 x 10^6 cfu, a clinical isolate) was inoculated intravenously. Shortly after inoculation, amphotericin B emulsion (1.25 mg/kg), amphotericin B (0.62 mg/kg) or lipid emulsion was injected once intravenously.

III RESULTS

A. THE SIZE OF AMPHOTERICIN B EMULSION

The size of amphotericin B emulsion is approximately 250 nm in diameter, and it was hardly changed by incubation time and temperature (Table 1).

Table 1 The change of size in amphotericin B emulsion by incubation time and temperature

	2	6	24 hours
4 C	229.5+19	289.1+43	266.8+36 nm
22 C	273.7+32	284.1+48	253.6+29 nm
45 C	269.6+31	242.8+26	254.8+27 nm

B. THE STABILITY OF AMPHOTERICIN B EMULSION

The stability of amphotericin B with the change of pH was examined. When incubated at 4 or 22 °C, it was quite stable between pH 4 and 10. Even at 37 °C, it was stable between pH 5 and 9. The stability with the change of temperature and storage duration was examined by HPLC. Amphotericin B emulsion was stable at 4 or 22 °C for at least 30 days(Fig. 1).

C. ACUTE TOXICITY OF AMPHOTERICIN B AND ITS EMULSION

The lethal dose 50 (LD50) was determined as shown in Table 2. DdY mice were the strongest among the three groups used, BALB/c mice were the weakest and ICR mice were intermediate. The younger the mice, the stronger they were.

The LD50 of amphotericin B emulsion was 7.8 mg/kg in 5-week-old BALB/c mice. The maximum tolerated dose of amphotericin B was 0.8 mg/kg and that of amphotericin B emulsion was 5.0 mg/kg. This reduction of toxicity was abolished completely by sonication. It was also affected

Fig. 1

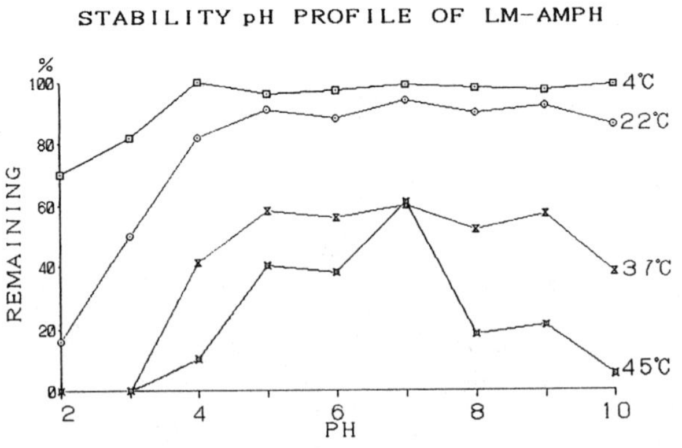

Table 2 Lethal dose 50 of amphotericin B in mice

	4	5	6	weeks-old
ddY	4.1	3.1	2.4	mg/kg
ICR	3.6	2.3	2.1	mg/kg
BALB/c	2.7	2.1	1.5	mg/kg

by the incubation time and temperature. Amphotericin B emulsion should be kept at 22 C at least 24 hours to reduce its toxicity (Fig. 2).

D. PHARMACOKINETICS OF AMPHOTERICIN B EMULSION

The serum concentrations of amphotericin B emulsion in mice were lower than that of amphotericin B (Fig. 3). This

Fig. 2

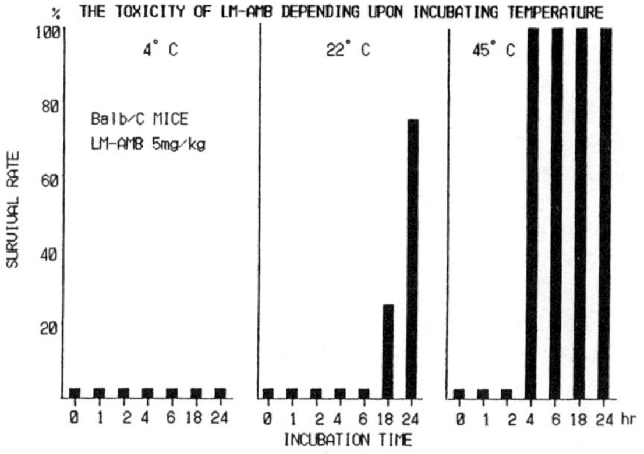

Fig. 3

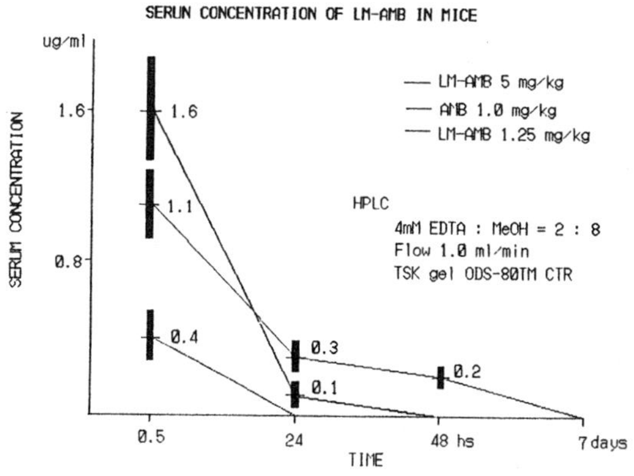

Fig. 4

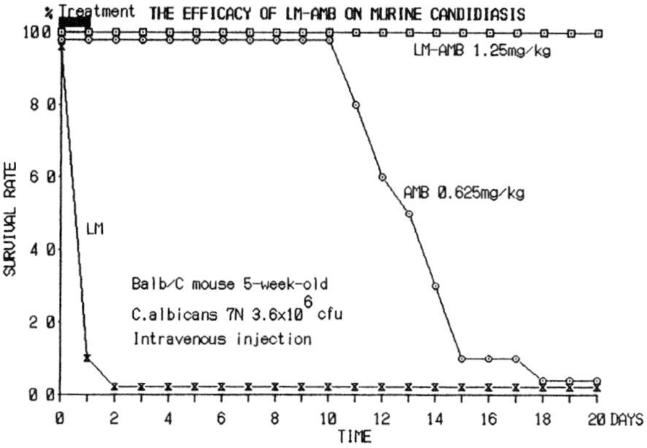

could be due to the predominant distribution of amphotericin B emulsion in reticuloendothelial systems.

E. THE EFFICACY OF AMPHOTERICIN B EMULSION AGAINST MURINE CRYPTOCOCCOSIS AND CANDIDIASIS

In murine cryptococcosis, all mice without therapy died within 13 days, all mice treated with 0.8 mg/kg of amphotericin B died within 18 days, and mice treated with amphotericin B emulsion died within 26 days. Pathological examination disclosed severe encephalitis and meningitis by cryptococcosis.

In murine candidiasis, all mice without therapy died within 2 days and mice treated with 0.625 mg/kg of amphotericin B also died within 18 days, while all mice treated with amphotericin B emulsion survived (Fig.4).

IV. DISCUSSION

Since amphotericin B has a strong acute toxicity, its clinical use is limited. However, vehicles such as liposomes reduced its toxicity and enabled clinical administration of an optimal amount of the drug(6). We have been using liposomes as a vehicle, but hesitated to use them in clinical trials for fear of instability and question about their safety.

Intralipid has been used for hyperalimentation and was proven to be safe. We applied this as a vehicle of amphotericin B following the methods of several authors(5,7,8). However, the data were quite variable and we failed to reproduce their results.

We did, however, discover the reason why they were so

variable. It is mandatory to keep amphotericin B emulsion at room temperature at least 24 hours, otherwise it does not reduce toxicity; sonication should also be avoided so that toxicity is not reduced. However, the reason for toxic reduction in response to temperature, incubation time and sonication is still obscure. No change of size, thermal transition or antimicrobial activity was observed.

In any event, the toxicity of amphotericin B emulsion was reduced so that it could be used in the treatment of murine cryptococcosis and candidiasis.

Further evaluation of amphotericin B emulsion could reveal the mechanism of toxicity reduction and allow future clinical use of the drug.

REFERENCES

1. J.R. Graybill, P.C. Craven, R.L. Taylor, D.M. Williams, W.E.Magee, Treatment of murine cryptococcosis with liposomal-associated amphotericin B. J. Infect. Dis.145:748-752(1982).
2. G. Lopez-Berestein, R.Mehta, R.L.Hopfer, K.Mills, L.Kasi, K.Mehta, V.Fainstein, M.Luna, E.M.Hersh, R.Juliano, Treatment and prophylaxis of disseminated infection due to Candida albicans in mice with liposomal-encapsulated amphotericin B. J. Infect. Dis. 147:939-944(1983).
3. S.Kohno, T.Miyazaki, K.Yamaguchi, H.Tanaka, T.Hayashi, M.Hirota, A.Saito, K.Hara, T.Sato, J.Sunamoto, Polysaccharide-coated liposomes with antimicrobial agents against intracytoplasmic pathogens and fungi. J.Bioact.Compat.Polym.3:137-147(1988).
4. Y.Mizusawa, T.Hamano, K.Yokoyama, Tissue distribution and anti-inflamatory activity of corticosteroid incorporated in lipid emulsion. Ann. Rem. Dis.41:263-267(1982).
5. R.Kirsh, R.Goldstein, J.Tarloff, D.Parris, J.Hook, N.Hannan, P.Bugelski, G.Poste, An emulsion formulation of amphotericin B improved the therapeutic index when treating systemic murine candidiasis. J. Infect. Dis. 158:1065-1070(1988).
6. G.Lopez-Berestein, V.Fainstein, R.Hopfer, et al. Liposomal amphotericin B for the treatment of systemic fungal infection in patients with cancer: a preliminary study. J. Infect. Dis.151:704-710(1985).
7. M.Singh, L.J.Ravin, Parenteral emulsions as drug carriers system. J. Parent. Science Technol.40:34-41(1986).
8. S.S.Davis, C.Washington, P.West, L.Illum, G.Liversidge, L.Sternson, R.Kirsh, Lipid emulsion as drug delivery systems. Ann. NY Acad. Scien.507:75-88,1988.

PART VII

INVESTIGATIONAL ANTIFUNGAL ANTIBIOTICS

30

Inhibitors of Cell Wall Synthesis

Nikkomycins

R.F. Hector[1], B.L. Zimmer[2], and D. Pappagianis[2]

Cutter Biological[1]
Berkeley, CA, 94710, USA

Dept. of Medical Microbiology[2], U.C. Davis School of Medicine,
Davis, CA, 95616, USA

I. INTRODUCTION

Chitin is a linear polymer of repeating N-acetylglucosamine units linked in a beta-1-4 fashion. The polymer confers rigidity to the exoskeleton of insects and crustaceans, and is found in the cell wall of most fungi. In the medically important fungi it is found in varying concentrations ranging from less than 1% in the case of the blastospore form of Candida albicans (1) to 10-20% in the dimorphic pathogenic fungi (2-8) and several filamentous fungi (9, 10). Because this polymer is not encountered in mammals, compounds which interfere with the synthesis of chitin could be useful as therapy of mycoses. The polyoxins, which are specific, competitive inhibitors of fungal chitin synthase due to their similarity in structure to UDP-N-acetylglucosamine (reviewed in reference 11), the substrate of chitin synthase, had previously been used in in vitro tests against Candida spp. (12-14) and dimorphic fungi with some success (15, 16). A related group of compounds is the nikkomycins, which are structurally similar to the polyoxins and are also competitive inhibitors of chitin synthase (17, 18). We employed nikkomycins X and Z (NX and NZ, respectively) in vitro against selected medically important fungi representing true yeast, dimorphic, and filamentous groups. Because of the high level of activity of these agents against the dimorphic pathogenic fungi, we subsequently evaluated them in mouse models of coccidioidomycosis, blastomycosis, and histoplasmosis, and these results are reported herein. In addition, data are provided on the pharmacokinetics and safety of these compounds.

II. IN VITRO TESTING

To obtain preliminary information about the spectrum of activity of the nikkomycins, susceptibility testing with NX and NZ against single isolates of diverse fungi was performed in broth using microtiter plates. Candida spp. were tested in yeast-nitrogen base (Difco) with glucose and asparagine, Blastomyces dermatitidis (yeast phase) and Aspergillus fumigatus were tested in Sabouraud's glucose broth, and Coccidioides immitis (spherule-endospore phase) was tested in modified Converse medium as previously described (19). All cultures were incubated at 37°C. MIC's were read at 48h for all but the dimorphic fungi, which were read at 96h, and the results are presented in Table 1 . As can be seen, NX and NZ showed the

TABLE 1. MICs OF NIKKOMYCINS AGAINST DIVERSE FUNGI

ORGANISM	MIC (ug/ml) NX	NZ
Coccidioides immitis	0.77	0.125
Blastomyces dermatitidis	8	30
Cryptococcus neoformans	125	250
Candida albicans	125	250
Candida tropicalis	>8000	>8000
Aspergillus fumigatus	>4000	>4000

greatest inhibition against the dimorphic pathogenic fungi, with values in the microgram per milliliter range. Both agents had a modest degree of activity against some yeasts but were inactive against Aspergillus in the milligram per milliliter range. The extreme resistance by C. tropicalis was an unexpected, but reproducible finding.

III. PHARMACOKINETICS

A bioassay for NZ was developed (20) and used for pharmacologic studies in outbred mice. Animals were treated either orally or intravenously with 100 mg/kg of NZ dissolved in phosphate-buffered saline. The results of intravenous administration indicated that after the initial serum concentration of 320 micrograms/ml the compound was rapidly eliminated, with a half-life of approximately 10-15 minutes (data not shown). Results from oral administration with 100 mg/kg, however, suggest that the compound is slowly absorbed, with a peak concentration of 10 micrograms/ml occurring approximately 45 minutes after administration. Though the number of data points are limited, the half life appears to be nearly one hour under these conditions. Because of the limited half-life of the NZ, mice were dosed orally on a b.i.d. schedule for all experiments.

IV. EFFICACY TESTING

To confirm the activity demonstrated in the susceptibility testing, a series of mouse models of mycoses were employed: either survival studies or organ-load assays. Experiments were conducted comparing orally administered NX with NZ, or in some cases, NZ was compared with various azole agents as well as amphotericin B (the latter agent given I.P.; see reference 20 for actual conditions of experiments).

A. COCCIDIOIDOMYCOSIS

In an organ load experiment with a pulmonary model in which mice were infected with Coccidioides immitis strain Silveira (ATCC 28868), NZ was compared to the azoles Bay R 3783 and fluconazole, with therapy administered over a five-day period. The results (Table 2) indicate that NZ at 50 mg/kg was able to eradicate nearly all of the fungus from the lungs of treated animals and was therefore comparable to 25 mg/kg of the triazole R 3783, and superior to fluconazole under the conditions employed. In a second experiment, 20 mg/kg of NZ given b.i.d. was compared with 50 mg/kg of the same drug given once daily. The data indicate that divided doses are more effective than one dose per day, which is likely a reflection of the short half-life of this drug.

TABLE 2. ORGAN LOADS IN COCCIDIOIDOMYCOSIS

EXPT.	TREATMENT GROUP	DOSE (mg/kg)	MEAN LOG CFU/gm±SEM
1	CONTROL	-	6.35±0.06
	R 3783	25 b.i.d.	0.00
	FLUCONAZOLE	25 b.i.d.	2.62±0.82
	NZ	50 b.i.d.	0.37±0.37
2	CONTROL	-	6.21±0.15
	NZ	20 b.i.d.	1.12±0.56
	NZ	50 q.d.	3.63±0.62

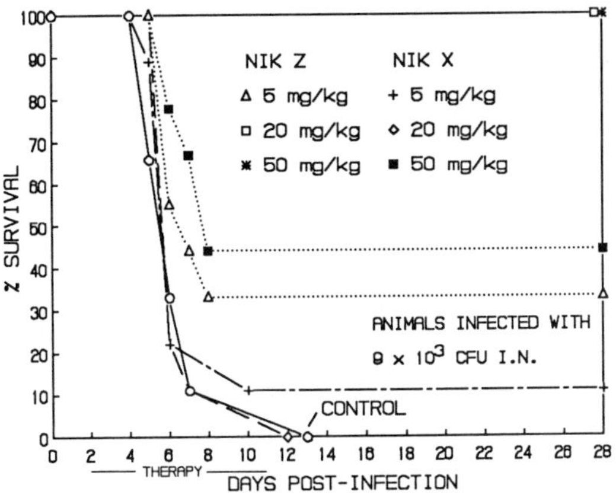

FIG. 1. Survival of mice with pulmonary coccidioidomycosis comparing controls with mice treated with NX and NZ.

In a survival experiment in which animals were infected by the intranasal route with a highly lethal challenge, three dose levels of NX and NZ (given b.i.d.) were administered after a 48h delay for 10 days. As can be seen in Figure 1, NZ was more active than NX, with the 20 and 50 mg/kg dosages of NZ resulting in complete protection while the 5 mg/kg dosage group had only slightly more deaths than the 50 mg/kg level of NX.

A model of meningocerebral coccidioidomycosis in mice was used to assess penetration into the CNS and combat the fungus in this deadly coccidioidal syndrome. Two dose levels of NZ given b.i.d. were compared to 10 mg/kg of R 3783 given once daily for 56 days. While the onset of mortalities was earlier in the nikkomycin groups (Fig. 2) than with the azole, the data suggest that R 3783 was acting in a fungistatic fashion in that deaths occurred in the latter group soon after cessation of therapy, whereas the numbers of deaths in the NZ group were ultimately fewer.

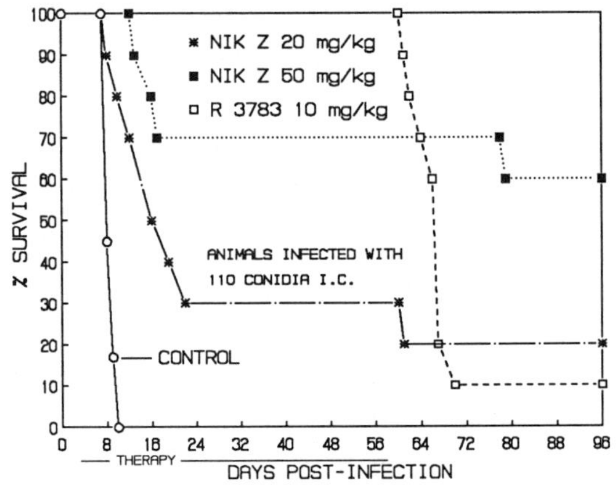

FIG. 2. Survival of mice with meningocerebral coccidioidomycosis comparing controls with NZ and the azole R 3783.

B. BLASTOMYCOSIS

A model of systemic blastomycosis was established in mice by intravenous infection with yeast-phase Blastomyces dermatitidis strain 1389 (obtained from University of Kentucky collection) which caused 100% mortality in control animals in less than 10 days. Again, both NX and NZ were employed at three dose levels. Both compounds demonstrated a good dose-response effect, with NZ again the more effective drug (Fig. 3). In a variation of this model, NZ at 20 mg/kg given b.i.d. was compared with four azoles and amphotericin B given at 1 mg/kg once daily, with therapy not administered until the first deaths had occurred on day 6. In this severe test of the ability of a drug to overcome advanced disease, the NZ group had the fewest mortalities, with no deaths occurring after day 8, i.e., two days after commencement of therapy (Fig. 4).

In an organ load experiment with the lungs as the target organ, three dose levels of NZ were compared with four azoles and amphotericin B given for five days. In this experiment the

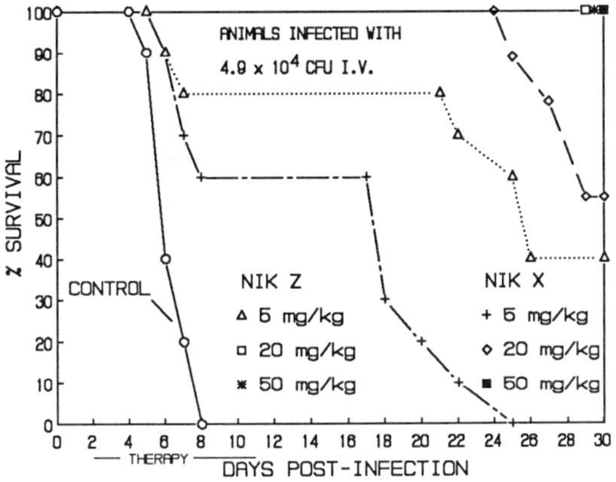

FIG. 3. Survival of mice with systemic blastomycosis comparing controls with NX and NZ.

lowest dose of NZ tested (5 mg/kg) was as active as amphotericin B at 1 mg/kg and the most active azole (R 3783) at 25 mg/kg (data not shown). The 50 mg/kg dose level of NZ resulted in the sterilization of the lungs of the majority of the animals.

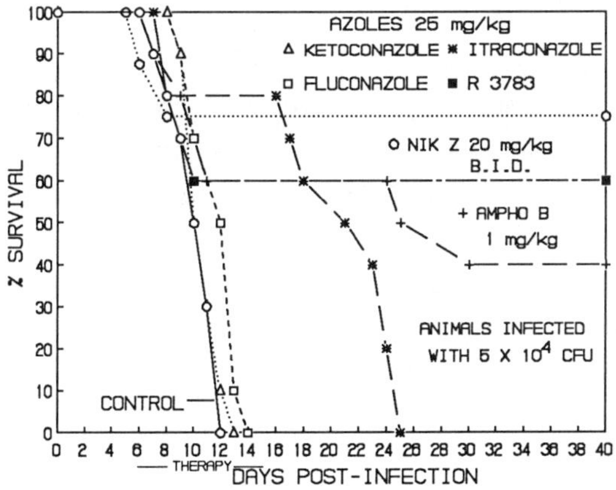

FIG. 4. Delayed-therapy study in systemic blastomycosis comparing controls with four azoles, amphotericin B, and NZ.

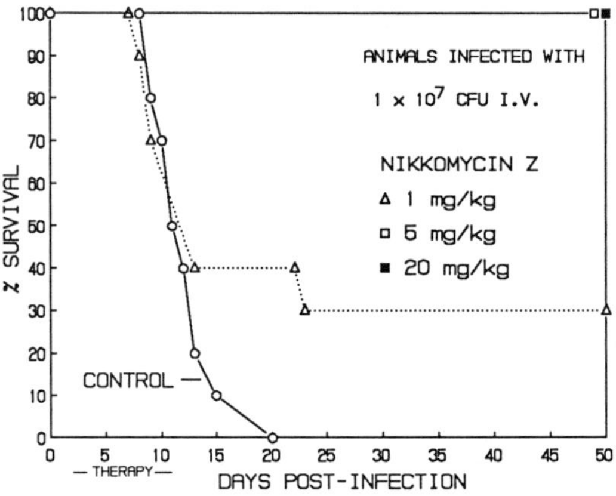

FIG. 5. Survival of mice with systemic histoplasmosis comparing controls with NZ at three dose levels.

C. HISTOPLASMOSIS

Three dose levels of NZ were used in a survival model in mice infected intravenously with Histoplasma capsulatum strain G217B (obtained from G. Kobayashi, Washington School of Medicine, St. Louis, MO). The results showed the effectiveness of NZ at dose levels of 5 and 20 mg/kg as all animals survived (Fig. 5). Results from an experiment for organ loads in animals treated for five days demonstrated that although a dose-response effect was seen, the moderate amount of clearance does not compare to that seen with the models of coccidioidomycosis and blastomycosis (data not shown). However, the reduction in cfu/gm was similar to that seen in animals receiving fluconazole.

D. CANDIDIASIS

A model of systemic candidiasis using inbred DBA/2N mice which were infected intravenously with Candida albicans strain

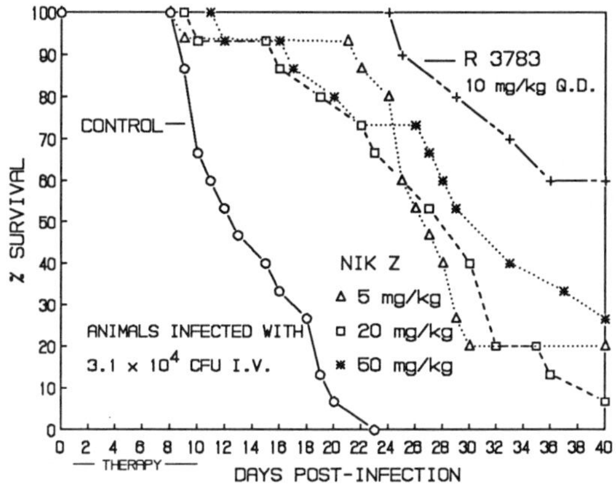

FIG. 6. Survival of mice with systemic candidiasis comparing controls with R 3783 and NZ at three dose levels.

B311 (originally obtained from H. Hasenclever, NIH) was employed to compare three dosage levels of NZ given b.i.d. with a single level of the azole Bay R 3783 administered once daily. Although NZ was able to delay the rate of mortality, no dose-response relationship was obvious, and the effect was inferior to that seen with the azole (see Fig. 6).

V. TOXICOLOGY

A limited safety trial was conducted in mice using agar vehicle or NZ given orally once daily at 100 or 400 mg/kg for a 28-day period in groups of 15 each. Weights were recorded twice-weekly, and showed no discernible differences over the test period among the three groups. At the end of the test period, 10 animals from each group were bled and necropsied. Routine blood counts and chemistry panels (the latter done on pools of three mice each for sufficient volume) revealed no differences among treated groups and untreated controls. Samples for pathology were sent to an independent pathology service for assessment, with the only unusual finding being a comparatively increased incidence of gliosis in the brains of mice receiving the 400 mg/kg dosage. Animals not sacrificed were held an additional 60 days for observation, with no outward differences apparent among the three groups.

VI. DISCUSSION

The potential for using chitin as a chemotherapeutic target in fungi had been recognized for a number of years (14, 17, 18), though the reports in the literature are largely limited to susceptibility testing. Previously, reports have shown that the specific chitin-synthase inhibitors known as polyoxins were highly active against dimorphic, highly-chitinous fungi (19, 21), and had some activity against C. albicans (12, 14, 22). We have demonstrated that the nikkomycins, in particular NZ, have fungicidal activity against selected dimorphic fungal pathogens in animal models of these mycoses. In particular, the experiment with delayed therapy in the blastomycosis model demonstrated the high level of activity of this agent in reversing advanced disease. However, NZ was less effective in the models of coccidioidal meningocerebral disease and systemic candidiasis.

Unlike the dimorphic fungal pathogens, in which chitin represents 10-20% of their cell walls in the parasitic phase (2-8), C. albicans has a much smaller component of chitin in its cell wall (1). Although small amounts of chitin can be found in the inner layers of the yeast cell wall (23), the highest concentration of the polymer is found in the yeast bud septum (24). This may partially explain the previous findings of Becker et al. (12) in which NZ was unable to prevent deaths in mice infected with a lethal challenge of C. albicans. However, the amount of chitin in the cell wall may not be the sole determinant of susceptibility. Indeed, the filamentous fungi often have as much of this polymer in the cell wall as the susceptible dimorphic pathogens (9, 10), but results of the MIC determination showed A. fumigatus to be refractory to the nikkomycins. Thus, in certain fungi, other wall polymers are likely able to substitute for any deficiencies created by inhibitors of cell-wall synthesis. This was demonstrated to be the case with the mycelial phase of Paracoccidioides brasiliensis, which synthesized additional alpha-glucan in response to treatment with papulacandin B, an inhibitor of beta-glucan synthesis (25). With the parasitic phases of C. immitis and B. dermatitidis, however, the need for chitin may be more critical. As has been previously shown, chitin is the first polymer synthesized in the cell wall during progressive cleavage of C. immitis spherules, part of the process involved in replication, with treatment by polyoxin D halting this process completely (16, 19). In the present study, NZ was found to have the same effect,with inhibition of progressive cleavage and lysis of cells evident. Interestingly, the MIC value for the nikkomycins versus C. immitis is approximately equal to the calculated K_i value for this agent against the isolated chitin synthase enzyme from diverse fungi (13, 17, 18, 21).

In conclusion, we have demonstrated that NX and NZ are efficacious against mycoses caused by the dimorphic fungal pathogens, exceeding the effectiveness of certain azoles and amphotericin B under the conditions employed. In the ranges tested the nikkomycins appear to have no adverse effects as assessed by a limited study, and thus may compare favorably to antifungal agents currently in use. Additionally, the findings confirm that the cell wall is a suitable and specific target for antifungal drugs, inviting continued efforts for development of effective and safe therapy of the mycoses.

VII. LITERATURE CITED

1. F.W. Chattaway, and M.R. Holmes, Cell wall composition of the mycelial and blastospore forms of Candida albicans, J. Gen. Microbiol., 51: 367-376. (1968).
2. T.E. Davis, Jr., J.E. Domer, and Y.T. Li, Cell wall studies of Histoplasma capsulatum and Blastomyces dermatitidis using homologous and heterologous enzymes, Infect.Immun., 15: 978-987. (1977).
3. J.E. Domer, Monosaccharide and chitin content of cell walls of Histoplasma capsulatum and Blastomyces dermatitidis, J. Bacteriol., 107: 870-877. (1971).
4. J.E. Domer, J.G. Hamilton, and J.C. Harkin, Comparative study of the cell walls of the yeastlike and mycelial phases of Histoplasma capsulatum, J. Bacteriol., 94: 466-474. (1967).
5. F. Kanetsuna, L.M. Carbonell, F. Gil, and I. Azuma, Chemical and ultrastructural studies on the cell walls of Histoplasma capsulatum, Mycopath. Mycol. Applicata, 54: 1-13. (1974).
6. E. Reiss, Serial enzymatic hydrolysis of cell walls of two serotypes of yeast-form Histoplasma capsulatum with alpha-(1-3)-glucanase, beta(1-3)-glucanase, pronase, and chitinase, Infect. Immun., 16: 181-188. (1977).
7. R. Wheat, T. Terai, A. Kiyomoto, N.F. Conant, E.P. Lowe, and J. Converse, Studies on the composition and structure of Coccidioides immitis cell wall, Coccidioidomycosis (L. Ajello, Ed.), Univ. of Arizona Press, Tucson, pp. 237-242. (1967).
8. R.W. Wheat, C. Tritschler, N.F. Conant, and E.P. Lowe, Comparison of Coccidioides immitis arthrospore, mycelium and spherule cells, and influence of growth medium on mycelial cell wall composition, Infect. Immunity, 17: 91-97. (1977).
9. J.H. Pollack, C.F. Lange, and T. Hashimoto, "Nonfibrillar" chitin associated with walls and septa of Trichophyton mentagrophytes arthrospores, J. Bacteriol., 154: 965-975. (1983).
10. C.A. Porter, and E. Jaworski, The synthesis of chitin by particulate preparations of Allomyces macrogynus, Biochem., 5: 1149-1154. (1966).
11. E. Cabib, The synthesis and degradation of chitin, Adv. Enzymol., 59: 59-101. (1988).
12. J.M. Becker, N.L. Covert, P. Shenbagmurthi, A.S. Steinfeld, F. Naider, Polyoxin D inhibits the growth of zoopathogenic fungi, Antimicrob. Agents Chemother., 23: 926-929. (1979.)
13. H. Mueller, R. Furter, H. Zahner, and D. Rast, Metabolic products of microorganisms. 203. Inhibition of chitosomal chitin synthetase and growth of Mucor rouxii by nikkomycin Z, nikkomycin X, and polyoxin A: a comparison, Arch. Microbiol., 130: 195-197. (1981).

14. J-C Yadan, M. Gonneau, P. Sarthou, and F. Le Goffic, Sensitivity to nikkomycin Z in Candida albicans: role of peptide permeases, J. Bacteriol., 160: 884-888. (1984).
15. U. Dahn, H. Hagenmaier, H. Hohne, W.A. Konig, G. Wolf, and H. Zahner, Nikkomycin, ein neuer Hemmstoff der Chitinsynthese bei Pilzen, Arch. Microbiol., 107: 143-160. (1976).
16. R.F. Hector, and D. Pappagianis, Inhibition of chitin synthesis in the cell wall of Coccidioides immitis by polyoxin D. J. Bacteriol., 154 :488-498. (1983).
17. G.U. Brillinger, Metabolic products of microorganisms. 181. Chitin synthase from fungi, a test model for substances with insecticidal properties, Arch. Microbiol., 121: 71-74, (1979)
18. J. Delzer, H.P. Fiedler, H. Muller, H. Zahner, R. Rathmann, K. Ernst, and W.A. Konig, New nikkomycins by mutasynthesis and directed fermentation, J. Antibiot.(Tokyo.), 37: 80-82. (1984).
19. R.F. Hector, B.L. Zimmer, and D. Pappagianis, Microtiter method for MIC testing with spherule-endospore-phase Coccidioides immitis, J. Clin. Microbiol., 26: 2667-2668. (1988).
20. R.F. Hector, B.L. Zimmer, and D. Pappagianis, Evaluation of nikkomycins X and Z in murine models of coccidioidomycosis, histoplasmosis, and blastomycosis, Antimicrob. Agents Chemother., 34: 587-593. (1990).
21. C.R. Cooper, J.L. Harris, C.W. Jacobs, and P.J. Szaniszlo, Effects of polyoxin AL on cellular development in Wangiella dermatitidis, Exp. Mycol., 8: 349-363. (1984).
22. P.J. McCarthy, P.F. Troke, and K. Gull, Mechanism of action of nikkomycin and the peptide transport system of Candida albicans, J. Gen. Microbiol., 131: 775-780. (1985).
23. G. Tronchin, D. Poulain, J. Herbaut, and J. Biguet, Localization of chitin in the cell wall of Candida albicans by means of wheat germ agglutinin. Fluorescence and ultrastructural studies, Eur. J. Cell Biol., 26: 121-128. (1981).
24. P.C. Braun and R.A. Calderone, Chitin synthesis in Candida albicans: comparison of yeast and hyphal forms, J. Bacteriol., 133: 1472-1477. (1978).
25. T. Davila, G. San-Blas, and F. San-Blas, Effect of papulacandin B on glucan synthesis in Paracoccidioides brasiliensis, J. Med. Vet. Mycol., 24: 193-202. (1986).

Cilofungin

John R. Perfect

Department of Medicine, Division of Infectious Diseases
Duke University Medical Center, Durham, North Carolina, U.S.A. 27710

INTRODUCTION

In the search for highly specific antifungal agents in treatment of deep-seated mycoses, the fungal cell wall has been an attractive target. This structure and its behavior distinguish fungi from other eucaryotic cells. First, it is logical to explore this site for antimicrobial attack since agents should display differential toxicity on fungi vs host cells. Second, the cell wall is involved in vegetative growth, substrate colonization, reproduction, dispersal, survival, host penetration and thus, represents a primary structure for fungal protection during host invasion (1). Fungal cell walls generally contain a majority of polysaccharides which are built from various sugars including glucose, N-acetylglucosamine, and mannose. However, the relative proportion of these sugars in the cell wall will vary within the various families of fungi. In a less prominent role glycoproteins and even fatty acids have been found in the walls of certain fungal species. The fungal cell wall becomes a complex macromolecular structure of interwoven fibrils containing chitin or cellulose cemented with various glucans, mannans, or galactans. The differences in cell wall composition have been used to develop taxonomic relationship between fungal species, but a further extension of these differences in cell wall composition allows chemists the ability to develop compounds which could interrupt formation of this unique structure.

Almost two decades ago, a group of polypeptide antifungal agents were discovered with potent and selective antifungal activity *in vitro*. The parent compounds for this group of new agents were Echinocandin B and aculeacin. Echinocandin B was a major lipopeptide produced by species of *Aspergillus nidulans* and *Aspergillus rugulosus*. These cyclopeptide antibiotics with long-chain fatty acids possessed antifungal activity *in vitro* against some yeasts and filamentous pathogenic fungi. In an attempt to improve on the original compound it was found that at the N-terminal end of the hexapeptide cyclized nucleus the linolenyl group could be removed and new chemical groups acylated onto this nucleus (2). These new semisynthetic analogs showed an array of *in vitro* antifungal activity against *Candida albicans*. Further investigations by the scientists at Lilly Laboratories found that a particular compound, 4-n-octyloxybenzoyl echinocandin (LY121019; Cilofungin) had less hemolytic potential in toxicology studies and greater *in vitro* antifungal activity than the parent Echinocandin B compound. This new analog of Echinocandin B with its improved therapeutic index received further testing. However, it should be pointed out that there were other Echinocandin B analogs made with similar *in vitro* antifungal potency to cilofungin. Cilofungin subsequently had further extensive investigations into its mechanisms of action, pharmacokinetics, *in vitro* antifungal activity, effects on treatment of animal and human mycoses.

MECHANISM OF ACTION

The effects of cilofungin on the cell wall structure of yeasts were vividly shown by scanning electron micrographs of *Candida albicans* blastospores exposed to low concentrations of cilofungin. These distorted and osmotically fragile yeasts suggested a major direct action on yeast cell wall metabolism by cilofungin. These observations plus the known inhibitory effect of Echinocandin B on beta-glucan synthesis of several fungi focused investigation on the glucan cell wall component (3,4). It was shown that cilofungin did not influence *C. albicans* DNA, RNA, or protein synthesis. At low concentrations (1-100 mcg/ml) cilofungin significantly inhibited labelled glucose into the glucan cell wall component of log phase cells. Further studies have shown cilofungin to be a noncompetitive and dose-dependent inhibitor of the (1-3)-beta-glucan synthase enzyme in *C. albicans* (5,6). Cilofungin did not have an effect on mannan or chitin synthesis and there has been only a minimal effect on sterol metabolism (7).

IN VITRO ANTIFUNGAL ACTIVITY

Potent *in vitro* activity against *Candida albicans* and *Candida tropicalis* has been confirmed by many laboratories (8-15). There has been a consensus that other candida species such as *C. parapsilosis* or *T. glabrata* are generally less susceptible. Other yeasts such as *Cryptococcus neoformans* or *Blastomyces dermatitidis* and dimorphic fungi such as Aspergillus species were not found to be susceptible. Our laboratory found the minimal inhibitory concentrations to cilofungin for *C. albicans* and *C. tropicalis* to be between 0.04-0.63 mcg/ml. Using 99% kill of original inoculum as a fungicidal endpoint, this compound had *in vitro* fungicidal activity similar to amphotericin B and remarkably different from the azole compounds which were fungistatic *in vitro*. During our examinations of fungicidal activity we did notice that certain strains were killed at low concentrations but growth paradoxically occurred in wells with higher concentrations of drug (10). This phenomenon described by Eagle for bacteria exposed to cell wall active antimicrobials has been described by other investigators with cilofungin and has an unknown clinical significance. Also, it may not occur in all medias and some investigators have suggested that micelle formation may inactivate high concentrations of the lipopeptide under certain conditions. Repeat testing of isolates continuously exposed to both high and low concentrations of cilofungin showed no significant change in susceptibility. Therefore, present data suggests that susceptible candida strains do not readily develop resistance *in vitro* to cilofungin on repeated exposure to the drug. However, no clinical data is available on *in vivo* resistance development. As predicted by its mechanism of action, the killing mechanism of cilofungin is generally delayed in stationary phase yeast cells, although some investigators have found significant killing of stationary cells suggesting other mechanisms of action for the drug (16). In rapidly dividing cells, killing by cilofungin is rapid and concentration dependent. Another potentially important feature of microbicidal agents is the presence of a post antibiotic effect on the microorganism after the drug levels have disappeared. In yeast strains examined in our laboratory a post antibiotic effect was not found with cilofungin treatment (10). However, others have reported a time and dose dependent postantibiotic effect in their assay system (17). Further studies will be needed to clarify this effect and its importance. The influence of media on the antifungal activity of cilofungin has been carefully studied (18). There may be slight differences between synthetic medias and yeast nitrogen base or Sabouraud but the main effect on *in vitro* results is explained by pH. With a drop in media pH, the minimum inhibitory concentration to cilofungin rises (11). Temperature and inoculum did not appear to significantly change *in vitro* results with this compound by one group (11), but another group found inoculum-dependent results (8).

The effect of cilofungin in combination with other antifungals on yeasts has been studied. Cilofungin has shown synergistic, antagonistic or no additive effects on certain strains with other antifungal agents such as amphotericin B, flucytosine, and azoles against Candida species. In general, the present *in vitro* combination tests do not predict a dramatic effect for combination chemotherapy *in vivo*. One report, however, showed impressive synergism with anticapsin which blocks chitin and manoprotein synthesis by inhibiting glucosamine-6-phosphate synthetase of Candida (16). We report in this symposium that cilofungin and nikkomycin (a chitin synthesis inhibitor) act together to inhibit hyphal growth and germination of diverse pathogenic dimorphic fungi such as Aspergillus, Fusarium, and Zygomycetes.

There has also been some data to address *in vitro* and *in vivo* correlation with cilofungin treatment. In one study *C. albicans* strains with high MICs (≥ 20 mcg/ml) were less effectively treated with cilofungin when compared to a susceptible strain (≤ 1 mcg/ml) (19). However, a second study was less precise in its ability to ascertain *in vitro*/*in vivo* correlations (11). A reasonable prediction from the present *in vitro* and *in vivo* studies is that certain highly cilofungin resistant strains of *C. albicans* may not respond to treatment, but these strains are relatively uncommon and should be identified during *in vitro* testing.

EFFECT ON HOST CELLS

Although the host immune responses are an important factor in the outcome of treatment for mycosis, the analysis of host cell and antimicrobial agent interaction is difficult to dissect. In general, cilofungin does not appear to adversely affect leukocyte function when tested *in vitro* (20). Intracellular yeasts can be reached and killed by this lipopeptide (21). The efficiency of intracellular phagocytic killing in the presence of cilofungin remains unclear but there is some data which finds that cilofungin interferes with opsonization of *C. albicans* by neutrophils (22). This interference could be relevant in tissue where antibodies and complement are limited during infection.

PHARMACOKINETICS

Dogs. Early studies in dogs found that serum concentrations of cilofungin were related to dose. Cilofungin serum concentrations at the end of an infusion of 10 mg/kg or 100 mg/kg dose ranged from 112-156 mcg/ml to 558-1064 mcg/ml, respectively, and at the end of 6 hours levels were still detectable in the 10 mg/kg/dose and between 50-100 mcg/ml with the 100 mg/kg/dose. There was no evidence of drug accumulation or altered peak serum concentrations with multiple dosing over 13 weeks. Cilofungin was not detectable in normal aqueous humor or cerebrospinal fluid during treatment (5,23).

Rabbits. In rabbits a 50 mg/kg intravenous dose will achieve peak serum levels of approximately 160 ug/ml but the drug is rapidly eliminated and there was no drug detectable in the serum after 90 min ($\leq$ 0.3 mcg/ml) (24). Beta-elimination half-life in rabbits is approximately 20 minutes (25). Although cilofungin levels were detected in the urine of some rabbits receiving treatment for one week, they were undetectable in others. Further studies showed that treatment of rabbits with high doses of cilofungin demonstrated a non-linear, saturable elimination pathway. If continuous infusion of cilofungin was given, significantly higher concentrations of drug were found in the bile and tissues. With sustained high plasma levels by continuous infusion, drug was measured within the central nervous system (25).

Humans. Single doses of cilofungin between 1-5 mg/kg dissolved in 26% polyethylene glycol showed peak concentrations at the end of infusion falling rapidly to undetectable levels after 3 hours. Multiple doses with 4 mg/kg showed a Cmax of 28.6 mcg/ml and C_{min} of 1.4 mcg/ml at steady state. Less than 2% of the cilofungin dose was recovered in the urine suggesting primary biliary excretion of drug (26).

TOXICITY

The toxicity of cilofungin was formally studied in dogs. Doses from 10-100 mg/kg/day five days a week for three months were given. Only dogs receiving the 100 mg/kg daily dose showed toxicity. These dogs had a 5% weight loss, and exhibited swelling and edema around the mouth and face, itching and decreased blood pressure. All effects reversed within several hours of dosing and suggested a histamine reaction. There was also elevation of liver enzymes during therapy with the high doses. Otherwise, no significant toxicity was noted. Early toxicology studies in normal human volunteers showed no significant toxicity with cilofungin infusions. However, during the initial evaluation of cilofungin treatment for deep-seated candidiasis seriously ill patients developed an anionic gap acidosis during treatment and evidence of acute nephrotoxicity (27). The investigation into this complication suggests that it may be caused by the high percentage of polyethylene glycol (26%) in the vehicle for cilofungin and its resultant effects on the kidney of seriously ill patients. However, these toxicology issues remain unresolved.

IN VIVO EFFICACY TRIALS

Antifungal activities of cilofungin on candida infections in murine models were generally found to be effective. Cilofungin orally administered against *C. albicans* infection of the gastrointestinal tract dropped viable yeast counts quicker than a nystatin-treated group. A general summary of the disseminated murine candidiasis models is that cilofungin can significantly reduce yeast counts in the kidney and improve survival (5,23,28-31). These effects are likely to be dose dependent with higher doses required for better clinical results. Cilofungin has also been shown to have anticandida activity in neutropenic animals. However, in its comparison with amphotericin B treatment, the majority of studies tend to find amphotericin B to be more potent than cilofungin but its dose range is limited by toxicity (32). A study compared cilofungin and amphotericin B treatment with the two drugs combined; it showed that the combination of cilofungin and amphotericin B was additive/synergistic in murine candidiasis (33).

In guinea pigs with a superficial *C. albicans* infection, a 5% cilofungin or 3% nystatin cream formulation cured all animals after a 5 day treatment regimen (23).

In rats with a vaginal candidal infection, a 3% cilofungin cream formulation was similar to a 2% miconazole preparation in reducing yeast counts. A 3% nystatin cream appeared to have a more prolonged suppressive effect compared to the other drugs used for this infection. Effects of cilofungin treatment on rat deep-seated candidiasis appears to be dose dependent with higher doses 50-100 mg/kg/d more effective than lower doses 6.25-25 mg/kg/d (11).

The rabbit models of disseminated candidiasis (endocarditis, pyelonephritis, endophthalmitis) have been used to study cilofungin treatment. The endocarditis model was used to determine if the *in vitro* fungicidal qualities of cilofungin would translate into effective treatment for an infection generally requiring cidal agents. Two studies using intermittent daily dosing of cilofungin did not find it successful in reducing viable yeast counts in the vegetations and definitely was less effective than amphotericin B treatment (24,34). A more recent study, however, did show treatment benefit in rabbit endocarditis with cilofungin if drug was given as a continuous infusion (35). In candida endophthalmitis, one study showed some benefit to cilofungin treatment (24) and another showed no benefit of treatment (36). Both studies, however, agree that amphotericin B treatment was more effective in the model when compared to intermittent dosing of cilofungin. In rabbit candida pyelonephritis, cilofungin treatment had a positive effect on reducing yeast counts in the kidney but was not an improvement over amphotericin B therapy. In a rabbit model using subcutaneous semipermeable chambers containing *C. albicans* and *C. parapsilosis* in serum, cilofungin treatment was not successful. Cilofungin was found to be greater than 90% protein bound and these results suggested that higher concentrations of drug were needed in protein-containing sites to enhance *in vivo* efficacy (37).

Both the marginal and lack of efficacy in the rabbit models of candidiasis for cilofungin may reflect the short exposure of the yeast to the drug in this species which rapidly eliminates the compound. Further studies into the efficacy of continuous drug administration with its non-linear kinetics in rabbits will help us appreciate the importance of high, prolonged drug levels of this cell-wall active agent at the site of a fungal infection.

One major criticism of this new antimicrobial agent is its limited spectrum. Although candida remains the major deep-seated mycoses, the commercial viability of a compound would be enhanced by a broader spectrum. A very recent study found remarkable activity of cilofungin treatment in an aspergillus model of infection (38). These findings suggest that the *in vitro* testing as presently performed may have missed a potential use for the beta glucan synthesis inhibitors. Another recent *in vivo* experiment found that a new beta glucan inhibitor was effective in treatment of *Pneumocystis carinii* infection (39). With further experience, we may find that this group of agents may not be so limited in their spectrum of *in vivo* antifungal activity.

Human clinical studies with cilofungin were begun for treatment of esophageal and invasive candidiasis. These studies have been terminated because of toxicity and complete analysis of efficacy was limited. Although cilofungin may never be used in clinical practice, its development has paved the way for studies of future cell-wall active antifungals and in particular other Echinocandin B analogs. This group of antifungals remains very attractive for therapeutic development.

REFERENCES

1. A. Cassone, Cell wall of pathogenic yeasts and implications for antimycotic therapy, Drugs Exp. Clin. Res., 12: 635. (1986).

2. M. Debono, b. J. Abbott, D. S. Fukuda, et al, Synthesis of new analogs of echinocandin B by enzymatic deacylation and chemical reacylation of the echinocandin B peptide: synthesis of the antifungal agent cilofungin (LY121019), J. Antibiot., 42: 389. (1989).

3. E. T. Sawistowska-Schroder, D. Kerridge and H Perry, Echinocandin inhibition of 1-3 beta-D-glucan synthase from *Candida albicans*, FEBS. Lett., 173: 134. (1984).

4. C. S. Taft and C. P. Selitrennikoff, LY121019 inhibits *Neurospora crassa* growth and (1-3)-beta-D-glucan synthase, J. Antibiot., 41: 697. (1988).

5. R. S. Gordee, D. J. Zeckner, L. C. Howard, W. E. Alborn and M. Debono, Anti-candida activity and toxicology of LY121019, a novel semisynthetic polypeptide antifungal antibiotic, Ann. N. Y. Acad. Sci., 544: 294. (1988).

6. C. S. Taft and C. P. Selitrennikoff, Cilofungin inhibition of (1-3)-beta-glucan synthase: the lipophilic side chain is essential for inhibition of enzyme activity, J. Antibiot., 43: 433. (1990).

7. M. Pfaller, J. Riley and T. Koerner, Effects of cilofungin (LY121019) on carbohydrate and sterol composition of *Candida albicans*, Eur. J. Clin. Microbiol. Infect. Dis., 8: 1067. (1989).

8. G. S. Hall, C. Myles, K. J. Pratt and J. A. Washington, Cilofungin (LY121019) an antifungal agent with specific activity against *Candida albicans* and *Candida tropicalis*, Antimicrob. Agents Chemother., 32: 1331. (1988).

9. L. H. Hanson and D. A. Stevens, Evaluation of cilofungin, a lipopeptide antifungal agent, *in vitro* against fungi isolated from clinical specimens, Antimicrob. Agents

Chemother., 33: 1391. (1989).

10. M. Hobbs, J. Perfect and D. Durack, Evaluation of *in vitro* antifungal activity of LY121019, Eur. J. Clin. Microbiol. Infect. Dis., 7: 77. (1988).

11. K. A. McIntyre and J. N. Galgiani, pH and other effects on the antifungal activity of cilofungin (LY121019), Antimicrob. Agents Chemother., 33: 731. (1989).

12. F. C. Odds, Activity of cilofungin (LY121019) against Candida species *in vitro*, J. Antimicrob. Chemother., 22: 891. (1988).

13. M. A. Pfaller, S. Wey, T. Gerarden, A. Houston and R. P. Wenzel, Susceptibility of nosocomial isolates of Candida species to LY121019 and other antifungal agents, Diagn. Microbiol. Infect. Dis., 12: 1. (1989).

14. E. D. Spitzer, S. J. Travis and G. S. Kobayashi, Comparative *in vitro* activity of LY121019 and amphotericin B against clinical isolates of candida species, Eur. J. Clin. Microbiol. Infect. Dis., 7: 80. (1988).

15. F. Meunier, C. Lambert and P. Van der Auwera, *In-vitro* activity of cilofungin (LY121019) in comparison with amphotericin B, J. Antimicrob. Chemother., 24: 325. (1989).

16. M. Pfaller, R. Gordee, T. Gerarden, M. Yu and R. Wenzel, Fungicidal activity of cilofungin (LY121019) alone and in combination with anticapsin or other antifungal agents, Eur. J. Clin. Microbiol. Infect. Dis., 8: 564. (1989).

17. W. A. Craig, J. Moffatt and W. Bayer, Post-antibiotic effect of LY121019 against *Candida albicans*, I. C. A. A. C., abs 1526. (1988).

18. M. A. Pfaller, T. Gerarden, M. Yu and R. P. Wenzel, Influence of *in vitro* susceptibility testing conditions on the anticandidal activity of LY121019, Diagn.

Microbiol. Infect. Dis., 11: 1. (1988).

19. J. R. Graybill and J. Ahrens, LY121019(LY) in murine candidiasis: *In vivo* and *in vitro* correlations, I. C. A. A. C., abstr 1526. (1988).

20. P. Van der Auwera and F. Meunier, *In vitro* effects of cilofungin (LY121019),amphotericin B and amphotericin B deoxycholate on human polymorphonuclear leukocytes, J. Antimicrob. Chemother., 24: 747. (1989).

21. M. D. Richardson and G. Scott, Effect of LY121019 in neutrophil monolayer assays on phagocytosis and intracellular killing of Candida albicans, I. C. A. A. C., Abstr 1519. (1988).

22. T. Meshulam, S. M. Levitz, R. D. Diamond and A. M. Sugar, Effect of cilofungin (LY121019), a fungal cell wall synthesis inhibitor, on interactions of *Candida albicans* with human neutrophils, J. Antimicrob. Chemother., 24: 741. (1989).

23. R. S. Gordee, D. J. Zeckner, L. F. Ellis, A. L. Thakkar and L. C. Howard, *In vitro* and *in vivo* anti-candida activity and toxicology of LY121019, J. Antibiot., 37: 1054. (1984).

24. J. R. Perfect, M. M. Hobbs, K. A. Wright and D. T. Durack, Treatment of experimental disseminated candidiasis with cilofungin, Antimicrob. Agents Chemother., 33: 1811. (1989).

25. J. Lee, R. Gordee, D. Coleman, et al, Cilofungin shows non-linear plasma pharmacokinetics and tissue penetration in rabbits, A. S. M., abstr F24. (1990).

26. H. R. Black, G. L. Brier, J. D. Wolny and S. H. Dorrbecher, Pharmacology and pharmacokinetics of cilofungin, I. C. A. A. C., abstr 1357. (1989).

27. B. N. Doebbeling, B. D. Fine,Jr., M. A. Pfaller, C. T. Sheetz, J. B. Stokes and R. P.

Wenzel, Acute tubular necrosis and anion-gap acidosis during therapy with cilofungin (LY121019) in polyethylene glycol, I. C. A. A. C., abstr 583. (1990).

28. L. M. Pope, K. Tanaka and G. T. Cole, Efficacy of LY121019 in clearance of *Candida albicans* from body organs of persistently-colonized immunocompromised mice, I. C. A. A. C., abstr 1528. (1988).

29. C. J. Morrison and D. A. Stevens, Effect of LY121019(LY) on experimental murine candidosis, I. C. A. A. C., abstr 1530. (1988).

30. N. Khardovi, L. Kalvakuntla, E. Wong, B. Rosenbaum and G. P. Bodey, Comparative activites of cilofungin (LY121019) and amphotericin B against disseminated *Candida albicans* infection in neutropenic mice, I. C. A. A. C., abstr 817. (1989).

31. N. Khardori, H. Nguyen, B. Rosenblaum, A. Khan, L. C. Stephens and L. A. Von Behren, Clearance of organisms in disseminated *Candida albicans* infection in mice treated with cilofungin LY121019, A. S. M., abstr A110. (1990).

32. K. R. Smith, K. M. Lank, C. G. Cobbs, G. A. Cloud and W. E. Dismukes, Comparison of cilofungin and amphotericin B for therapy of murine candidiasis, Antimicrob. Agents Chemother., 34: 1619. (1990).

33. L. H. Hanson, A. M. Perlman, K. V. Clemons and D. A. Stevens, Synergy between cilofungin (C) and amphotericin B (AMB) in a murine model of candidosis, I. C. A. A. C., abstr 818. (1989).

34. A. Padula and H. F. Chambers, Evaluation of cilofungin (LY121019) for treatment of experimental *Candida albicans* endocarditis in rabbits, Antimicrob. Agents Chemother., 33: 1822. (1989).

35. M. S. Rouse, B. M. Tallan, J. M. Steckelberg, N. K. Henry and W. R. Wilson, Continuous-intravenous-infusion cilofungin is effective treatment of *Candida albicans*

experimental Candidiasis, I. C. A. A. C., abstr 187. (1990).

36. M. A. Crislip, S. G. Filler, C. L. Mayer and J. E. Edwards,Jr., Comparison of cilofungin and amphotericin B for the treatment of disseminated candidiasis with endophthalmitis in rabbits, A. S. M., abstr F78. (1990).

37. R. Chapman, J. Moody, . Fasching, L. Sinn, D. Gerding and L. Peterson, *In vitro* and *in vivo* activity of Cilofungin (Cilo) against clinical isolates of *Candida albicans* (A) and *Candida parapsilosis* (CP), I. C. A. A. C., abstr 819. (1989).

38. D. W. Denning and D. A. Stevens, Cilofungin treatment of disseminated aspergillosis in a murine model, I. C. A. A. C., abstr 286. (1990).

39. D. M. Schmatz, M. A. Romancheck, L. A. Pitatrelli, K. Nollstadt, K. Bartizal and M. J. Turner, Use of B-1,3 glucan synthesis inhibitors for treatment and prevention of *Pneumocystis carinii* pneumonia, I. C. A. A. C., abstr 585. (1990).

Synergistic Interaction of Nikkomycin and Cilofungin Against Diverse Fungi

J. R. Perfect[1], K. A. Wright[1] and R. F. Hector[2]

Department of Medicine, Division of Infectious Diseases[1]
Duke University Medical Center
Durham, North Carolina, 27710, USA

Cutter Biological[2]
Berkeley, California, 94710, USA

I. INTRODUCTION

The role of the cell wall in the life cycle of fungi is as dynamic as it is complex. While the cell wall provides the architectural framework for the fungus, it also changes during the morphological development of the organism. In the past, studies of fungal cell wall chemistry and morphology were used as a tool for the taxonomy of fungi (1). More recently, studies have focused on the fungal cell wall as a selective target for antifungal compounds, as this organelle differentiates the eukaryotic fungi from their host cells (2).

To date, most antifungal compounds whose target is the cell wall inhibit one of two crucial cell wall components. The first category of compounds is inhibitors of chitin synthesis; the second category is inhibitors of ß-glucan synthesis.

Inhibitors of chitin synthesis include the polyoxins and nikkomycins. The nikkomycins have a high level of activity against dimorphic fungi (3). Inhibitors of ß-glucan synthesis include echinocandin B, aculeacins and papulacandin. An analog of echinocandin B, cilofungin (LY121019), has received a great deal of attention in recent years. Cilofungin has potent fungicidal activity against Candida (4). The efficacy of both of these antifungal agents has been shown in a variety of animal models (3,5).

Various combinations of chitin and ß-glucan inhibitors have been considered, because none of the aforementioned compounds has the ideal antifungal profile. For instance, nikkomycin is not fungicidal, while cilofungin is. However, the nikkomycins have inhibitory activity against filamentous fungi, while cilofungin has a very limited spectrum of activity. It is known that for most fungi, the makeup of the cell wall varies during the life cycle (1). It has been previously shown in *Candida albicans* that the inhibition of ß-glucan synthesis results in increased production of chitin (6). It is also possible that different mechanisms for chitin synthesis are active during different growth phases, as suspected in *Coccidioides immitis* (7). Thus, the combination of a chitin and a ß-glucan inhibitor would seem likely to have synergistic activity. It is thought that perhaps one drug would complement deficiencies in the other.

Indeed, such combinations of chitin and ß-glucan inhibitors have shown synergy against *Candida albicans*. The combination of cilofungin and anticapsin produced rapid and sustained fungicidal in vitro activity, as well as eliminated the Eagle's effect noted with cilofungin alone (8). Both combinations of nikkomycin X or Z with papulacandin B were also synergistic against *Candida albicans* (6).

In the present study, we begin to evaluate the synergistic activity of nikkomycin Z and cilofungin against diverse dimorphic fungi. These include: *Aspergillus fumigatus, Cunninghamella bertholletiae, Fusarium oxysporum, Fusarium solani, Rhizopus arrhizus and Trichophyton rubrum.* These organisms were chosen for three important reasons. First, none of these organisms is susceptible to either single drug when tested *in vitro*. Second, these organisms represent a variety of cell wall compositions. Finally, antifungal therapy of infections caused by these fungi remains particularly limited.

II. MATERIALS AND METHODS

A. ORGANISMS

Recent clinical isolates of the following organisms were obtained from the Clinical Mycology Laboratory, Duke University Medical Center, Durham, NC: *Aspergillis fumigatus* (DUMC 131.90), *Cunninghamella bertholletiae* (DUMC 138.90), *Fusarium oxysporum* (DUMC 165.89), *Fusarium solani* (DUMC 152.89), *Rhizopus arrhizus* (DUMC 170.89), and *Trichophyton rubrum* (DUMC 149.90). A stock isolate of *A. fumigatus* (ATCC 13073) was also used.

Cultures were maintained at 30°C on slants of potato dextrose agar (Difco Laboratories, Detroit, MI). Cultures between five and ten days old were used for susceptibility testing. Conidia were recovered from the slant cultures using a wetting solution of 0.05% Tween 80 (J.T. Baker Chemical Co., Phillipsburg, N.J.) in phosphate buffered saline (PBS). The conidia suspension was counted using a hemacytometer, and diluted in Yeast Nitrogen Base (Difco Laboratories, Detroit, MI), buffered with PBS, pH 7.4 (bYNB).

B. ANTIFUNGAL AGENTS

Each drug was prepared at a concentration four times the final well concentration. Cilofungin (LY 121019, Eli Lilly and Co., Indianapolis, IN), was first dissolved at a 40x concentration in 95% ethanol, and then diluted 1:10 in bYNB. Nikkomycin Z (Miles Pharmaceuticals, West Haven, CT), was dissolved directly in bYNB.

For each assay, a 96-well Falcon microtiter plate (Becton Dickinson Co. USA) was prepared using a checkerboard dilution scheme. Each plate included a single growth control well to which no drugs were added. Eleven wells contained serial two-fold dilutions of nikkomycin alone, with the final well concentrations ranging from 4000 to 4 μg/ml. Seven wells contained serial two-fold dilutions of cilofungin alone, with final well concentrations ranging from 250 to 4 μg/ml. The remaining seventy-seven wells contained combinations of all dilutions of the two drugs.

C. SUSCEPTIBILITY TESTING

1. Determination of fractional inhibitory concentrations. A basic broth microdilution technique was used (9). Inoculum size was 1 x 10^4 conidia/ ml. In the initial assay for antifungal susceptibility, the drugs and conidia suspension were added simultaneously. To determine the antifungal effects on actively growing fungi, separate microtiter plates were seeded with conidia and incubated for a period of time, appropriate for each species. After germination of at least 50% of the conidia, the drug dilutions were added to the wells.

Antifungal activity was determined by observing morphological alterations of cell growth, using an inverted phase contrast microscope (Nikon Diaphot-TMD) with a camera attachment. The effects of nikkomycin and cilofungin on cell wall synthesis were manifested in two ways: the development of large, refractile vacuolated cells, previously determined to be osmotically sensitive, and the inhibition of filamentous growth. While degrees of inhibition of filamentous growth were discernible, the chosen endpoint criteria was the absence of all filamentous growth. In the experiments where conidia were allowed to germinate before adding drugs, filamentous growth was compared to the growth at the time the drugs were added.

As a quantitative determination of synergy, the fractional inhibitory concentration index (FIC index) was calculated wherever possible, using the equation below (10). The combination value was derived from the lowest concentration of each of the drugs in antifungal combinations permitting no growth. An FIC index of 0.5 was used as the cut-off point for synergism.

$$\text{FIC Index:} \quad \frac{\text{MIC}^{N}\ \text{comb}}{\text{MIC}^{N}} + \frac{\text{MIC}^{C}\ \text{comb}}{\text{MIC}^{C}}$$

2. Assay for fungicidal activity. From each microtiter plate, twenty representative wells were cultured, including the growth control, selected drug dilutions, and the corresponding combinations. Ten microliter aliquots were dropped onto Sabouraud dextrose agar plates (Difco Laboratories) and incubated at 30°C for 24-48 hr. Growth was scored as either positive or negative when compared to the control. In this assay, no growth indicated 95% kill or better.

III. RESULTS AND DISCUSSION

A. ASPERGILLUS FUMIGATUS

When the conidia and the drug combinations were incubated for 24 hr at 37°C, the synergy was obvious to the unaided eye. Figure 1 shows the concentration combinations at which nikkomycin and cilofungin inhibited visible growth of *A. fumigatus* (ATCC 13073). Cilofungin alone inhibited filamentous growth at 125 μg/ml; nikkomycin alone was not inhibitory when tested up to 4000 μg/ml. However, combinations of the drugs were synergistic. The FIC index (0.07) is well below the cut-off for synergistic activity.

When aliquots were plated on agar for determination of fungicidal activity, results were ambiguous. Many aliquots representing synergistic drug combinations were positive when subcultured. They were, however, significantly smaller than the growth control.

In another experiment, microtiter wells were seeded with conidia 24 hr prior to the addition of drugs. Figure 2 illustrates the synergistic effects on actively growing fungi. In this and all subsequent experiments, filamentous growth was observed with an inverted microscope, thus making the endpoint criteria even stricter. The FIC index for this experiment was 0.04.

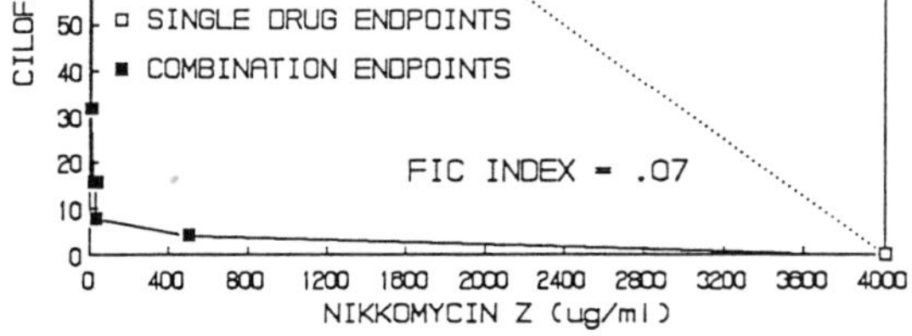

Figure 1. Synergistic effects of nikkomycin and cilofungin on conidia of *Aspergillus funigatus* (ATCC 13073). Endpoints represent complete inhibition of visible growth.

A final observation was consistent for these and all experiments performed. At high concentrations of cilofungin (250 μg/ml), alone and in combination with nikkomycin, deposits of yeast-like cells filled the bottom of the wells. These have been previously described and determined to be viable in cilofungin susceptibility studies {1366}. The cells from the cilofungin well (250 μg/ml) were viable on Sabouraud agar, but combinations with increasing concentrations of nikkomycin proved to be fungicidal.

B. CUNNINGHAMELLA BERTHOLLETIAE

Under a variety of experimental conditions, nikkomycin and cilofungin proved to be synergistic against *C. bertholletiae*. In a series of experiments incubating drugs and conidia from 18 to 24 hr at 30°C, the resultant FIC indices ranged from 0.07 to 0.27. When aliquots were plated at 24 hr for a measure of fungicidal activity, the results correlated well with the microscopic observations: aliquots from any wells originally scored as negative for filamentous growth, were completely negative when subcultured in the absence of drugs. In one experiment, the original microtiter plates were incubated for an additional 24 hr. The FIC index (0.14) remained well within the synergistic range, suggesting fungicidal activity for many of the drug combinations.

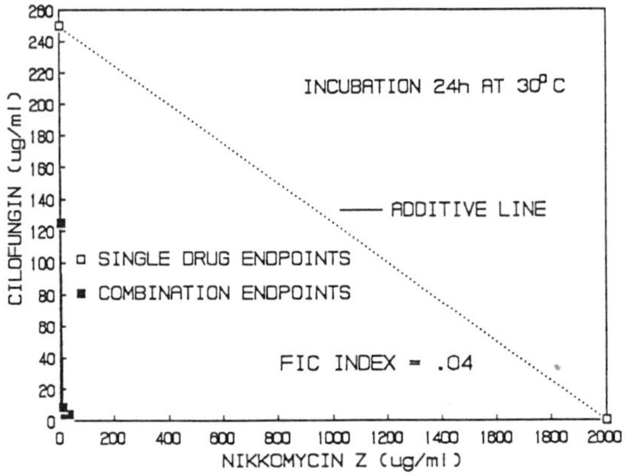

Figure 2. Synergistic effects of nikkomycin and cilofungin on actively growing *Aspergillus fumigatus* (DUMC 131.90). Endpoints represent complete inhibition of filamentous growth.

A separate assay for inhibition of actively growing fungus also showed excellent synergy. Conidia of *C. bertholletiae* were incubated for 6-8 hr, until filamentous growth was detected. After an additional 24 hr incubation with the drugs, the FIC index was 0.02. Selected aliquots from this plate were also subcultured on agar, and again, the synergistic combinations were also fungicidal.

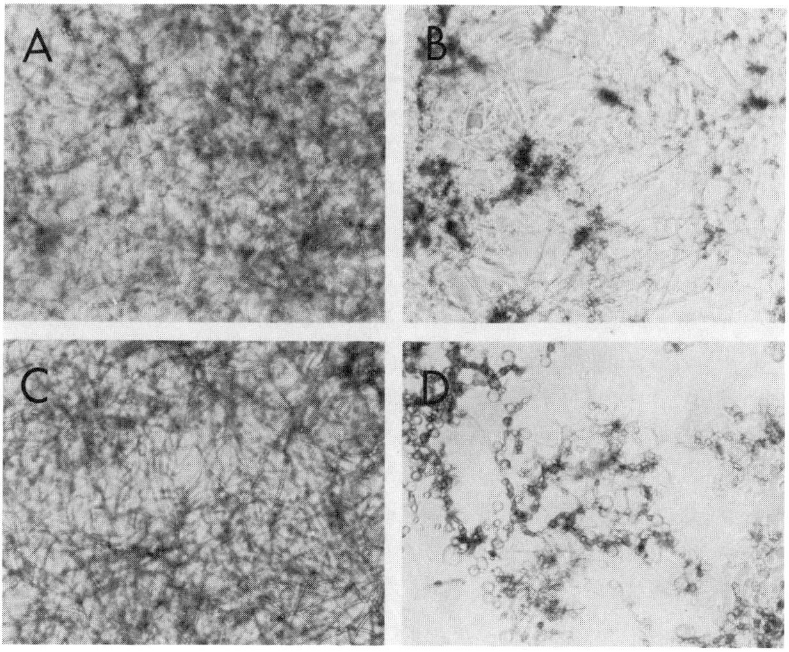

Figure 3. Synergistic effects of nikkomycin and cilofungin on *Fusarium oxysporum*. Inhibition of filamentous growth, and development of large, refractile vesicles were observed at 24 hr. A. Growth control; B. Nikkomycin, 4 μg/ml; C. Cilofungin, 4 μg/ml; D. Nikkomycin, 4 μg/ml + cilofungin, 4 μg/ml.

C. FUSARIUM SPP.

The *Fusarium* species proved to be more difficult to evaluate with the endpoint defined. for this study. In a single experiment, complete inhibition of filamentous growth was noted only at the highest concentration for both drugs (250 μg/ml cilofungin or 4000 μg/ml nikkomycin). In repeated experiments, though, filamentous growth was observed for both drugs singly, and at all combinations tested. Even though there was never complete inhibition, it was possible to discern varying degrees of filamentous growth. Additionally, the large refractile vesicles were noted at even the lowest combination concentration. Figure 3 dramatically illustrates the combined effects of the two drugs on the morphology of *Fusarium oxysporum*. Aliquots were not subcultured on agar. Fungicidal activity was suggested in the first experiment, though, after the microtiter plate was incubated for an additional 24 hr at 30°C. Filamentous growth was observed at the highest concentrations tested for both cilofungin (250 μg/ml) and nikkomycin (4000 μg/ml), which had been negative 24 hr earlier. However, all that could be seen in the combination well for the same drug concentrations was the remains of hyphal fragments and lysed cells.

D. RHIZOPUS ARRHIZUS

A definite conclusion could not be made about synergistic activity of the combination against *Rhizopus arrhizus*. In repeated experiments, the FIC index (0.53) was borderline for synergistic activity. However, incubating the conidia for 12 hr, and allowing them to germinate prior to the addition of drugs, appeared to improve the synergistic antifungal activity. After an additional 12 hr incubation period, the FIC index was 0.25. It should be noted, though, that the inhibitory concentrations were still high (62.5 μg/ml cilofungin, 1000 μg/ml nikkomycin).

E. TRICHOPHYTON RUBRUM

Again, the choice of endpoint criteria prohibited quantitative determination of synergy. After 72 hr incubation, there was very little filamentous growth in the control well. Germination had occurred, but hyphae were very short. A few small foci of filamentous growth were observed, but nothing like the overgrown filamentous network seen with other fungi. Thus it was more difficult to describe antifungal effects based on inhibition of filamentous growth. However, at 72 hr, antifungal effects were clearly noted by the presence of the large, refractile vesicles. It was difficult to assess synergy, but the higher concentrations of nikkomycin clearly enhanced antifungal effects. At low concentrations of both drugs, there were some vesicles present among the germinated conidia, and with higher concentrations, increasing numbers of larger vesicles and ungerminated cells were observed. At the highest concentrations, many of the vesicles were lysed.

IV. CONCLUSION

In these preliminary experiments, we have explored the possible synergistic interaction of nikkomycin and cilofungin. For *Aspergillis fumigatus, Cunninghamella bertholletiae*, and *Rhizopus arrhizus*, we were able to assess synergistic effects quantitatively. For other fungi, this was not possible, but we can confidently report our observations of the morphological effects of nikkomycin and cilofungin on the filamentous fungi. To a great extent, this analysis was impeded by the difficulties associated with antifungal susceptibility testing. Only recently has progress been made towards adopting a standard, reproducible method for single drug susceptibility testing of yeast (12). Even so, the present study was further complicated by the analysis of two antifungal agents against six filamentous fungi with different growth characteristics. Methods such as the quantitation of hyphal mass, agar dilution (13), and broth macro- and micro-dilution techniques (14) have been employed with filamentous fungi, but there is not agreement on a standard method. Most techniques rely on visual observation of growth, which is a very subjective endpoint criteria. With microscopic observations of filamentous growth, and a strict endpoint, the calculation of an FIC index was possible as well as reproducible. In other cases, though, a criteria based on the proliferation of the large refractile vesicles might have been a useful index of antifungal effects. Even considering the practical difficulties, the observed synergistic effects of nikkomycin and cilofungin are exciting. Further investigation of the mechanisms of their action and interaction against the fungal cell wall will certainly be a significant contribution to the development of new antifungal agents.

ACKNOWLEDGMENT

We are especially grateful to Wiley Schell of the Clinical Mycology Laboratory, Duke University Medical Center, for his expert advice and assistance.

REFERENCES

1. S. Bartnicki-Garcia, Cell wall chemistry, morphogenesis, and toxonomy of fungi, Ann. Rev. Microbiol., 22: 87. (1968).

2. S. Cassone, Cell wall of pathogenic yeasts and implications for antimycotic therapy, Drugs Under Expt. Clin. Res., 12: 635. (1986).

3. R. F. Hector, B. L. Zimmer and D. Pappagianis, Evaluation of nikkomycins X and Z in murine models of Coccidioidomycosis, Histoplasmosis and Blastomycosis, Antimicrob. Agents Chemother., 34: 587. (1990).

4. M. Pfaller, J. Riley and T. Koerner, Effects of cilofungin (LY121019) on carbohydrate and sterol composition of *Candida albicans*, Eur. J. Clin. Microbiol. Infect. Dis., 8: 1067. (1989).

5. R. S. Gordee, D. J. Zeckner, L. F. Ellis, A. L. Thakkar and L. C. Howard, *In vitro* and *in vivo* anti-candida activity and toxicology of LY121019, J. Antibiot., 37: 1054. (1984).

6. R. F. Hector and P. C. Braun, Synergistic action of nikkomycins X and Z with papulacandin B on whole cells and regenrating protoplasts of Candida albicans, Antimicrob. Agents Chemother., 29: 389. (1986).

7. R. F. Hector and D. Pappagianis, Inhibition of chitin synthesis in the cell wall of Coccidioides immitis by polyoxin D, J. Bacteriol., 154: 488. (1983).

8. M. Pfauer, R. Gordee, T. Gerarden, M. Yu and R. Wenzel, Fungicidal Activity of cilofungin (LY121019) alone and in combination with anticapsin or other antifungal agents, Eur. J. Clin. Microbiol. Infect. Dis., 8: 564. (1989).

9. M. G. Rinaldi and A. W. Howell, Antifungal susceptible testing, Diagnostic Procedures for Mycotic and Parasitic Infections (B. Wentworth, ed.), American Public Health Association, Washington, p. 338. (1988).

10. H. O. Hallander, K. Dornbusch, L. Gezelius, K. Jacobson and I. Karlsson, Synergism between aminoglycosides and cephalosporins with antipseudomonal activity: interaction index and killing curve method, Antimicrob. Agents Chemother., 22: 743. (1982).

11. M. G. Rinaldi, D. A. McGough and J. L. Anderson, In vitro evaluation of LY121019, a recent, semi-synthetic, lipopeptide antifungal agent, I. C. A. A. C., abstr 267. (1987).

12. M. A. Pfaller, M. G. Rinaldi, J. N. Galgiani, et al, Collaborative investigation of variables in susceptibility testing of yeasts, Antimicrob. Agents Chemother., 34: 1648. (1990).

13. J. C. Christenson, I. Shalit, D. F. Welch, A. Guruswamy and M. I. Marks, Synergistic action of amphotericin B and rifampin against Rhizopus species, Antimicrob. Agents Chemother., 31: 1775. (1987).

14. A. Reuben, E. Anaissic, P. E. Nelson, et al, Antifungal susceptibility of 44 clinical isolates of Fusarium species determined using a broth microdilution method, Antimicrob. Agents Chemother., 33: 1647. (1989).

31

A New Family of Antibiotics: Benzo[*a*] Naphthacenequinones

A Water-Soluble Pradimicin Derivative, BMY-28864

T. Oki

Bristol-Myers Squibb Research Institute, Bristol-Myers Squibb K.K., 2-9-3 Shimo-Meguro, Meguro-ku, Tokyo 153, Japan

I. INTRODUCTION

A number of antifungal agents have been discovered and developed, but only a few are active in both *in vitro* and *in vivo* systems. The primary fungicidal drug used to treat systemic mycoses is amphotericin B. Despite its general effectiveness, amphotericin B is associated with a number of complications and unique toxicities that limit its usage. Azoles and triazoles have been extensively synthesized in the 1970's and 1980's, and itraconazole and fulconazole appear to have the most potential for the treatment of superficial and deep mycoses in humans with less toxicity than currently available azoles. On the other hand, an increasing number of invasive fungal infections have been reported in patients who are severely immunocompromised by AIDS, organ and bone marrow transplantations and cancer chemotherapy. The problems faced under such circumstances have stimulated a search for new antifungal agents that are active against a wide range of fungal pathogens, have new mechanisms of action, and are less toxic.

In the course of screening microbial metabolites, two unique antifungal agents, pradimicin A [1,2, Fig. 1] and cispentacin [3,4, Fig. 1] were discovered in 1987.

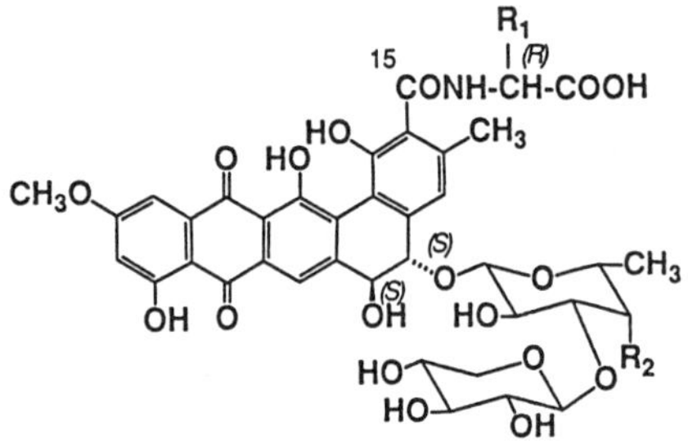

	R_1	R_2
Pradimicin A	CH_3	$NHCH_3$
Pradimicin FA-1	CH_2OH	$NHCH_3$
Pradimicin FA-2	CH_2OH	NH_2
BMY-28864	CH_2OH	$NH(CH_3)_2$

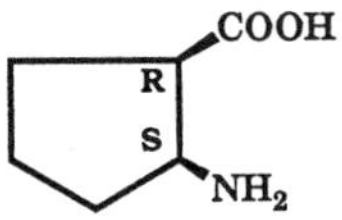

Cispentacin
[(1R,2S)-2-Aminocyclopentane-1-carboxylic acid]

Fig. 1 Chemical structures of pradimicin and cispentacin

II. PRADIMICIN A AND ITS MODIFICATION

A novel antifungal antibiotic pradimicin A is produced by *Actinomadura hibisca* sp. nov. No. P157-2 (ATCC 53557) and *Actinomadura verrucosospora* subsp. *neohibisca* sp. nov. No. R103-3. The antibiotic has been recovered from the fermentation broth supernatant by precipitation at pH 5.0, purified by a combination of solvent partition and chromatography, and isolated as amphoteric red crystals of the monosodium salt. D-Alanine, D-xylose, 4,6-dideoxy-

4-methylamino-D-galactose and a substituted 5,6-dihydro-benz[a] naphthacenequinone have been identified as chemical degradation products, and the complete structure for pradimicin A was assigned after NMR spectral studies as shown in Fig. 1. Pradimicin A, while relatively non-toxic and quite broadly active against human fungal pathogens, had very poor solubility, making both treatment and toxicological assessments somewhat problematical. In order to improve the water solubility, the microbial modification has primarily been focused on the D-alanine moiety to be replaced with other amino acids [5]. Pradimicins FA-1 and FA-2, D-serine congeners of pradimicin A and C, were predominantly produced by feeding DL-serine to the growing culture of a variant strain A2493 of *A. hibisca* [6]. Reductive alkylation of pradimicin FA-2 (solubility 0.03 mg/ml in Dulbecco's phosphate buffered saline containing 0.9 mM Ca^{++} and 0.5 mM Mg^{++}, pH 7.2, at 25°C) with $NaBH_3CN$ and formaldehyde yielded a water soluble derivative BMY-28864 (solubility; >20 mg/ml) [7].

III. ANTIFUNGAL ACTIVITY AND ACUTE TOXICITY

Comparative *in vitro* studies, as shown in Tables 1 and 2, indicated that pradimicin A and BMY-28864 show limited antibacterial activity against *Micrococcus luteus* and *Mycobacteria*, yet are significantly more active than ketoconazole against a wide variety of yeasts and fungi including clinically important pathogens and azole resistant *Candida* on Sabouraud dextrose agar medium.

BMY-28864 has a broader antifungal spectrum than pradimicin A against a variety of strains of *Candida*, *Cryptococcus*, *Aspergillus*, *Sporothrix* and *Trichophyton*, but is not susceptible to *A. flavus* and *Mucor spinosus*. *In vitro* anti-*Candida* activity of BMY-28864 was not influenced by the medium pH, inoculum size and serum concentration in the medium. The cidal action of BMY-28864 against *Candida albicans* and *Saccharomyces cerevisiae* was demonstrated at about MIC concentration.

As shown in Table 2, 17-epipradimicin A has no *in vitro* antifungal activity indicating that the change in stereo-chemistry at the C-17 position results in a complete loss of activity [8]. Accumulated results demonstrate that the D-amino acid moiety of pradimicins plays an important role in the expression of antifungal activity.

TABLE 1

In Vitro Antibacterial Activity

Test organism	MIC (μg/ml)		
	BMY-28864	Pradimicin A	Kanamycin A
Staphylococcus aureus FDA 209P	>100	>100	0.8
Staphylococcus epidermidis D153	>100	>100	0.8
Enterococcus faecalis A9612	-	>100	50
Micrococcus luteus PCI1001	12.5	3.1	3.1
Micrococcus luteus ATCC9341	3.1	3.1	12.5
Bacillus subtilis PCI219	>100	>100	0.1
Escherichia coli Juhl	>100	>100	6.3
Enterobacter cloacae A9659	>100	>100	3.1
Klebsiella pneumoniae D11	>100	>100	0.8
Pseudomonas aeruginosa A9930	>100	>100	25
Proteus vulgaris A9436	>100	>100	1.6
Morganella morganii A9553	>100	>100	6.3
Serratia marcescens A20222	>100	>100	6.3
Mycobacterium 607	-	25	0.8
Mycobacterium 607 KM-R*	-	25	>100
Mycobacterium 607 KM/SM-R**	-	25	>100
Mycobacterium phlei	-	12.5	0.4
Mycobacterium ranae	-	25	0.8

* Kanamycin-resistant strain
** Kanamycin & Streptomycin-resistant strain
Nutrient agar (Eiken), and 1001 agar for *Mycobacterium*

TABLE 2

Comparative *In vitro* Antifungal Activities of BMY-28864, Pradimicin A, Amphotericin B and Ketozonazole Against Yeasts, and Filamentous, Dimorphic and Dematiaceous Fungi

Test organism	MIC (μg/ml)*			
	BMY-28864	Pra-A	Amph-B	KCZ
Saccharomyces cerevisiae ATCC9763	3.1	12.5(>100)	0.2	50
Candida albicans A9540	6.3	50 (>100)	0.8	25
Candida albicans ATCC38247	0.8	3.1	25	12.5
Candida albicans YA22851 (5-FC R)	3.1	12.5	1.6	6.3
Candida albicans 83-2-14	12.5	>100	0.8	6.3
Candida tropicalis IFO10241	50	>100	0.8	12.5
Candida tropicalis CS-07	6.3	25	1.6	50
Candida tropicalis 85-130	12.5	>100	1.6	12.5
Candida parapsilosis CS-08	3.1	>100	1.6	<0.05
Candida parapsilosis IFM40088	3.1	6.3	0.8	<0.05
Candida glabrata IFM40065	0.8	0.8	0.8	0.8
Candida glabrata IFM40091	1.6	1.6	0.8	0.1
Candida krusei A15052	3.1	25	1.6	50
Candida krusei 85-12-19	1.6	1.6	1.6	0.8
Cryptococcus neoformans D49	1.6	1.6	0.4	0.2
Cryptococcus neoformans IAM4514	1.6	0.8	0.4	0.2
Cryptococcus neoformans CS-01	1.6	1.6	1.6	0.8
Cryptococcus neoformans IFM40046	1.6	0.8	0.8	0.8
Aspergillus niger van Tieghem	50	>100	0.8	1.6
Aspergillus fumigatus IAM2034	3.1	1.6	0.8	1.6
Aspergillus fumigatus IAM2530	3.1	1.6	1.6	3.1
Aspergillus fumigatus IFM40775	3.1	1.6	1.6	3.1
Aspergillus flavus FA21436,NRRL484	25	25	1.6	0.4
Aspergillus flavus CS-18	100	25	6.3	1.6
Fusarium moniliforme A2284	12.5	3.1	3.1	6.3
Mucor spinosus IFO5317	>100	>100	1.6	50
Sporothrix schenckii IFO8158	3.1	1.6	3.1	6.3
Sporothrix schenckii IFM40750	3.1	1.6	0.8	1.6
Trichophyton mentagrophytes #4329	3.1	1.6(>100)	0.8	0.2
Trichophyton mentagrophytes D155	3.1	1.6	0.8	0.2

Determined on Sabouraud dextrose agar, pH 7.0
Inoculum size: $2x10^6$ cells/ml (5 μl/spot)
Pra-A: Pradimicin A
( ): MICs of 17-Epipradimicin A

The *in vivo* efficacy of BMY-28864 was assessed in experimental infections of mice produced by intravenous inoculation of *C. albicans*, *C. neoformans* and *A. fumigatus* in comparison with pradimicin A, amphotericin B and ketoconazole. Male ICR mice weighing 20 to 25 g were infected with 10 times the median lethal inoculum size of the test fungi. The agent at various dose levels was administered to groups of 5 mice each once a day, twice daily for 2 days or once for 5 consecutive days, and the dose that protects 50% of the mice from infection (PD_{50}; mg/kg) was calculated from survival rates on day 20 after fungal infection. As shown in Table 3, BMY-28864 exhibits pronounced therapeutic efficacy, equal to pradimicin A, curing mice from these fungal systemic infections.

TABLE 3

Comparative *In Vivo* Efficacy of BMY-28864

Organism		Intravenous dosing	PD50 (mg/kg/inj.) BMY-28864	Pra-A	Amph-B	KCZ
C. albicans	A9540	single	12.0	7.5	0.35	40.0
	"	bidx2	2.7	3.6	0.19	>100
	"	qdx5	7.5	3.5	0.12	-
	A25928	bidx2	10.9	12.5	0.08	50.0
	A25942	bidx2	14.4	25.0	0.25	-
	A26090	bidx2	6.3	3.1	0.13	>100
	A15051	bidx2	6.3	>25	0.06	-
C. neoformans	IAM4514	single	11.0	11.0	0.36	>100
	"	qdx5	2.8	0.95	0.18	-
A. fumigatus	IAM2034	single	36.0	16.0	0.28	45.0
	"	qdx5	15.0	7.2	0.09	-
Acute toxicity (LD_{50}, mg/kg)			>600	120	4.5	-

Intravenous infection with $10LD_{50}$ in ICR mice
Determined on day 20

Against *Candida* and *Aspergillus* lung infections in immunocompromised mice, BMY-28864 showed as good PD_{50} values as in normal mice. The LD_{50} value of pradimicin A was 120 mg/kg following intravenous administration to mice, and that of BMY-28864 increased favorably up to more than 600 mg/kg. The ratio between acute toxicity and efficacy (LD_{50}/PD_{50}) is much better for BMY-28864 (>60∿>16) than for amphotericin B (15∿12).

IV. ANTIVIRAL ACTIVITY

Pradimicin A shows selective anti-influenza A activity in MDCK cells by both dye-uptake and plaque reduction assays, while its derivative BMY-28864 does not exhibit antiviral activity against HSV-1 and influenza A viruses and cytotoxicity in Vero and MDCK cells, as shown in Table 3. Interestingly, it was found that pradimicin A effectively suppressed the human T-lymphotropic virus type IIIB (HTLV-IIIB)-induced cytopathic effects of MT-4 cells, and also showed inhibitory activity at 12.5 μg/ml to the syncytia formation in the cocultures of MOLT-4 and MOLT-4/HIV_{HTLV}-IIIB cells [9, 10]. It is noticeable that various mammalian cells in culture tolerated up to 500 μg/ml of pradimicins.

TABLE 4

Comparative Antiviral Activity of BMY-28864

Virus/ Host cells	ID50/TD50 (μg/ml) BMY-28864	Pra-A	Ribavirin	Acyclovir	AZT
Herpes Simplex Virus-1/Vero cells					
-Dye uptake	>400/>400	12.8/12.8	-	0.27/>200	-
-Plaque reduction	>200/>200	>200/>200	-	0.22/>200	-
Influenza A virus/MDCK cells					
-Dye uptake	>400/>400	8.7/>200	4.0/>50	-	-
-Plaque reduction	>200/>200	6.8/>200	1.6/>200	-	-
HIV/HTLV type 1-carrying T cells					
	70/>500	3.1/>100	-	-	0.03/133

V. MODE OF ACTION

Pradimicin A showed cidal activity at 10 μg/ml against *C. albicans* both under growing and non-growing conditions in Difco yeast nitrogen base containing 1% glucose (pH 7.0) and Dulbecco's phosphate buffered saline containing 0.9 mM Ca^{++} and 0.5 mM Mg^{++} (pH 7.2), followed by rapid induction of K^{+} leakage from the cells. Another significant observation was the substantial binding of pradimicin A to the cells of *C. albicans* in the presence of calcium ion [11]. These interesting phenomena relating to the action mechanism were confirmed by using a water soluble derivative BMY-28864. As shown in Table 5, BMY-28864 requires calcium ion for expressing its antifungal activity and for binding to susceptible microorganisms such as *Candida*, *Saccharomyces*, *Cryptococcus* and *Trychophyton*. BMY-28864 cannot bind to unsusceptible *Mucor* and bacteria even in the presence of 200 μM Ca^{++}.

TABLE 5

Binding of BMY-28864 to Various Microorganisms and Its MIC in the Presence and Absence of Ca^{2+}

Microorganism	Amount of bound BMY-28864 (μg/mg dried cells)		MIC (μg/ml)	
	$+CaCl_2$	$-CaCl_2$	$+CaCl_2$	$-CaCl_2$
Saccharomyces cerevisiae ATCC9763	52	6	3.1	>100
Candida albicans A9540	41	3	6.3	>100
Cryptococcus neoformans IAM4514	12	4	1.6	>100
Trychophyton mentagrophytes No. 4329	14	6	12.5	>100
Mucor spinosus IFO5317	7	6	>100	>100
Escherichia coli NIHJ JC-2	0	0	>100	ND
Bacillus subtilis ATCC6633	0	0	>100	ND

Dried cells (1 mg/ml) were mixed with 60 μg/ml BMY-28864 in the presence and absence of 200 μM calcium chloride in 50 mM sodium phosphate, pH 7.0. The amount of BMY-28864 which bound to the cells was determined by spectrophotometry at 498 nm. MICs were determined on YNBG-PB agar for fungi, and on nutrient agar for bacteria.

As shown in Table 6, antifungal activity can be antagonized by mannan and dried yeast cells, but not by mannose, chitin and glucan. It was demonstrated that BMY-28864 binds rapidly and substantially to yeast mannan to yield an insoluble complex in the presence of Ca^{++}. The killing effect, binding to cell surface mannan and potassium leakage from *C. albicans* was completely reversed with 2 mM EGTA. Human erythrocytes and various mammalian cells showed neither binding of BMY-28864 nor potassium leakage or cell death in the presence of a large amount of calcium ion. The calcium dependent action of BMY-28864 is considered to be mediated primarily by mannan residues on the cell surface and plasma membrane which hence bring about the selective action on yeasts and fungi leading to a perturbation of membrane function. Electron microscopic observations supported the unique mode of action of BMY-28864: invagination and detachment of cell membrane, nuclear membrane damage, delocalization of nuclei and damaged microtubules.

TABLE 6

Antagonistic Effect of Various Substances on Antifungal Activities of Pradimicin A and BMY-28864

Antagonist	50% Antagonistic conc. (μg/ml)* BMY-28864	Pradimicin A
Yeast mannan (Sigma, M7504)	17	6
Acetone powder of *C. albicans* cells	1300	690
Acetone powder of *S. cerevisiae* cells	530	490
Mannose	>4000	>4000
Chitin	>4000	>4000
Yeast glucan (Sigma, G5011)	>4000	>4000

Reaction: Pradimicin derivative (100 μg/ml) and Antagonist (<4 mg/ml) in 10mM PB (pH 7.0) supplemented with 0.02mM $CaCl_2$, for 15 min at room temperature

*Assay: Minimum concentration required to antagonize 50% of the antifungal activity of pradimicin A or BMY-28864 against *Asp. niger* by the agar well diffusion method on MA medium

VI. PHARMACOKINETICS

Blood level, urinary excretion and tissue distribution of BMY-28864 were investigated in male ddY mice. After intravenous administration of 20 mg/kg, plasma concentrations of BMY-28864 and pradimicin A declined with a half-life of about 10 min and 2.6 hrs, respectively, as shown in Table 7. The plasma level of BMY-28864 was retained at a level greater than 10 μg/ml for 16 hours with 570 μg.hr/ml of AUC. Excellent urinary recovery (92% of dose for 24 hrs) and favorable tissue distribution were observed in BMY-28864, while pradimicin A showed characteristic kidney accumulation and poor urinary recovery (42% for 24 hrs). A high level of pradimicin A was retained in the kidney for 24 hrs. No metabolites were detected in the tissue, urine or plasma of mice given 100 mg/kg of pradimicin A and BMY-28864. The unexpected metabolic stability of this type of molecule is characteristic.

TABLE 7

Pharmacokinetics in Mice (20 mg/kg iv, n=6)

	BMY-28864	Pradimicin A
Plasma level		
$T_{1/2}$ (hr) α	0.2	2.6
ß	4.6	20
AUC (μg.hr/ml)	570	331
Urinary recovery (%)		
7 hrs/24 hrs	69 / 92	18 / 42
Tissue level (μg/g or ml)		
Liver 7 hrs/24 hrs	5.1 / ND	32.1 / 29.1
Kidney "	12.6 / 7.8	361 / 192
Lung "	8.5 / ND	10.0 / 6.6
Spleen "	ND / ND	11.5 / 10.6
Plasma "	29.0 / 1.4	9.5 / 4.5

ND: Not detectable Assay: HPLC

REFERENCES

1. T. Oki, M. Konishi, K. Tomatsu, K. Tomita, K. Saitoh, M. Tsunakawa, M. Nishio, T. Miyaki, and H. Kawaguchi, Pradimicin, A Novel class of potent antifungal antibiotics, J. Antibiotics, 41:1701 (1988).

2. M. Tsunakawa, M. Nishio, H. Ohkuma, T. Tsuno, M. Konishi, T. Naito, T. Oki, and H. Kawaguchi, The structures of pradimicin A, B and C: a novel family of antifungal antibiotics, J. Org. Chem., 54:2532 (1989).

3. M. Konishi, M. Nishio, K. Saitoh, T. Miyaki, T. Oki, and H. Kawaguchi, Cispentacin, a new antifungal antibiotic, I. Production, isolation, physico-chemical properties and structure, J. Antibiotics, 42:1749 (1989).

4. T. Oki, M. Hirano, K. Tomatsu, K. Numata, and H. Kawaguchi, Cispentacin, a new antifungal antibiotic, II. *In vitro* and *in vivo* antifungal activities, J. Antibiotics, 42:1756 (1989).

5. M. Kakushima, Y. Sawada, M. Nishio, T. Tsuno, and T. Oki, Biosynthesis of pradimicin A, J. Org. Chem., 54:2536 (1989).

6. Y. Sawada, M. Hatori, H. Yamamoto, M. Nishio, T. Miyaki, and T. Oki, New antifungal antibiotics pradimicins FA-1 and FA-2: D-serine analogs of pradimicins A and C, J. Antibiotics, 43(10), in press (1990).

7. T. Oki, M. Kakushima, M. Nishio, H. Kamei, M. Hirano, Y. Sawada, and M. Konishi, Water-soluble pradimicin derivatives, synthesis and antifungal evaluation of *N,N*-dimethyl pradimicins, J. Antibiotics, 43(10), in press (1990).

8. M. Kakushima, M. Nishio, K. Numata, M. Konishi, and T. Oki, Effect of stereochemistry at the C-17 position on the antifungal activity of pradimicin A, J. Antibiotics, 43:1028 (1990).

9. A. Tanabe, H. Nakashima, O. Yoshida, N. Yamamoto, O. Tenmyo, and T. Oki, Inhibitory effect of new antibiotic, pradimicin A on infectivity, cytopathic effect and replication of human immunodeficiency virus *in vitro*, J. Antibiotics, 41:1708 (1988).

10. A. Tanabe-Tochikura, T. Tochikura, O. Yoshida, T. Oki, and N. Yamamoto, Pradimicin A inhibition of human immuno-deficiency virus: Attenuation by mannan, J. Virology, 176:467 (1990).

11. Y. Sawada, K. Numata, T. Murakami, H. Tanimichi, S. Yamamoto, and T. Oki, Calcium-dependent anticandidal action of pradimicin A, J. Antibiotics, 43:715 (1990).

A Novel Antifungal Antibiotic, Benanomicin A

H. Yamaguchi, S. Inouye*, Y. Orikasa*, H. Tohyama*, K. Komuro*, S. Gomi*, S. Ohuchi*, T. Matsumoto*, M. Yamaguchi, T. Hiratani, K. Uchida, Y. Ohsumi**, S. Kondo*** and T. Takeuchi***

Research Center for Medical Mycology, Teikyo University, Tokyo, Pharmaceutical Research Center, Meiji Seika Kaisha, Ltd., Yokohama, University of Tokyo, Tokyo** and Institute of Microbial Chemistry, Tokyo, Japan****

INTRODUCTION

A novel antifungal antibiotic benanomicin A (abbreviated as BNM-A) was produced by *Actinomadura* sp. MH193-16F4 and isolated as a dark red powder (1). The structure of BNM-A (Fig. 1) possessing a unique benzonaphthacene chromophore was elucidated (2), and the biosynthetic studies indicated that the aglycone of BNM-A was derived from a dodecaketide, methionine and alanine (3). BNM-A inhibited *de novo* infection of T-cells with human immunodeficiency virus type 1 (HIV-1) and syncytium formation of T-cells by co-cultivation with the virus producing cells (4).

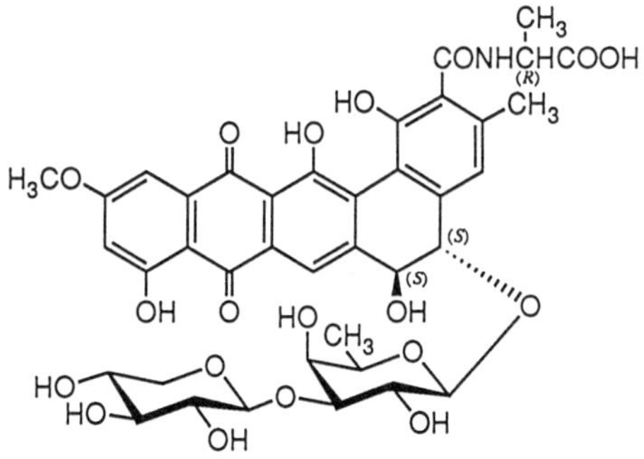

Sodium salt

Appearance : dark red powder
Molecular formula : $C_{39}H_{40}NO_{19}\cdot Na$
Molecular weight : 849
Solubility : *ca.* 10% in water

FIG. 1. Structure of benanomicin A

TABLE 1

In vitro activity of benanomicin A against major pathogenic fungi

Organism	(No. of strains)	MIC (μg/ml) Benanomicin A range	geometric mean	Amphotericin B range	geometric mean
Candida albicans	(6)	5-10	7.08	0.63-2.5	1.32
Candida glabrata	(4)	1.25-2.5	1.78	0.63-2.5	2.49
Candida tropicalis	(3)	10-40	15.9	2.5	2.5
Candida parapsilosis	(2)	10	10	10	10
Aspergillus fumigatus	(5)	5-20	7.59	1.25-10	3.79
Cryptococcus neoformans	(5)	1.25-5	2.18	0.63-2.5	1.44
Trichophyton mentagrophytes	(4)	10-20	16.8	0.63-20	4.22

Medium: Kimmig agar
Inoculum: 10^6 CFU/ml

IN VITRO ACTIVITY

BNM-A sodium salt is soluble in water, is stable at pH 2 - 11 and also stable to heat. BNM-A showed no antibacterial activity except in a few strains, but potent antifungal activity against a wide range of fungi including pathogens of endemic and opportunistic mycoses. Table 1 shows MIC values against major pathogenic fungi. When geometric means of MIC values were compared, BNM-A was more

TABLE 2

Structure-activity relationships of benanomicin A and related compounds against three fungal strains

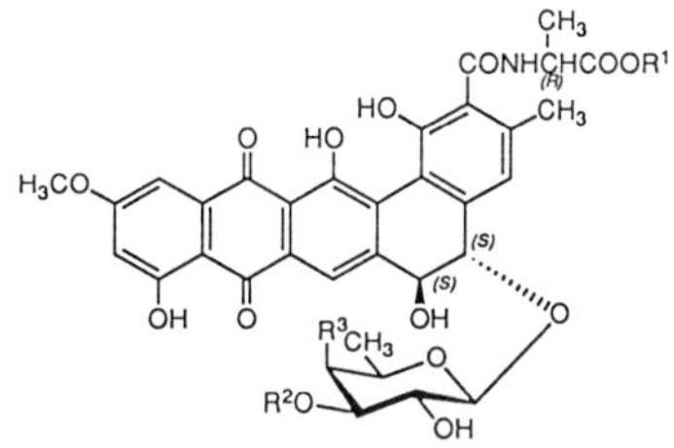

Compound	R^1	R^2	R^3	MIC (μg/ml)		
				C.albicans TIMM1768	*C.neoformans* Cr-1	*A.fumigatus* TIMM1775
A	H	xylosyl	OH	6.25	3.13	12.5
A-ME	CH_3	xylosyl	OH	>100	100	>100
A-DX	H	H	OH	3.13	3.13	>100
A-DX-ME	CH_3	H	OH	>100	>100	>100
B	H	xylosyl	NH_2	12.5	3.13	6.25
B-AC	H	xylosyl	NHAc	12.5	12.5	>100
Aglycone	H	without sugar moiety		>100	>100	>100

Medium: Kimmig agar
Inoculum: 10^5 CFU/ml

active than amphotericin B against *Candida glabrata*, equal to *C. parapsilosis*, but less active against *C. albicans*, *C. tropicalis*, *Aspergillus fumigatus*, *Cryptococcus neoformans* and *Trichophyton mentagrophytes*. The MIC values obtained in agar and broth dilution methods were slightly affected by inoculum sizes in the range of 10^4 to 10^7 CFU/ml.

Structure-activity studies were conducted using seven compounds related to BNM-A and three fungal strains, as shown in Table 2. Replacement of hydroxyl group by amino group caused no essential change in the activity, but *N*-acetylation of amino group resulted in a reduction of the activity against *Cryptococcus* and especially *Aspergillus* strains. Esterification of the carboxyl group or removal of two sugar moieties resulted in a reduction or a loss of the activity. When the xylose moiety was removed, the activity against yeasts was maintained, but the activity against filamentous fungi was reduced.

IN VIVO ACTIVITY

The *in vivo* activity of BNM-A was examined using systemic infection models of mice inoculated intravenously. BNM-A showed *in vivo* efficacy by oral

TABLE 3

In vivo efficacy of benanomicin A against systemic fungal infections in mice

Organism	Inoculum (CFU/mouse)	ED_{50} (mg/kg/day) Benanomicin A sc	iv	Amphotericin B sc	iv	Fluconazole sc	iv
Candida albicans TIMM 1768	10^6	1.3	0.96	0.034	0.032	3.4	3.7
Aspergillus fumigatus TIMM 1775	10^6	19	56	0.076	0.042	-	>50
Cryptococcus neoformans TIMM 1855	10^6	18	-	1.8-7.5	-	-	-

Treatment was started 1 h after intravenous inoculation by parenteral administration once a day for 5 days.

administration, but more effectively by parenteral administration. As judged from ED_{50} values, the *in vivo* activity of BNM-A was enhanced by repeated administrations rather than a single one. This is in sharp contrast to amphotericin B, which showed lower ED_{50} value by a single than repeated administrations. By administration subcutaneously or intravenously once daily for 5 days against three fungal infections, BNM-A showed the least ED_{50} value against *C. albicans* TIMM1768, followed by *C. neoformans* TIMM1855 and *A. fumigatus* TIMM1775 (Table 3). The ED_{50} values of BNM-A were intermediate between those of amphotericin B and fluconazole which were determined simultaneously.

Interestingly, the *in vivo* efficacy of BNM-A against *C. albicans* and *A. fumigatus* remained unchanged or slightly increased on treatment 24 h after inoculation as compared with treatment 1 h after inoculation. The *in vivo* activity of amphotericin B also remained unchanged in 1h and 24 h, but fluconazole showed more than twofold increase in ED_{50} value after 24 h (*C. albicans*). In order to confirm the *in vivo* efficacy, clearance of *C. albicans* from main organs of the surviving mice was examined (Table 4). The *Candida* cells tend to remain in kidney, and BNM-A showed nearly complete clearance of the pathogen from kidney, which was comparable to amphotericin B and better than fluconazole. Also, BNM-A and amphotericin B showed better gain of body weight than fluconazole.

PHARMACOKINETICS AND TOXICITY

The pharmacokinetics of a single dosing of BNM-A (20 mg/kg, iv) in rats showed plasma half-life 2.26 h and AUC 360 μg·h/ml (0 - ∞). Mice and dogs showed

TABLE 4
Clearance of *Candida albicans* from kidneys of surviving mice

Drug	Dose (mg/kg/day)	Survival rate	Colonies in kidney
Benanomicin A	62.9	5/5	-
	31.5	5/5	-
	15.8	5/5	+
	7.9	5/5	+++
Amphotericin B	5.0	0/5	toxic
	0.63	5/5	-
	0.31	5/5	-
	0.16	5/5	++
Fluconazole	50	4/5	++
	20	5/5	+++
	10	2/5	++
	5	1/5	+++

Intravenous treatment was started 1 h after intravenous inoculation once a day for 5 days.

similar half-lives (1.85 and 2.13 h, respectively). BNM-A was mainly excreted through kidney in rats and dogs, and urinary excretion ratio was 70.0% (24 h) in rats and 68.2% (5 h) in dogs.

BNM-A was well tolerated by experimental animals; mice, rats and dogs survived by intravenous dosing of 600 mg/kg. No clinical symptom has been observed so far by repeated administration of 100 mg/kg per day for 28 days in rats in the general toxicity test and 150 mg/kg per day in the reproduction test. No mutagenicity was observed by reversion, chromosomal aberration and micronucleus tests.

Since BNM-A has some structural similarity to anthracycline antibiotics, the cytocidal effect was examined using cultured animal cells. BNM-A showed no inhibitory activity against P388 leukemia and L5178Y lymphoma cells at 100 μg/ml. When chemotherapeutic indexes were calculated from acute toxicity and *in vivo* efficacy, the LD_{50}/ED_{50} values were >125 for BNM-A, 28.1 for amphotericin B and >10.8 for fluconazole.

MODE OF ACTION

When BNM-A was brought into contact with yeasts, red coloring of the fungal cells with partial coagulation in broth or formation of a red ring at the outskirts of the inhibition zone on an agar plate was most characteristic, indicating binding of BNM-A to the fungal cells. Using BNM-A and related compounds, the relationships between activity and cell binding were examined in *C. albicans* Y-2 and *Saccharomyces cerevisiae* X2180-1A. Upon exposure to 100 μg/ml for 30 min, bioactive BNM-A and BNM-B showed binding of 13 - 18 μg per 10^7 *Candida* cells and 25 - 30 μg per 10^7 *Saccharomyces* cells, whereas inactive methyl ester and aglycone showed negligible binding. The role of Ca^{2+} on the binding was indicated on pradimicin A having similar structure to BNM-A (5). Ca^{2+} was also shown to be important in the binding of BNM-A. BNM-A bound to the *Candida* cells was hardly extracted with acetone, slightly with water, moderately with *N,N*-dimethylformamide and 5 mM EGTA, and most efficiently with dimethyl sulfoxide. Interestingly, BNM-A showed negligible binding to mouse erythrocytes and rat kidney cells. Selective binding of BNM-A to fungal cells but not to mammalian cells may be the origin of selective toxicity.

BNM-A showed a fungicidal action toward *C. albicans* TIMM1768 in a dose-dependent manner. When the *Candida* cells surviving after treatment with 31 μg/ml of BNM-A for 2 h were cultured in a fresh medium, regrowth was started only 8 h after cultivation, and postantibiotic effect was 2.75 h. Amphotericin B used as a reference showed suppression of regrowth even after 24 h. When the dimethyl sulfoxide extract of the *Candida* cells was analyzed by HPLC using a reversed phase C_{18} column and a 1:1 mixture of 0.5% KH_2PO_4 aq solution and methanol as a mobile phase, BNM-A bound on the cells was recovered intact, and no metabolite was observed.

BNM-A was bound to the *Saccharomyces* cells under either growing or non-growing conditions, but killing action was observed only in a medium fed with glucose, namely under growing condition, and killing of the non-growing cells in a medium without glucose was very small (Fig. 2). This indicates that binding is essential but not enough for expression of the fungicidal activity, and that energy metabolism after binding is important for the activity.

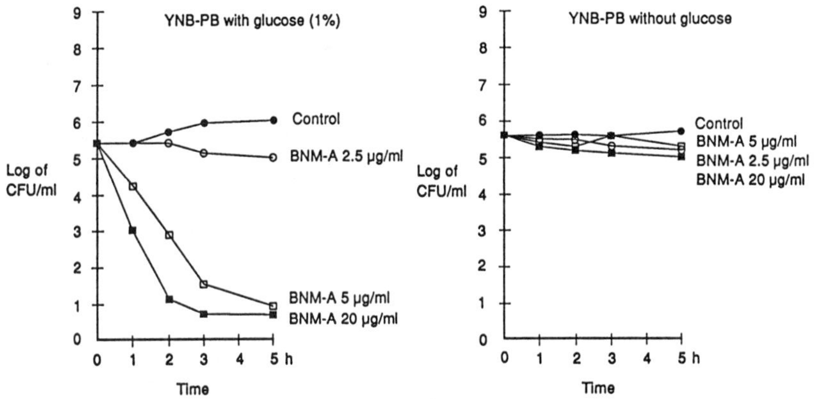

FIG. 2. Effect of glucose on viable counts in *Saccharomyces cerevisiae* X2180-1A

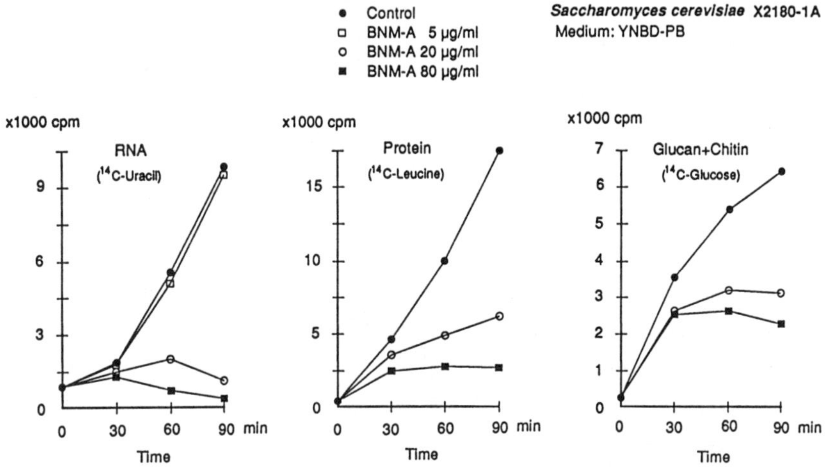

FIG. 3. Effect of benanomicin A on incorporation of radioactive precursors

BNM-A suppressed RNA synthesis from ^{14}C-uracil, protein synthesis from ^{14}C-leucine or glucan + chitin synthesis from ^{14}C-glucose at 20 and 80 μg/ml in a dose-dependent manner in *S. cerevisiae* (Fig. 3). But, non-specific suppression was observed. Moreover, BNM-A at 5 μg/ml showed no suppression on RNA and protein synthesis, suggesting that BNM-A does not primarily affect synthesis of macromolecules. When the *Saccharomyces* cells were treated with BNM-A, a leakage of ATP from fungal cells occurred 30 min later, and increased time-dependently in growing condition. Again, no leakage occurred in non-growing

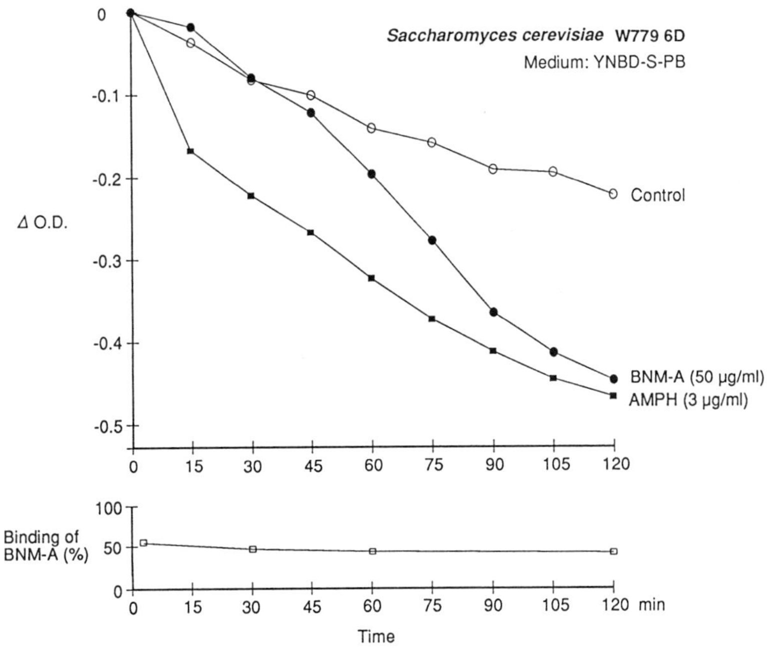

FIG. 4. Time course of protoplast lysis and cell binding

condition. These results suggested that a primary target of BNM-A may not be the synthesis of high molecular components, but fungal cell membrane. Therefore, in the following experiments, protoplast lysis was studied in detail, using *S. cerevisiae* as a main test organism.

Similar to the effect on intact cells, BNM-A and BNM-B bound to protoplasts and caused lysis, but methyl ester and aglycone showed negligible binding and no protoplast lysis. The protoplast lysis caused by BNM-A occurred only when glucose, or other metabolizable carbon source such as mannose or glycerol was present in YNB-PB medium, similar to the intact cell killing. Removal of glucose or addition of 2-deoxyglucose as a carbon source induced no lysis. When a time course of protoplast lysis and cell binding was followed (Fig. 4), the binding occurred immediately after addition of BNM-A to the *Saccharomyces* cells, and remained around the 50% level. But the lysis occurred after a lag (*ca.* 45 min), and reached a maximum after 120 min. This indicates that BNM-A caused time-dependent

TABLE 5
Inhibitory activity of benanomicin A on yeast ATPases

Time (min)	Inhibition of ATPase (%)		
	Plasma membrane	Vacuolar membrane	Mitochondrial membrane
2	58.5	-4.4	7.6
5	50.0	-5.0	10.6
10	41.4	0	5.9

ATPases were prepared from *Saccharomyces cerevisiae* X2180-1A.
Concentration of benanomicin A: 20 µg/ml

damage to the cell membrane. Unlike BNM-A, amphotericin B showed rapid lysis without a lag under either growing or non-growing conditions.

Detailed mechanism of the perturbation of the fungal cell membrane by BNM-A is not known. A fungal cell possesses various ATPases, of which plasma membrane ATPase of *S. cerevisiae* was moderately inhibited by 20 µg/ml of BNM-A, but vacuolar membrane ATPase and mitochondrial membrane ATPase were not (Table 5). Although the inhibitory activity of BNM-A is not strong enough to be a primary target, the selective effect on the cell membrane function may be related in some way with cell membrane perturbation.

In summary, 1) BNM-A is active against a wide range of fungi *in vitro*. A carboxylic acid and at least one sugar moiety are essential for the activity. 2) The *in vivo* activity was demonstrated by parenteral administration against systemic infections due to *Candida albicans*, *Cryptococcus neoformans* and *Aspergillus fumigatus* in mice. 3) BNM-A is well distributed and shows very low toxicity, being tolerated by intravenous dosing of 600 mg/kg in animals. 4) The fungicidal activity was shown on the growing intact cells and glucose-fed protoplasts in yeasts, and correlated with the cell binding and the membrane damage depended on energy metabolism.

BNM-A is a promising candidate for a chemotherapeutic agent against deep-seated mycoses.

REFERENCES

1) Takeuchi T.; T. Hara, H. Naganawa, M. Okada, M. Hamada, H. Umezawa, S. Gomi, M. Sezaki and S. Kondo: New antifungal antibiotics, benanomicins A and B from an Actinomycete. J. Antibiotics **41**: 807-811, 1988
2) Gomi S.; M. Sezaki, S. Kondo, T. Hara, H. Naganawa and T. Takeuchi: The structures of new antifungal antibiotics, benanomicins A and B. J. Antibiotics **41**: 1019-1028, 1988
3) Gomi S.; M. Sezaki, M. Hamada, S. Kondo and T. Takeuchi: Biosynthesis of benanomicins. J. Antibiotics **42**: 1145-1150, 1989
4) Hoshino H.; J. Seki and T. Takeuchi: New antifungal antibiotics, benanomicins A and B inhibit infection of T-cell with human immunodeficiency virus (HIV) and syncytium formation by HIV. J. Antibiotics **42**: 344-346, 1989
5) Sawada Y.; K. Numata, T. Murakami, H. Tanimichi, S. Yamamoto and T. Oki: Calcium-dependent anticandidal action of pradimicin A. J. Antibiotics **43**: 715-721, 1990

32

RI-331 and Other Amino Acid Analogs

H. Yamaki, M. Yamaguchi*, and H. Yamaguchi*

Institute of Applied Microbiology, University of Tokyo, 113 Tokyo, Japan

**Research Center for Medical Mycology, University of Teikyo, 359 Otsuka, Hachioji City, 192 Tokyo, Japan*

ABSTRACT

We reviewed some antifungal amino acid antibiotics including recently developed RI-331 and cispentacin which are possibly useful in systemic Candidiasis, concentrating on the mechanism by which (S) 2-amino-4-oxo-5-hydroxypentanoic acid coded as RI-331 preferentially inhibits the protein biosynthesis in Saccharomyces cerevisiae by inhibiting the biosynthesis of the aspartate family of amino acids methionine, isoleucine and threonine. This inhibition was effected by impeding the biosynthesis of their common intermediate precursor, homoserine. The target enzyme of the antibiotic was homoserine dehydrogenase (EC.1.1.1.3). Inhibition by this antibiotic of biosyntheses of methionine, isoleucine and threonine which are essential for animals clearly elucidates the mechanism of selective toxicity against fungi.

INTRODUCTION

The recent increase of opportunistic fungal infection prompted us to search for new types of antifungal agents. Recent papers describe the possible usefulness of amino acid antibiotics including RI-331 (1) and cispentacin (2). We review here some properties of these antifungal antibiotics and other amino acid analogues which have been characterized as antimetabolites.
Our study concentrating on the antifungal mechanism of action of RI-331 is presented in this paper.

MECHANISM OF ACTION OF RI-331

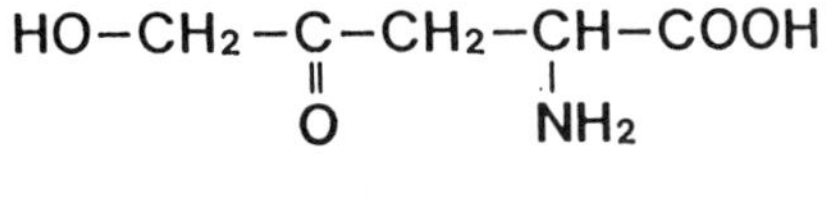

FIG. 1. The chemical structure of RI-331

In our program for screening of antifungal agents, we isolated an amino acid analog, (S)-2-amino-4-oxo-5-hydroxypentanoic acid (Fig. 1) coded as RI-331 from a culture broth of Streptomyces sp. The antibiotic was active against several pathogenic fungi of medical importance including Candida albicans and Cryptoccocus neoformans, was also effective in treating systemic Candidiasis in mice, and was highly tolerated by experimental animals. Our major concern was to understand on a biochemical basis the selective toxicity of the antibiotic toward such fungi. The mechanism of action of the antibiotic explored using susceptible Saccharomyces cerevisiae is described.

EFFECT ON GROWTH

The antibiotic at concentrations above 0.1 mM almost completely inhibited the yeast growth within 2 hours after the onset of incubation. RI-331 exerts essentially a static action toward the tested Sacch.cerevisiae strain.

EFFECT ON BIOSYNTHESES OF DNA, RNA AND PROTEIN

Effect of RI-331 on the biosyntheses of DNA, RNA and protein in growing Sacch.cerevisiae was explored by determination of the counts taken up from the specific radioactive precursors in the medium. The antibiotic significantly inhibited the incorporation into protein of labelled amino acids, [^{14}C]asparagine and [^{14}C]glutamine by more than 90% at 150 ug/ml of RI-331, but to a lesser extent the incorporation of [^{3}H]adenine into DNA and RNA fractions: 20% and 30% at 150 µg/ml, respectively. The antibiotic primarily inhibits the protein synthesis of yeast cells (Table 1). In order to examine whether RI-331 affects the protein-synthesizing machinery itself, its effect on the cell-free system from Sacch.cerevisiae which are capable of synthesizing polypeptides with native messengers was studied.

TABLE 1.

Effect of RI-331 on protein, RNA and DNA syntheses in growing Sacch.cerevisiae cells measured by the radioactivity of [^{14}C] Asn or [^{14}C] Gln taken up into protein, and [^{3}H] adenine into RNA and DNA

RI-331 (μg/ml)	[^{14}C] Asn	[^{14}C] Gln
0	17,264 (100)	16,773 (100)
15	5,796 (34)	5,282 (32)
150	1,407 (8)	1,032 (6)

RI-331 (μg/ml)	Radioactivity (dpm) of [^{3}H] adenine taken up into	
	RNA	DNA
0	10,457 (100)	3,543 (100)
15	9,775 (93)	2,930 (83)
150	7,014 (67)	1,956 (55)

Numbers in the brackets represent % incorporation.

The incorporation of [^{3}H] leucine into peptides by the cell-free system was completely refractory to RI-331 even at concentrations as high as 1500 μg/ml, leading to the possibility that the biosynthesis of certain intracellular amino acids is blocked by the antibiotic.

EFFECT ON INTRACELLULAR AMINO ACID POOL

Intracellular amino acid fraction was prepared from Sacch. cerevisiae cells incubated with RI-331, and the relative amount of each amino acid was determined by amino acid autoanalyzer. The antibiotic induced a remarkable change in the size and composition of the amino acid pool. It was characterized by a marked decrease in the level of threonine, methionine, isoleucine and glutamate that was accompanied by a somewhat lesser decrease in the level of histidine and proline, and an increase in the level of alanine, valine, leucine, phenylalanine, tyrosine, serine and aspartate (Table 2).

TABLE 2.

The change of composition of amino acid pools induced by RI-331 in <u>Sacch.cerevisiae</u> cells.

Amino acid	Control (C)	+ RI-331 (R)	R/C
Gly	1.499	1.139	0.76
Ala	5.665	12.237	2.16
Val	1.153	12.949	11.23
Leu	0.207	0.597	2.88
Ile	0.315	0.015	0.05
Met	0.064	0.007	0.11
Cys	0.025	0.017	0.68
Phe	0.096	0.151	1.57
Tyr	0.088	0.939	10.67
Pro	1.075	0.381	0.35
His	65.274	33.158	0.51
Ser	1.619	14.804	9.14
Thr	11.217	1.257	0.11
Glu	52.523	8.552	0.16
Asp	4.579	11.758	2.57
Lys	2.885	3.604	1.25
Arg	42.149	40.592	0.96

The values of (C) and (R) represent the amounts of intracellular amino acids expressed as nmol per 2×10^8 cells without and with RI-331 (15 μg/ml)-treatment, respectively. The number of R/C represents the ratio of (R) to (C) value.

TABLE 3.

The antagonistic effect of several amino acids on the growth inhibiting activity of RI-331 against Sacch.cerevisiae.

Amino acid added	IC_{50} of RI-331 (μg/ml)	Degree of reversion
None (control)	1.7	1.0
Gly	2.5	1.5
Ala	2.4	1.4
Val	2.9	1.7
Leu	2.1	1.2
Ile	6.3	3.7
Met	12.5	7.4
Phe	2.8	1.6
Pro	2.0	1.2
Ser	4.8	2.8
Thr	9.9	5.8
Homoserine	50.0	29.4
Asp	2.0	1.2
Asn	6.6	3.9
Glu	2.4	1.4
Gln	3.7	2.2
Arg	1.9	1.1
Lys	1.9	1.1

IC_{50} value was determined on the basis of optical density.

REVERSAL BY AMINO ACIDS

The question arises whether the exhaustion of some intracellular amino acids induced by the antibiotic is responsible for the RI-331 activity. To gain a better understanding to the answer to this question, the antagonistic effect of each amino acid was examined.
For brevity, the reversal activity is expressed by the

degree of reversion of the increase in IC_{50} values when 200 μg/ml of the testing antagonist was added.
Among 18 amino acids or metabolites, homoserine was the most potent antagonist inducing a 29-fold increase in the IC_{50} value, and the order of the next most significantly antagonistic was methionine, threonine, isoleucine, asparagine, serine and glutamine. Other amino acids were ineffective or only slightly effective.

FIG. 2. Biochemical pathway involved in metabolism of the aspartate family of amino acids in prototrophic micro-organisms and an assumed site of action of RI-331.

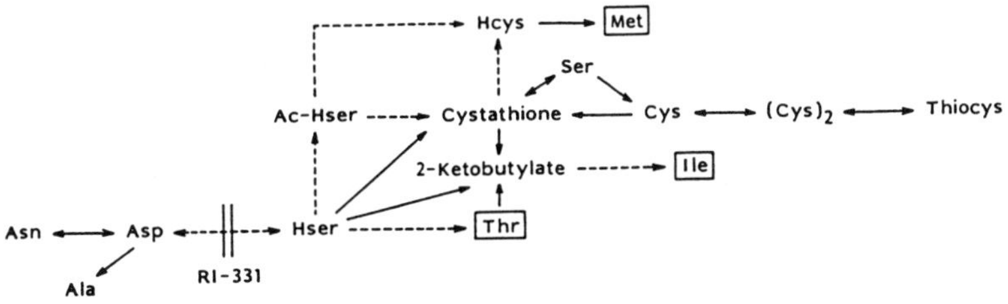

Indications: ——› General, ----› defective in animals, amino acids essential for animals are boxed.
Abbreviations: Hser, homoserine; Hcys, homocysteine; $(Cys)_2$, cystine; Thiocys, thiocysteine.

These results led us to postulate that the antifungal activity of RI-331 is mainly due to the inhibition of protein biosynthesis caused by the decreased rate of biosyntheses of threonine, methionine and isoleucine.
The most potent action of homoserine as the antagonist of RI-331 action led us to the possibility that the exact site of action of the antibiotic might be on the metabolic step(s) involved in biosynthesis of homoserine or its precursor(s) (3,4) (Fig. 3). Confirmation of the validity

of our theory awaits further studies using yeast cell-free systems capable of converting aspartate to homoserine.

FIG. 3. The pathway converting aspartate to homoserine, and the target site of RI-331.

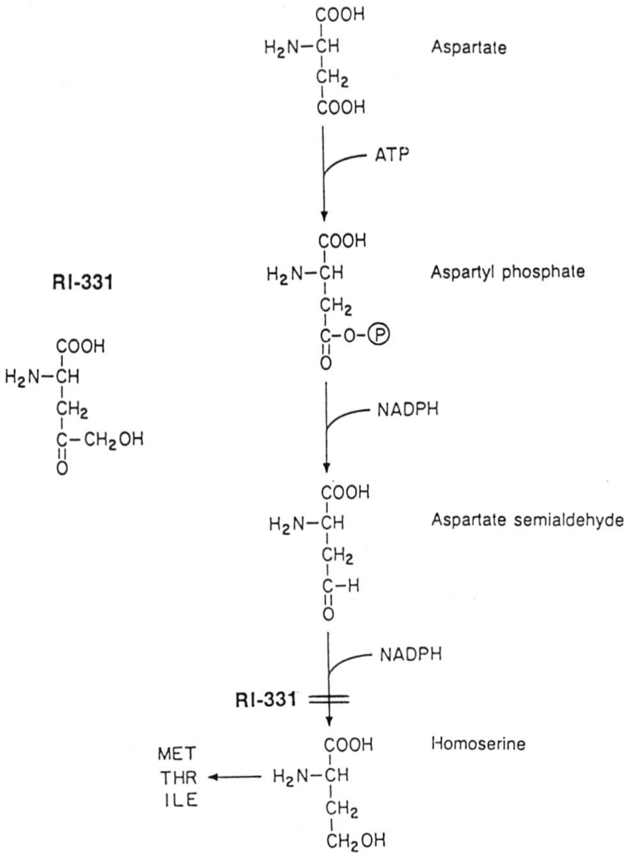

THE CONVERSION OF ASPARTATE TO HOMOSERINE IN CELL-FREE SYSTEM.

In the conversion of aspartate to homoserine three enzymes, aspartate kinase, aspartate semialdehyde dehydrogenase and homoserine dehydrogenase are involved. The enzymatic conversion of aspartate into homoserine using a crude enzyme fraction containing these three enzymes was significantly inhibited by RI-331. We then searched for an enzyme susceptible to the antibiotic using the purified preparations of each enzyme (5,6,7). The former two enzymes were refractory, and the last, homoserine dehydrogenase, was susceptible to the antibiotic, substantiating that the enzyme involved in the biosynthesis of homoserine should be subjected to study as a primary target of RI-331 (8). The mechanism of inactivation by the antibiotic of homoserine dehydrogenase is under investigation.

OTHER AMINO ACID ANALOGS

A large number of amino acid analogs have been developed as antimetabolites to date, some of which exhibit antifungal activity. The majority of effective compounds described have been chemically synthesized, and some compounds were isolated from their natural origin as antibiotics or substances toxic to animals (9,10). We will review here the compounds which are possibly available against fungal infections. A recent paper describes a promising antifungal antibiotic, cispentacin which is effective in treating Candidiasis in mice and has low toxicity to these animals (2). The chemical structure and protective effect of cispentacin are shown in Fig. 4.

FIG. 4. Protection from lung Candidiasis by cispentacin administration to immunocompromised mice.

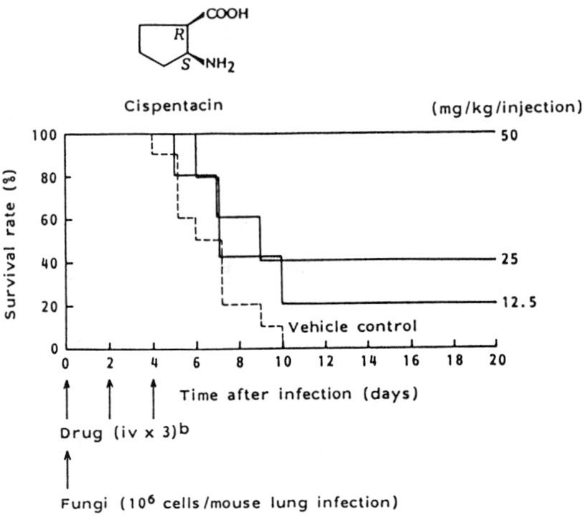

(From Ref. 2, with permission)

The mechanism of antifungal action and the mode of protection from Candidiasis by this substance are unknown as yet.

As described in the previous section, an inhibitor of yeast homoserine dehydrogenase, RI-331 has been a candidate useful as an antifungal agent. We referred to an inhibitor of homoserine dehydrogenase and some inhibitors which possibly block the biosynthesis of homoserine in Escherichia coli.
The chemically synthesized compound 2-amino-4-oxo-5-chloropentanoate has been reported to inhibit homoserine dehydrogenase in Escherichia coli (11). The antimicrobial

activity of β-hydroxynorvaline, O-methylthreonine and O-methylserine is reversed by the addition of methionine, isoleucine, threonine or homoserine, suggesting that these compounds inhibit the pathway from aspartate to homoserine (10). The target site of these compounds may be aspartate kinase, aspartate semialdehyde dehydrogenase or homoserine dehydrogenase. If the compounds are able to inactivate fungal enzymes involved in the biosynthesis of homoserine, they may be inhibitors hopeful as antifungal agents. Other types of inhibitors which interfere with the pathway of biosyntheses of essential amino acids other than threonine, isoleucine and methione may also possibly be available for antifungal chemotherapy.

REFERENCES

1. H. Yamaguchi, K. Uchida, T. Hiratani, T. Nagate, N. Watanabe, and S. Omura, RI-331, a new antifungal antibiotic. Ann. N. Y. Acad. Sci., 544: 188 (1988)

2. T. Oki, M. Hirano, K. Tomatsu, K. Numata, and H. Kamei, Cispentacin, a new antifungal antibiotic. II. In vitro and in vivo antifungal activities. J. Antibiotics, 42: 1756 (1989)

3. H. Yamaki, M. Yamaguchi, T. Nishimura, T. Shinoda, and H. Yamaguchi, Unique mechanism of action of an antifungal antibiotic RI-331. Drugs Expl. Clin. Res., 14: 467 (1988)

4. M. Yamaguchi, H. Yamaki, T. Shinoda, Y. Tago, H. Suzuki, T. Nishimura, and H. Yamaguchi, The mode of antifungal action of (S)2-amino-4-oxo-5-hydroxypentanoic acid, RI-331. J. Antibiotics, 43: 411 (1990)

5. S. Black, and N. G. Wright, β-Aspartokinase and β-aspartyl phosphate, J. Biol. Chem., 213: 27 (1955).

6. S. Black, and N. G. Wright, Aspartic β-semialdehyde dehydrogenase and aspartic β-semialdehyde, J. Biol. Chem., 213: 39 (1955)

7. S. Black, and N. G. Wright, Homoserine dehydrogenase, J. Biol. Chem., 213: 51 (1955)

8. H. Yamaki, M. Yamaguchi, H. Imamura, H. Suzuki, T. Nishimura, H. Saito, and H. Yamaguchi, The mechanism of antifungal action of (S) 2-amino-4-oxo-5-hydroxypentanoic acid, RI-331. The inhibition of homoserine dehydrogenase in Saccharomyces cerevisiae. Biochem. Biophys. Res. Commun., 168: 837 (1990)

9. W. Shive, and C. G. Skinner, Amino acid analogues. Metabolic Inhibitors I. (R. M. Hochster and J. H. Quastel, ed.) p. 1. Academic Press, New York. (1963)

10. L. Fowden, D. Lewis, and H. Tristram, Toxic amino acids. Their action as antimetabolites. Advances in Enzymology (F. F. Nord, ed.) p. 89. Interscience Publishers, New York. (1967)

11. C. G. Hirth, M. Veron, C. Villar-Parasi, N. Hurion and G. N. Cohen, The threonine-sensitive homoserine dehydrogenase and aspartokinase activities of Escherichia coli K12. Eur. J. Biochem. 50: 425 (1975)

PART VIII

NEW PROSPECTS IN THE USE OF ANTIFUNGAL AGENTS

33

Antifungal Susceptibility Testing: *In Vitro* and *in Vivo*

Michael A. Pfaller, M.D.

Department of Pathology
273 MRC
University of Iowa College of Medicine
Iowa City, IA 52242

I. INTRODUCTION

Opportunistic fungal infections are becoming increasingly important causes of morbidity and mortality in the hospitalized patient. In addition to the well-known opportunistic pathogens such as Aspergillus spp and Candida spp, serious infections are being reported with increasing frequency due to Fusarium spp, the zygomycetes, demateaceous fungi, and other usually "non-pathogenic" fungi (1-3). A major part of this increase has been attributed to use of newer and more effective antibacterial agents, aggressive surgical procedures, bone marrow and solid organ transplantation, immunosuppressive and cytotoxic therapy for malignancies and other diseases, and the emergence of AIDS (1,3-7). Paralleling the increase of fungal infections over the last decade has been an increase in the usage of systemic antifungal agents worldwide (7) and the introduction of a number of new antifungal agents with systemic activity. With the increased use of both established and investigational agents has come the recognition of resistance in selected isolates to one or more antifungal agents (4-6,8-16). As a result of these developments, increased attention is now being paid to methods of *in vitro* and *in vivo* susceptibility testing of antifungal agents. Not only are these methods potentially useful in the development and preclinical evaluation of new antifungal agents, but now the clinical laboratory is being asked to assume a greater role in the selection and monitoring of antifungal chemotherapy for clinical purposes. Thus, it is clear that efforts must now be made to standardize laboratory tests with antifungal agents and to establish the clinical relevance of these measures (4,5,9,10,12,16-25).

II. IN VITRO SUSCEPTIBILITY TESTS WITH ANTIFUNGAL AGENTS

Susceptibility tests with antifungal agents are preformed for the same reason that tests with antibacterial agents are preformed. Ideally the *in vitro* susceptibility tests will i) provide a reliable measure of the relative activity of two or more antifungal agents, ii) correlate with *in vivo* activity and predict the outcome of therapy, iii) provide a means with which to monitor the development of resistance among a normally susceptible population of organisms, and iv) predict the therapeutic potential of newly discovered investigational agents (4,,5,9,10,16,18,20,24). Unfortunately current *in vitro* test methods are non-standardized, unreliable, and lack documented clinical predictive value (9,10,12,16,18,21,23,24). Efforts are now being made to address these issues and will be discussed below.

A. IN VITRO TESTING VARIABLES

In vitro susceptibility test procedures with antifungal agents are similar in design to those employed with antibacterial agents and are influenced by a number of technical variables including inoculum size and preparation, medium formulation and pH, and duration and temperature of incubation (4,5,9,10,12,16-20, 24,25,26). The methods which have been applied to antifungal susceptibility testing include broth dilution (macro and micro), agar dilution, and disk diffusion. An additional variable which has been particularly problematic is the method of endpoint determination. A number of different methods of endpoint determination have been applied in efforts to develop a test method which would be objective and easy to perform and interpret in the clinical laboratory including visual, turbidimetric, colorimetric, radiometric, dry weight determination, and the use of ATP photometry (5,9,12,20,25). In addition, antifungal susceptibility testing is complicated by problems unique to fungi which include slow growth rate (relative to bacteria) and the ability of certain (dimorphic) fungi to grow either as a unicellular (yeast) form which produces blastospores or as a hyphal (mold) form which may produce asexual spores depending on the conditions of pH, temperature, and medium composition. Finally, the basic properties of the antifungal agents themselves such as solubility, chemical stability, and the tendency to produce partial inhibition of growth over a wide range of concentrations, must be taken into account.

Given the increasing number of antifungal agents and the perceived need for *in vitro* susceptibility testing to assist in their clinical application, it has become apparent that efforts are needed to standardize antifungal susceptibility testing just as they were for antibacterial testing previously (4,5,9,10). With this in mind the National Committee for Clinical Laboratory Standards (NCCLS) has established a subcommittee to coordinate work on antifungal susceptibility tests with a goal of developing a reliable reference method for *in vitro* susceptibility testing of yeasts and other fungi and ultimately to correlate the results of this method with clinical effectiveness. Due to the complex nature of this problem the initial efforts of the NCCLS subcommittee have focused on testing methods for yeasts and yeast-like fungi with particular emphasis on C. albicans.

B. *ACTIVITIES OF THE NCCLS SUBCOMMITTEE ON ANTIFUNGAL SUSCEPTIBILITY TESTING*

Since 1983 the NCCLS subcommittee has been involved in several studies concerning antifungal susceptibility testing. These studies have included i) a survey of antifungal susceptibility testing practices among the NCCLS membership, ii) multicenter studies of the precision of non-standardized test methods, iii) a study to determine the most reliable method of inoculum preparation, and iv) a multicenter study to define the medium and set of incubation conditions for yeast susceptibility testing which would optimize reproducibility within and among laboratories while maintaining the reference rank order of susceptibility of a panel of isolates to commonly used antifungal agents.

1. *Survey of antifungal susceptibility testing practices.* A questionnaire survey was conducted nationwide and included approximately 350 hospitals, with a bed-size of 300 or greater. The results of the survey indicated a significant interest in antifungal susceptibility testing for clinical purposes among hospital-based laboratories (16); however, the majority of the laboratories (72%) tested 20 or fewer isolates per year and 40% performed five or fewer tests per year. The general lack of experience in most laboratories coupled with test variability and lack of published data correlating test results with clinical response calls into question the predictive value of test results

from such low volume laboratories.

2. *Multicenter studies of the precision of non-standardized test methods.* Two multicenter studies were conducted using either the broth dilution method of Shadomy et al. (20) or multiple non-standardized methods in order to determine the intra- and inter-laboratory variation in MIC values for amphotericin B, 5-fluorocytosine (5-FC), and ketoconazole (16,18). Although both studies documented excellent intra-laboratory reproducibility, differences in MIC values of 16-fold to several thousand-fold were observed for a given isolate tested in different laboratories. Despite this variation in endpoint values the relative susceptibilities of a panel of isolates within an individual laboratory generally agreed with the reference rank order. Based on these findings it was felt that the lack of agreement among laboratories was likely due to problems in uniform execution of test procedures and lack of standards designed to facilitate agreement among methods. Thus, it was suggested that analysis and standardization of each of the key technical steps including inoculum preparation, medium composition and pH, and temperature and duration of incubation might increase the reproducibility of the broth dilution method for yeast susceptibility testing.

3. *Inoculum preparation.* The first of the test variables, inoculum preparation, was addressed in a multicenter study in which the precision of four methods of inoculum preparation was evaluated in three different laboratories (19). The methods of inoculum preparation included in the study were the spectrophotometric method, the Wickerham card method, the hemocytometer count method, and the Prompt inoculation system (3M, St. Paul, MN). Overall, the most reproducible method of inoculum preparation, both within a given laboratory and among laboratories, was the spectrophotometric method. The method was simple and objective and was not significantly affected by the genus or species tested. This method has been adopted as the standard method of inoculum preparation by the NCCLS subcommittee.

4. *Test medium and incubation conditions.* Recently a multicenter study was performed to evaluate the effect of media, incubation time (24h vs 48h), and temperature (30 C vs 35 C) on intra- and inter-laboratory variation in yeast MIC results for amphotericin B, 5-FC, and ketoconazole (26). Testing was performed on coded isolates with a previously established rank order of antifungal susceptibilities using a single macrobroth dilution method in 11 laboratories. Four completely defined media were evaluated including yeast-nitrogen base (YNB; Difco Laboratories, Detroit, MI), Synthetic Amino Acid Medium-Fungal (SAAMF; American Biorganics, North Tonawanda, NY), RPMI-1640 (Sigma Chemical Company, St. Louis, MO), and HR Antifungal Assay Medium (Oxoid LTD., Basingstoke, Hampshire, England). All media were buffered to pH 7.0 using 3-[N-morpholino]-propanesulfonic acid (MOPS; Sigma, St. Louis, MO) as the buffering agent (final concentration 0.165M).

The goal of this study was to be able to identify the medium and set of incubation conditions for yeast susceptibility testing which would adequately support the growth of the test isolates and optimize reproducibility within and among laboratories while maintaining the reference rank order of susceptibilities for each antifungal agent.

The results of this study provide further documentation of the excellent intra-laboratory reproducibility of macrobroth antifungal susceptibility testing regardless of antifungal agent or test medium. Furthermore, the study demonstrated improved inter-laboratory agreement in MIC results when a standardized macrobroth dilution testing method was employed. Incubation at 35 C for 24h (5-FC and ketoconazole) or 48h (amphotericin B) appeared optimal for the organisms and antifungal agents evaluated in this study. Based on the overall agreement among laboratories and agreement with the reference rank order, it appeared that RPMI-1640 performed slightly better than the other defined antifungal testing media.

Thus, significant progress has been made in developing a standardized method for *in vitro* susceptibility testing of antifungal agents. Future studies by the NCCLS subcommittee using RPMI-1640 medium, 35 C and 24-48h incubation will include larger numbers of yeast isolates and examine the issues of inoculum size and the correlation between macro-and micro-dilution methods. Despite this progress the clinical relevance of *in vitro* antifungal susceptibility testing remains unclear. Obviously this issue must be resolved before fungal susceptibility testing can be offered routinely in the clinical microbiology laboratory.

III.CORRELATION OF IN VITRO TEST RESULTS WITH CLINICAL OUTCOME

Ideally *in vitro* susceptibility testing should give a reliable prediction of *in vivo* response in animal models at the very least and ultimately in human infections. Unfortunately, the evidence for a clinical correlation with *in vitro* test results is limited at best. The important studies by Stiller et al. (22) and Polak and Dixon (21) have demonstrated that general predictions of outcome can be made based upon the *in vitro* susceptibility of C. albicans to 5-FC; however, these investigators were unable to make individual predictions of outcome due to the considerable overlap among the different susceptibility categories. Similar data has been even more difficult to generate with the azole class of antifungals (12,24). Recently, Boyle et al. (27) demonstrated a significant correlation between the *in vitro* activity of a series of bis-triazole tertiary alcohols and *in vivo* response in a murine model of candidiasis. They emphasized that prediction of *in vivo* efficacy of antifungal drugs from their *in vitro* activity should take into account i) the intrinsic antimicrobial activity, ii) the metabolic stability of the compound, iii) the serum concentration-time profile, iv) protein binding, and v) host defenses. Clearly this is a tall order for most *in vitro* test systems. Although improved *in vitro* test systems that correlate well with *in vivo* outcome may be developed, the *in vitro* conditions still may have to vary with the type of antifungal agent being evaluated (28). Given these qualifications it is not surprising that numerous investigators have found little or no correlation between *in vitro* susceptibility results and *in vivo* outcome with the various antifungal agents (4,5,9,12,23,24). This is especially marked with the newer triazoles such as fluconazole and SCH39304 (12,24).

Although a small amount of evidence for *in vivo* correlation of *in vitro* test results has been generated by carefully performed experimental studies such as those mentioned above, similar data for naturally acquired (human) infection is even less common. This is not surprising given the problems with the *in vitro* susceptibility testing methods and the difficulties encountered in interpreting the outcome of therapy in these extremely complex patients (4,5,24). In addition, therapeutic failures due to resistant organisms appear to be rare. Although clinical failures due to the development of amphotericin B resistance in isolates of C. lusitaniae are well known (8,11), it has been considerably more difficult to ascribe clinical failure to the development of resistance to the azoles or other antifungal agents with a variety of etiologic agents.

Perhaps the best documented examples of azole-resistant organisms associated with clinical treatment failure are C. albicans strains AD and KB (15,29). These isolates were obtained from patients with chronic mucocutaneous candidiasis who relapsed following protracted courses (17-23 months) of therapy with ketoconazole. The *in vitro* resistance of these isolates to ketoconazole, and cross-resistance to other azole antifungals, has been documented by extensive tests in several laboratories (15,29-32). *In vitro* susceptibility results also predicted the (lack of) *in vivo* response of these strains to ketoconazole and fluconazole in two different experimental models of disseminated candidiasis (24,30,31). The mechanism of resistance was attributed to decreased uptake of azoles, presumably due to an altered phospholipid to sterol ratio (32).

Aside from the clinical experience with C. albicans strains AD and KB, the data correlating the results of *in vitro* susceptibility testing and clinical outcome with azoles has not been favorable (12,24). A comparison of macrobroth MICs and clinical response to ketoconazole in patients with histoplasmosis, blastomycosis, cryptococcosis and sporotrichosis was conducted by the NIAID Mycoses Study Group (33). Although clinical isolates of H. capsulatum and B. dermatitidis were uniformly susceptible, there were no major differences in MIC values among isolates from patients who responded to therapy versus those who failed. In contrast, strains of C. neoformans from responding patients appeared resistant to ketoconazole, whereas the MICs for many isolates from non-responding patients were low (susceptible). Certainly one can explain a low MIC associated with therapeutic failure by a number of factors including poor drug penetration, lack of fungicidal activity, or compromised host defenses; however, it is more difficult to rationalize a high MIC associated with therapeutic success. Such paradoxical findings suggest that the *in vitro* susceptibility testing conditions may not be physiologically (or clinically) relevant (24).

Despite the widespread use of amphotericin B as the therapy of choice for serious fungal infections there is very little documented correlation between *in vitro* susceptibilities and *in vivo* response to this useful but toxic agent. Recently, Powderly et al. (14) related the *in vitro* susceptibility to amphotericin B of *Candida* spp causing fungemia to therapeutic outcome in patients undergoing bone marrow transplantation and/or myelosuppressive chemotherapy. They found a strong association between the *in vitro* susceptibility to amphotericin B and the clinical outcome in the immunocompromised patients. One hundred percent (10/10) of the episodes of candidemia caused by isolates with MICs greater than 0.8 μg/ml were fatal infections, compared with eight of 17 (47%) episodes caused by *Candida* spp with MICs of 0.8 μg/ml or less (p=0.04). They related these findings to the peak serum levels of amphotericin B which are obtained following a dose of 0.5 mg/Kg (1.2 0.3 μg/ml) or 1 mg/Kg (2.4 0.97 μg/ml) and noted that many of the patients in their series may have had serum levels of amphotericin B less than the MICs of the fungal isolates for much of the time they were being treated. This may explain why patients with fungemia due to *Candida* spp with MICs greater than 0.8 μg/ml were more likely to die because of that infection than patients with infection due to *Candida* spp whose *in vitro* susceptibility to amphotericin B was 0.8 μg/ml or less. They suggested that for clinical purposes if decreased susceptibility to amphotericin B is documented that alternative treatment strategies need to be developed to manage fungal infection in immunocompromised patients. Presently, they recommend the combination of amphotericin B plus 5-FC as the probable therapy of choice for fungemia or disseminated infection with such organisms.

The recommendations of Powderly et al. (14) are rational given the data presented; however, they imply that a much greater reliance should be placed on *in vitro* antifungal susceptibility test results than is warranted at the present time. Although these and other studies (34) suggest some correlation with MIC results for amphotericin B and clinical outcome, the general applicability of these results remains confused by i) the retrospective nature of the studies, ii) the documented variability of the non-standardized *in vitro* test methods employed, and iii) the difficulty in defining fungal diseases and their response to therapy. Given these reservations it seems unlikely that a discrete MIC breakpoint (>0.8 μg/ml) will be predictive of outcome in all institutions. Several key issues will need to be addressed in order to generate clinically useful data from *in vitro* test procedures including (24): i) whether MIC values have sufficient reproducibility to establish interpretive breakpoints; ii) whether there are clinical isolates in which treatment failure can be correlated with *in vitro* resistance; and iii) whether *in vitro* test procedures are predictive of all mechanisms of antifungal resistance seen *in vivo*. Some of these issues are currently being addressed by the NCCLS and other organizations; however, much work remains to be done in order to develop simple *in vitro* testing procedures for antifungal agents that have predictive value for *in vivo* efficacy.

IV. IN VIVO MODELS FOR EVALUATION OF ANTIFUNGAL AGENTS

Animal models have been used extensively by mycologists and microbiologists for determining the relative efficacy of antifungal agents *in vivo* as well as in studies of pathogenesis, virulence factors, and host defenses. Although *in vitro* test systems offer a simple and convenient means of comparing various antifungal agents, their results are not always predictive of *in vivo* efficacy and they do not take into account the toxicity, the susceptibility to metabolism, or the dynamic effects of the drug on both the host and pathogen and their interrelationship (28,35). Analysis of such complex interactions clearly can only be performed using appropriate animal models. Rinaldi has extensively reviewed several *in vivo* models of mycotic diseases currently used in assessing the activity of antifungal drugs (35). These models have been developed in an effort to duplicate a disease process in humans by using an experimental animal to receive a fungal challenge with a known or suspect human pathogen. These models may not always predict the clinical response to therapy with a specific antifungal agent; however, they do serve as a reasonable guide in assessing the microbe-drug-host interaction (28,35,36). Although clearly not practical for clinical susceptibility testing, *in vivo* models are invaluable in the screening and development of new antifungal compounds and in designing better treatment strategies for specific fungal infections.

Currently model fungal infections have been established in at least 11 different animal species (28,35). Useful models of disseminated infection due to Candida spp, Aspergillus spp, and other systemic pathogens have been developed in mice, rats, rabbits, and guinea pigs. The hamster, mouse, and rat have proven useful in studies of vaginal candidiasis. The guinea pig has proven to be a reproducible and reliable model for dermatophytosis and has been utilized to test both topical and systemic antifungal agents including ketoconazole, miconazole, fluconazole, and itraconazole. Given the large number of fungal pathogens, separate infection models must generally be developed for each of the genera (28). Likewise, the models should take into account the different patterns of fungal infection (superficial, mucosal, disseminated, localized) and mimic the clinical presentation (acute, subacute, chronic) whenever possible. Thus, for the evaluation of a given antifungal agent several different animal models may need to be employed.

Experimental animal model systems may vary widely in their

level of sophistication; however, all model systems should have several features in common (36): i) uniform inoculum size, ii) the infection mimics human infection, and iii) the system is reproducible from experiment to experiment. Furthermore, models designed to evaluate antifungal compounds should allow quantitative assessment of antifungal activity (fungicidal vs fungistatic), evaluate the effects of timing and duration of therapy, and take into account the effect of host defenses (immunocompromised) on the outcome of therapy. Hare and Loebenberg (28) have suggested the use of multiple strains of recent clinical isolates, sufficient numbers of animals and experiments, and the use of several different models of infection as a means of enhancing the clinical predictive value of animal models in the assessment of antifungal activity.

There are of course limitations in the use of animal models to predict the clinical efficacy of antifungal agents. Although conscientious efforts are made to mimic human infection in the animal model this may not be entirely possible due to differences in routes and sites of infection, course and severity of disease, or differences in the pathogenicity of the etiologic agent in the various hosts. Likewise, differences in host defenses and the immune response to the infection may clearly influence the results of therapy. The choice of timing, route of administration, and dosage of drug can influence results profoundly in the experimental model and may not approximate the realities of patient care closely enough to be of any clinical relevance. Finally, the toxicologic and pharmacokinetic properties of an antifungal agent in animal models may not always coincide with those in humans. Despite these limitations, animal models of fungal infection provide a useful and reliable method for the pre-clinical evaluation of antifungal drugs.

V. SUMMARY AND CONCLUSIONS

The increasing demand for new, effective therapeutic options for serious fungal infections has resulted in an increased interest in methods of *in vitro* and *in vivo* susceptibility testing of antifungal agents. Antifungal susceptibility testing is of potential value as a means of i) predicting the likely outcome of therapy, and ii) predicting the therapeutic potential of newly discovered investigational agents. Unfortunately, the current applicability of *in vitro* antifungal susceptibility tests is limited by inadequate standardization and insufficient correlation of *in vitro* test results with clinical outcome. Efforts by the NCCLS Subcommittee on Antifungal Susceptibility Testing to develop a standardized *in vitro* testing method have resulted in the development of a macrobroth dilution method with improved intra- and inter-laboratory reproducibility which may provide a standardized means of assessing the relative *in vitro* activities of commonly used antifungal agents against clinical yeast isolates. The clinical correlation of the test results with this method remains to be established. Although *in vivo* animal models for antifungal testing are not practical for clinical testing, they are extremely useful for screening antifungal compounds, designing and evaluating new therapeutic strategies, and for validation of *in vitro* test methods. Efforts to develop additional clinically relevant models of fungal infection are important and should be encouraged.

ACKNOWLEDGEMENTS

This work was supported in part by the Department of Veterans Affairs. The secretarial assistance of Ruth Kjaer is greatly appreciated.

VI.REFERENCES

1. E.J. Anaissie, G.P. Bodey, and M.G. Rinaldi, Emerging fungal pathogens, Eur. J. Clin. Microbiol. Infect. Dis., 8:323 (1989).
2. T. Horan, D. Culver, W. Jarvis, G. Emori, S. Banerjee, W. Martone, and C. Thornsberry, Pathogens causing nosocomial infections: Preliminary data from the National Nosocomial Infections Surveillance System, Antimicrob. Newsletter, 5:65 (1988).
3. M.A. Pfaller, Opportunistic fungal infections: The increasing importance of Candida species, Infect. Cont. Hosp. Epidemiol., 10:270 (1989).
4. D.J. Drutz, *In vitro* antifungal susceptibility testing and measurement of levels of antifungal agents in body fluids, Rev. Infect. Dis., 9:392 (1987).
5. D.A. Stevens, Problems in antifungal chemotherapy, Infection, 15:87 (1987).
6. T.J. Walsh, and A. Pizzo, Treatment of systemic fungal infections: Recent progress and current problems, Eur. J. Clin. Microbiol. Infect. Dis., 7:460 (1988).
7. T.J. Walsh, P.F. Jarosinski, and R.A. Fromtling, Increasing usage of systemic antifungal agents, Diag. Microbiol. Infect. Dis., 13:37 (1990).
8. J.D. Dick, W.G. Merz, and R. Saral, Incidence of polyene-resistant yeasts recovered from clinical specimens, Antimicrob. Agents Chemother., 18:158 (1980).
9. J.N. Galgiani, Antifungal susceptibility tests, Antimicrob. Agents Chemother., 31:1867 (1987).
10. J.N. Galgiani, The need for improved standardization in susceptibility testing, Recent Trends in the Discovery, Development and Evaluation of Antifungal Agents (R.A. Fromtling, ed.), J.R. Prous Science, Publishers, Barcelona, p. 15 (1987).
11. T.L. Hadfield, M.B. Smith, R.E. Winn, M.G. Rinaldi, and C. Guerra, Mycoses caused by Candida lusitaniae, Rev. Infect. Dis., 9:1006 (1987).

12. F.C. Odds, Laboratory tests for the activity of imidazole and triazole antifungal agents *in vitro*, Sem. Dermatol., 4:260 (1985).
13. A. Polak, and H.J. Scholer, Mode of action of 5-fluorocytosine and mechanisms of resistance, Chemotherapy, 21:113, (1975).
14. W.G. Powderly, G.S. Kobayashi, G.P. Herzig, and G. Medoff, Amphotericin B-resistant yeast infection in severely immunocompromised patients, Am. J. Med., 84:826 (1988).
15. J.F. Ryley, R.G. Wilson, and K.J. Barrett-Bee, Azole resistance in Candida albicans, Sabouraudia, 22:53 (1984).
16. D.L. Calhoun, G.D. Roberts, J.N. Galgiani, J.E. Bennett, D.S. Feingold, J. Jorgensen, G.S. Kobayashi, and S. Shadomy, Results of a survey of antifungal susceptibility tests in the United States and interlaboratory comparison of broth dilution testing of flucytosine and amphotericin B, J. Clin. Microbiol., 23:298 (1986).
17. G.V. Doern, T.A. Tubert, K. Chopin, and M.G. Rinaldi, Effect of medium composition on results of macrobroth dilution antifungal susceptibility testing of yeast, J. Clin. Microbiol., 24:507 (1986).
18. J.N. Galgiani, J. Reiser, C. Brass, A. Espinel-Ingroff, M.A. Gordon, and T.M. Kerkering, Comparison of relative susceptibilities of Candida species to three antifungal agents as determined by unstandardized methods, Antimicrob. Agents Chemother., 31:1343 (1987).
19. M.A. Pfaller, L. Burmeister, M.S. Bartlett, and M.G. Rinaldi, Multicenter evaluation of four methods of yeast inoculum preparation, J. Clin. Microbiol., 26:1437 (1988).
20. S. Shadomy, A. Espinel-Ingroff, and R.Y. Cartwright, Laboratory studies with antifungal agents: Susceptibility tests and bioassays, Manual of Clinical Microbiology 4th ed. (E.H. Lennette, A. Balows, W.J. Hausler, Jr., and H.J. Shadomy, ed.), American Society for Microbiology, Washington, D.C., p. 991 (1985).
21. A. Polak, and D.M. Dixon, *In vitro/in vivo* correlation of antifungal susceptibility testing using 5-fluorocytosine and ketoconazole as examples of two extremes, Recent Trends in the Discovery, Development and Evaluation of Antifungal Agents (R.A. Fromtling, ed.), J.R. Prous Science Publishers, Barcelona, p. 45 (1987).
22. R.L. Stiller, J.E. Bennett, H.J. Scholer, H.J. Wall, A. Polak, and D.A. Stevens, Correlation of *in vitro* susceptibility test results with *in vivo* response: Flucytosine therapy in a systemic candidiasis model, J. Infect. Dis., 147:1070 (1983).
23. A. Espinel-Ingroff, and S. Shadomy, *In vitro* and *in vivo* evaluation of antifungal agents, Eur. J. Clin. Microbiol. Infect. Dis., 8:352 (1989).
24. G. Kobayashi, and E.D. Spitzer, Testing of organisms for susceptibility to triazoles: Is it justified?, Eur. J. Clin. Microbiol. Infect. Dis., 8:387 (1989).

25. M.R. McGinnis, and M.G. Rinaldi, Antifungal drugs: Mechanisms of action, drug resistance, susceptibility testing, and assays of activity in biological fluids, Antibiotics in Laboratory Medicine (V. Lorian, ed.), The Williams & Wilkins Co., Baltimore, p. 223 (1986).
26. M.A. Pfaller, M.G. Rinaldi, J.N. Galgiani, M.S. Bartlett, B.A. Body, A. Espinel-Ingroff, R.A. Fromtling, G.S. Hall, C.E. Hughes, F.C. Odds, and A.M. Sugar, Collaborative investigation of variables in antifungal susceptibility testing of yeasts, Antimicrob. Agents Chemother., 34:in press (1990).
27. F.T. Boyle, J.F. Ryley, and R.G. Wilson, *In vitro-in vivo* correlations with azole antifungals, Recent Trends in the Discovery, Development and Evaluation of Antifungal Agents (R.A. Fromtling, ed.), J.R. Prous Science Publishers, Barcelona, p. 31 (1987).
28. R.S. Hare, and D. Loebenberg, Animal models in the search for antifungal agents, ASM News, 54:235 (1988).
29. C.R. Horsburgh, and C.H. Kirkpatrick, Long-term therapy of chronic mucocutaneous candidosis with ketoconazole: Experience with twenty-one patients, Am. J. Med., 74:23 (1983).
30. C.E. Hughes, R.L. Bennett, and W.H. Beggs, Broth dilution testing of Candida albicans susceptibility to ketoconazole, Antimicrob. Agents Chemother., 31:643 (1987).
31. T.E. Rogers, and J.N. Galgiani, Activity of fluconazole (UK 49,858) and ketoconazole against Candida albicans *in vitro* and *in vivo*, Antimicrob. Agents Chemother., 30:418 (1986).
32. C.A. Hitchcock, K.J. Barrett-Bee, and N.J. Russell, The lipid composition of azole-sensitive and azole-resistant strains of Candida albicans, J. Gen. Microbiol., 132:2421 (1986).
33. S. Shadomy, S.C. White, H.P. Yu, W.E. Dismukes, and the NIAID Mycoses Study Group, Treatment of systemic mycoses with ketoconazole: *In vitro* susceptibilities of clinical isolates of systemic and pathogenic fungi to ketoconazole, J. Infect. Dis., 152:1249 (1985).
34. M. Radetsky, R.C. Wheeler, M.H. Roe, and J.K. Todd, Microtiter broth dilution method for yeast susceptibility testing with validation by clinical outcome, J. Clin. Microbiol., 24:600 (1986).
35. M.G. Rinaldi, *In vivo* models of the mycoses for the evaluation of antifungal agents, Recent Trends in the Discovery, Development and Evaluation of Antifungal Agents (R.A. Fromtling, ed.), J.R. Prous Science Publishers, Barcelona, p. 11 (1987).
36. A.B. Onderdonk, Use of an animal model system for assessing antimicrobial activity, Antimicrob. Newsletter, 7:9 (1990).

34

Future Prospectives and Concluding Remarks

George S. Kobayashi

Department of Internal Medicine
Washington University School of Medicine
St. Louis, Missouri, USA 63110

This volume contains the papers presented at the First International Conference on Antifungal Chemotherapy held September 24-26, 1990 in Oiso, Japan. In his opening remarks, Dr. Hideyo Yamaguchi emphasized that the incidence of opportunistic fungal infections is increasing particularly in patients who are receiving intensive antineoplastic, immunosuppressive, and antibacterial therapy for severe underlying conditions such as leukemia, acquired immunodeficiency diseases (AIDS) and those undergoing bone marrow or other organ transplantation. These views were echoed in the Plenary Session by Dr. Soroku Yamagata in his lecture on "Recent Trends of HIV Infections in Japan". This session was concluded by Dr. Vassil St. Georgiev who reviewed the current status of available antifungal agents and our knowledge of their mechanisms of action. These opening talks set the theme for the scientific session of the First International Conference on Antifungal Chemotherapy by stressing the need for novel

[1]Portions of this report were supported by USPHS grants AI 07015, AI 29609 and NO1-AI72640 from the National Institutes of Health.

antifungals as well as development of newer innovative strategies to treat these diseases.

In their presentations, Drs. Berg, Hiruma, Conti Diaz, and Hay introduced their sessions by focusing on the historical aspects of the problem and discussing projected needs. They emphasized repeatedly that in order to establish with certainty that a specific fungus is the cause of a disease, the same organism must be isolated from serial specimens cultured at well-spaced intervals of time, and fungal elements that are morphologically consistent with the isolate should be observed in tissue specimens taken from the lesion. While these procedures constitute good mycological practices it is often not possible to establish with certainty that a fungus is responsible for the clinical situation that is being managed and therapy is occasionally instituted empirically without benefit of culture or pathologic confirmation. This was emphasized in the session "Problems in the Treatment of Fungal Infections in Immunocompromised Hosts" chaired by Drs Troke and Ikemoto. Specific problems in the clinical management of patients that are at high risk of developing opportunistic life-threatening fungal infections such as those undergoing aggressive therapy to treat neoplastic diseases, those who are being given immunosuppressive drugs for organ transplantation, those who are being managed through the use of supportive measures such as intravenous catheters for parenteral hyperalimentation, and the population of patients with AIDS were discussed by Drs. Stevens, Dismukes, Oka, and Armstrong in their presentations. It is predictable that this problem will continue to grow as the number of patients undergoing organ transplantation and immunosuppressive therapy increases, and the incidence of individuals afflicted with the human immunodeficiency virus (AIDS) escalates.

Paralleling the growing incidence of life-threatening fungal infections, particularly in patients who are at high risk, and efforts to devise tests that rapidly diagnose and monitor these diseases has been the need for and development of new antifungal agents, elucidation of their mechanism of action, and novel strategies for their delivery. As discussed in the presentations by Drs. Vanden Bossche, Ryder, Nozawa, Brajtburg, Ito, Feczko, Hector, Perfect and Van Cutsem, most of the presently available agents are targeted to interfere with the synthesis of chitin, cell wall polysaccharides and ergosterol. The major categories of useful antifungals are the polyene macrolides, the azole derivatives, pyrimidine nucleoside peptide derivatives, the cyclic lipopeptides, and the allylamines. During this Conference Drs. Oki, Inouye, Yamaki, Takahashi, Nishikawa, and Polak discussed several promising compounds that have recently been isolated, identified, and chemically characterized. These presentations were followed by discussions on novel strategies for use of biological response modifiers by Drs. Otani, Fukuzawa, Bolard, Anaissie, and Yamamoto as well as drug delivery systems by Drs. Hay, Bonner, Brajtburg, and Kohno.

It was apparent that even with these advances, there still remains a critical need for newer classes of antifungals that are effective and specific against the fungus and nontoxic to the host. The question is, how do we go about this? The ideal strategy for developing new antifungals is to study the biochemistry or physiology of the organism in question and then design compounds or ways that will specifically interfere with vital processes of the organism and kill it without affecting host functions. Not only must the compound be innocuous to the host but it must have the right pharmacological properties. It must reach the fungus at the site of parasitization without being metabolized or inactivated. While this may be the ideal way to develop new antifungals it is extremely expensive and time consuming, and there is no assurance that positive results will accrue. As a result, most discoveries still rely on random screening of natural products, chemical modifications of existing agent, and classical enrichment technics involving bacteria.

The procedures most often used to evaluate antifungal activity are various in vitro susceptibility screens followed by in vivo evaluations in infected animals to determine efficacy and toxicity. One must keep in mind that both procedures go hand in hand. Since there are no standard procedures for in vitro susceptibility testing, results that are generated from such tests may not reflect what will happen in the in vivo model. To illustrate this point, I would like to describe a study that we recently published. In this study, 12 clinical isolates of Histoplasma capsulatum were tested against two triazoles, Sch39304 and fluconazole using amphotericin B as a comparative standard. The minimum inhibitory concentration (MIC) of the two triazoles were identical against the same isolates and ranged from 2.95 to >1,000 ug/ml. The MIC against amphotericin B ranged from 0.3 to 1.09 ug/ml and exhibited sharp endpoints compared to the triazoles. In experimental therapy studies using a "susceptible" strain of H. capsulatum as infecting organism and treatment regimens that started 24 hours after infection both triazoles were effective in treating the infections but amphotericin B was the best. Since two strains of H. capsulatum exhibited a high degree of tolerance (resistance) to the two triazoles, we decided to infect mice with one of these strains to see if resistance would also be reflected in vivo. Here again both triazoles were effective in treating the infected mice which indicated that in this case in vitro testing was misleading since mice treated with both traizoles responded to the regimens we tested. This poses a dilemma and suggests the possibility that some very promising agents will be overlooked if in vitro screening procedures are relied upon as sole method to evaluate antifungal activity. In the final session, Dr. Michael Pfaller discussed problems and efforts that are currently being expended to develop standardized testing procedures that will be more predictive of in vivo activities.

At the present time, several investigators are approaching the subject of fungal control using the technics of molecular biology. While a great deal of information is available concerning the molecular basis of bacterial, viral, and even protozoal pathogenesis little is known about mechanisms of fungal pathogenesis. Inroads however are being made by investigators such as KJ Kwon-Chung, and Jeffrey Edman who have cloned the genome of Cryptococcus neoformans, developed a transformation system and are looking for virulence factors at the gene level by focusing on the organisms ability to grow at 37C, phenoloxidase activity, and the production of an acidic mucopolysaccharide capsule.

Phenoloxidase activity and the ability to synthesize melanin is distributed among other fungi such as the dematiaceous fungi, in addition to C. neoformans, and believed to be a virulence factor. The genetic studies with Wangiella dermatitidis by Paul Szaniszlo, Chester Cooper, and Dennis Dixon have contributed a great deal to our understanding of the biochemical pathway of melanogenesis in this important agent of phaeohyphomycosis. They have isolated an albino mutant that has reduced virulence for mice and speculate that defects in the pentaketide pathway of melanin production contribute to the loss of virulence. Studies at the gene level are being conducted by other workers on such subjects as the mechanisms of surface adherence, filamentation, and switching in Candida albicans and those pertaining to the production of elastase and other proteases and the role they play in virulence of Aspergillus.

Our research concerning antifungal strategies have focused on H. capsulatum as a laboratory model because it is the most common respiratory mycosis in the world, endemic in the Ohio and Mississippi Valley region of the United States where our institution is located, and therapy for disseminated disease is far from ideal. An important feature of this fungus is its property of dimorphism. In nature it resides in the soil as mycelia producing characteristic macro- and microconidia. Primary infection occurs in the lung when spores or hyphal fragments are inhaled, phagocytosed, and then convert to a yeast morphology whereupon they replicate within nonimmune macrophages. The mycelial and yeast phases of H. capsulatum can be reproduced in the laboratory by controlling the temperature of incubation. Mycelia grow at 25C and yeasts at 37C. The ability of H. capsulatum to convert from the mycelial to yeast morphology is required for progressive infection. This conclusion is based on several observations. Examination of histopathologic sections reveal that only yeasts are seen in infected tissues. Secondly, there is a correlation between sensitivity of the fungus to elevated temperatures and virulence for mice. Finally, mycelia that are unable to undergo the transition to yeast are not virulent. Strong support for this concept was provided by our studies with mycelia treated with the sulfhydryl blocking agent p-chloromercuriphenolsulphonic acid (pcms). Mycelia treated with pcms fail to undergo the transition to yeast; they are viable but not virulent. We have further shown that mice immunized with these preparations are protected from lethal challenge with H. capsulatum.

Recently, our efforts have been focused on the molecular biology of the phase transition in H. capsulatum. It is our notion that the mycelium to yeast transition involves alterations in the pattern of gene expression, which leads to expression of specific regulatory genes. These genes, control changes in many features of the metabolic processes of cells and the morphology of the organism. Our efforts have been directed at isolating members of both types of genes active in either the mycelial or yeast phase or early during the phase transition. We have initiated studies to analyze structural genes, eg, tubulin and actin, phase specific genes, eg, genes that are expressed only in the yeast phase, and genes that potentially have regulatory function, eg, heat shock genes.

Since the mycelium to yeast transition is induced by heat and conversion to the yeast morphology is required for pathogenicity, we felt that the early events of the phase transition were part of a heat shock response which is followed by adaptation of the organism to the elevated temperature. This notion was supported by observations that synthesis of new proteins occurred soon after the shift from 25C to temperatures between 34C and 40C. Confirmation of these findings have been supported by the recent work of Bruno Maresca and his colleagues who have cloned, sequenced and characterized the hsp70 and hsp83 genes from H. capsulatum and studied expression of these genes in strains that differed in virulence and sensitivities to heat. We are currently studying the phenomenon of heat shock response with the intent to find unique gene sequences or proteins that can be attacked pharmacologically.

The molecular biological approach to the study of medically relevant fungi is still in a developmental stage and current research efforts still rely on traditional approaches for the discovery and development of better antifungals. It is evident from the proceedings of this meeting that a number of advances have been made in the development of new antifungals and strategies to treat fungal diseases and that interest in these subjects is currently at peak level. From the published text of this Conference, the speakers met the challenge made by Dr. Yamaguchi at the beginning of this Conference and the goals were successfully achieved.

PART IX

APPENDIX: POSTER PRESENTATIONS

A1

In Vitro and *in Vivo* Antifungal Activities of M-732, a New Thiocarbamate Derivative

T. Inoue, Y. Oku, K. Yokoyama*, H. Kaji*, K. Nishimura*, M. Miyaji*

Research Laboratory, Zenyaku Kogyo Co., Ltd., Ohizumi-machi, Nerima-ku, Tokyo, 178, Japan

** Research Center for Pathogenic Fungi and Microbial Toxicoses, Chiba University, Inohana, Chiba, 280, Japan*

INTRODUCTION

M-732 [O-(5,6,7,8-tetrahydro-2-naphthyl) N-(6-methoxy-2-pyridyl)-N-methylthiocarbamate ($C_{18}H_{20}N_2O_2S$); Mol. wt. 328.44] is a new thiocarbamate antifungal agent developed by Tosoh Corp. and Zenyaku Kogyo Co., Ltd., Tokyo, Japan. Iwata *et al.* earlier reported a marked antidermatophytic activity of M-732.[1)]

To evaluate its clinical application, the antifungal activity of M-732 was tested against several fresh clinical isolates and stock cultures of dermatophytes as well as some other pathogenic fungi.

In addition, the topical therapeutic effect of this compound was examined using an experimentally induced dermatophytosis in guinea pigs.

MATERIALS AND METHODS

The *in vitro* antifungal sensitivity testing was done by determining the MIC values with the agar dilution method using Sabouraud dextrose (2 %) medium (pH 6.0, Difco). Tolciclate and bifonazole were used as references.

Hartley guinea pigs were infected with *Trichophyton mentagrophytes* IFM 40769. The topical treatment with 1 % and 2 % M-732 creams as well as 1 % tolciclate cream (Toskil^{TM}) was started 3 days after the inoculation. The creams were applied once a day for 14 days. Lesions ranged from 1+ to 4+ depending on the degree of papule, erythema, scale, crust, or bleeding. Two days after the last treatment, the infected areas were cut into small pieces and cultured. The percentage of negative cultures was determined by the number of skin pieces without fungal growth.

RESULTS AND CONCLUSION

M-732 showed an excellent antidermatophytic activity to both the clinical isolates and the stock cultures of the dermatophytes (Table 1). In particular, it was highly effective on *T. rubrum*, the most common human dermatophyte. The MIC_{90} values of M-732, tolciclate and bifonazole were 0.078, 0.313, and 2.5 μg/ml, respectively. Regarding the antidermatophytic activity *in vitro*, M-732 was superior to tolciclate and bifonazole. The clinical isolates were slightly more resistant to all three antifungal agents than the stock cultures (Table 1). *Hortaea werneckii*, *Blastomyces dermatitidis*, *Paecilomyces lilacinus*, *Aspergillus* spp. and *Cryptococcus neoformans* were highly sensitive to M-732. On the contrary, *Sporothrix schenckii* and *Candida* spp. were highly resistant to both M-732 and tolciclate.

Table 1. *In vitro* antifungal activities of M-732, tolciclate and bifonazole against the stock cultures and the fresh clinical isolates* of dermatophytes

Organism (no. of strains)	MIC (μg/ml) range of :		
	M-732	Tolciclate	Bifonazole
Trichophyton mentagrophytes (23)	0.019 - 0.156	0.078 - 0.625	0.313 - 5.0
*T. mentagrophytes** (43)	0.078 - 0.313	0.156 - 0.625	2.5 - 20
T. rubrum (20)	0.004 - 0.039	0.019 - 0.313	0.313 - 5.0
*T. rubrum** (32)	0.019 - 0.078	0.078 - 0.313	0.313 - 2.5
T. tonsurans (4)	0.009 - 0.039	0.039 - 0.156	2.5
*T. tonsurans** (2)	0.019 , 0.039	0.078 , 0.156	2.5 , 10
T. violaceum (7)	0.019 - 0.078	0.078 - 0.156	0.313 - 10
*T. violaceum** (3)	0.078 - 0.156	0.156 - 0.313	2.5 - 5.0
T. verrucosum (3)	0.009 - 0.019	0.039 - 0.156	1.25 - 2.5
T. schoenleinii (1)	0.019	0.078	0.156
Microsporum audouinii (2)	0.078 , 0.313	0.156 , 0.313	0.625 , 10
M. canis (8)	0.009 - 0.078	0.039 - 0.156	0.078 - 5.0
*M. canis** (15)	0.039 - 0.156	0.078 - 0.313	1.25 - 20
M. gypseum (15)	0.039 - 0.156	0.078 - 0.313	0.625 - 20
*M. gypseum** (6)	0.078 - 0.313	0.156 - 0.313	2.5 - 10
Epidermophyton floccosum (10)	0.009 - 0.078	0.039 - 0.313	0.039 - 5.0
*E. floccocum** (4)	0.039 - 0.078	0.156 - 0.313	0.078 - 0.156

* All the strains were isolated from clinical cases within the past year.
Inoculum size: 1 x 10^3 conidia (or CFU)/spot
Inoculation was performed with a microplanter MIT-P (Sakuma Co., Ltd., Japan).
The MICs were read after 14 days of incubation at 27°C.

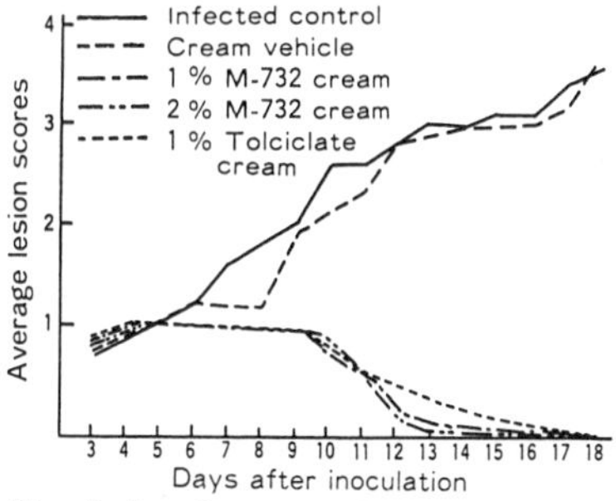

Fig. 1. Development of lesion scores in guinea pigs infected with *T. mentagrophytes* IFM 40769
Topical treatment of 0.2g of each cream was started 3 days after the inoculation. The creams were applied once a day for 14 days.

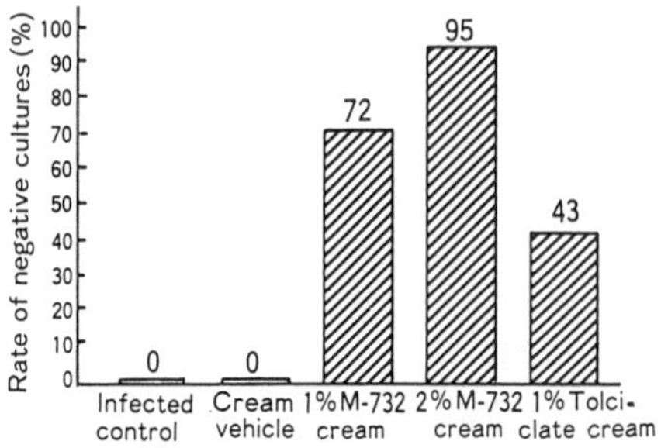

Fig. 2. Rate of negative cultures from the infected skin
Two days after the last treatment, the infected areas were cut into small pieces and cultured.

All three different topical creams used showed a remarkable therapeutic effect on the improvement of the lesions in the animal experiment. However, the M-732 cream seemed to cure the lesions a little more quickly than the 1 % tolciclate cream (Fig. 1). M-732 cream eliminated the dermatophyte from the skin lesions more effectively than the tolciclate cream (Fig. 2). Also, the toxicity of M-732 was low. These results suggest that M-732 cream would be very effective on human dermatophytoses.

1) Iwata *et al.*, Antimicrobial Agents and Chemotherapy, Vol. 33: p. 2118-2125, 1989.

A2

Comparative Studies of the Influence of Amorolfine and Oxiconazole on the Ultrastructure of *Trichophyton mentagrophytes*

W. Melchinger, A. Polak*, and J. Müller

Mycology Section, Institute for Medical Microbiology and Hygiene, University of Freiburg, Germany FR.
* Hoffmann-La Roche Ltd., Basel, Switzerland

SUMMARY

Amorolfine applied in concentrations of 0.1-100 µg/ml caused the following damages to the ultrastructure of *Trichophyton mentagrophytes*: Electron-transparent areas appeared in the cytoplasma. The cell walls increased in thickness. Extracytoplasmic membrane vesicles were formed and deposited in the cell wall. Starved fungal cells, with normal ultrastructure, could be found. Lysed, dead cells demonstrated the process of final, vigorous ultrastructural damages.

INTRODUCTION

Amorolfine (Roche 24-4767/002 = (4-(3-(p(1,1-dimethylpropyl)-phenyl) 2-methylpropyl-2,6-cis dimethylmorpholine hydrochloride)) exhibits a broad spectrum of antifungal activity and is particularly effective in the topical therapy of superficial mycoses caused by yeasts and dermatophytes (1, 2, 3, 4). The mode of action has been described by Polak-Wyss (5, 6). Amorolfine inhibits as fenpropimorph and fenpropidine the biosynthesis of ergosterol, an essential constituent of the fungal cytoplasmic membrane. In all fungal species ignosterol or ergosta-8,14,24(28)-trienol is accumulated; in *Trichophyton* species at high concentrations of amorolfine (> 10 µg/ml) squalene is also accumulated. The drug is fungicidal against dermatophytes and yeasts (4). The effect of amorolfine on the ultrastructure of the yeast species *Candida albicans* has been studied by Müller et al. (7). The aim of the present study was to investigate the ultrastructural changes in the dermatophyte *Trichophyton mentagrophytes* caused by amorolfine compared with those by oxiconazole.

MATERIAL AND METHODS

Trichophyton mentagrophytes, strain No. 109 Roche, was grown, for comparison in two different media: a. Sabouraud (2 %) glucose broth, 30°C for 5 d, or b. Tryptone yeast extract (2 %) glucose broth, 30°C, for 3 d, until micromycelia had been formed. These were transferred into fresh media to which 0.1, 1, 10, or 100 µg amorolfine/ml, or oxiconazole respectively, had been added. After incubation for 6, 24, and 48 h at 30°C aliquots were harvested, fixed in glutaraldehyde (2 %) and osmium tetroxide (2 %) and processed for electronmicroscopic examination.

RESULTS

The type of the growth medium had no obvious influence on the nature of ultrastructural damage caused by amorolfine or oxiconazole. The ultrastructural damage caused by azoles is well documented and has been reviewed by Müller (8). The ultrastructural oxiconazole-related changes observed in the present study are qualitatively the same as found with amorolfine. They differ, however, with respect to the intensity and to the kinetics during the observation time.

In comparison with the controls and increasing with the length of exposure time amorolfine causes the following damage to *Tr. mentagrophytes*:

1. Cloddy, electron-dense degeneration of the cytoplasma.
2. Appearance of electron-transparent areas which are not surrounded by membranes.
3. The cells increase in size and the cell walls increase considerably in thickness compared with non-treated fungus cells.
4. Extracytoplasmic phospholipid bodies surrounded by membranes are formed and deposited in the cell wall.
5. More cytoplasmic vacuoles are formed indicating a premature ageing of the fungus cell.
6. Starved fungus cells can be found which are normal in their ultrastructure, but obviously exhausted in cellular substance.
7. Electron-dense material is deposited on the external cell wall surface representing cytoplasmic constituents released in the course of the damaging process.
8. Final necrosis of the total *Trichophyton* protoplasts with persistance of the cell wall is observed.

These results documented by electronmicrographs will be described in detail elsewhere (9).

DISCUSSION

The molecular weights of both antifungals are in the same range (amorolfine 317, oxiconazole 429). It is, therefore, legitimate to compare the antifungal activities on the base of the same concentrations of weight per volume. Since fungicidal activity is observed after 48 h of exposure to 0.001 µg/ml with both drugs (4) the drug concentrations as well as the exposure times used in the present study are appropriate to elucidate drug-related ultrastructural changes in fungal pathogens.

The individual aspects of ultrastructural damage cited in the paragraph Results mark their succession in the course of the observation time. Some characters of ultrastructural damages are observed even with the highest drug concentration after 24-48 h exposure. The interpretation is that about 90 % of the fungus cells die rapidly from high drug concentrations, the remaining cells, however, need up to 2 d until death. These persisters, responsible for the late fungicidal action, are not lysed quickly, but may pass different stages of damage until their late death.

Comparing the two antifungals one can recognize that electron-transparent areas in the cytoplasma appear earlier under the influence of oxiconazole, while extracytoplasmic membrane vesicles are more pronounced when the fungus was exposed to amorolfine. Furthermore, the character of the damage due to amorolfine found in *Tr. mentagrophytes* resembles that observed in the yeast species *C. albicans* (7). The amorolfine-related increase of the cell wall thickness, however, was markedly more pronounced in *Tr. mentagrophytes* than in *C. albicans*.

REFERENCES

1. A. Polak-Wyss, Experimental activity of a new antimycotic. Current Chemotherapy & Immunotherapy, Proc. 12th Int. Congr. of Chemotherapy, Florence (Italy), p. 1023-1025 (1981).
2. A. Polak-Wyss, Antifungal activity in vitro of Ro 14-4767/002, a phenylpropylmorpholine, Sabouraudia 21, 205-213 (1983).
3. A. Polak-Wyss, H. Lengsfeld, and G. Oesterhelt, Effect of oxiconazole and Ro 14-4767/002 on sterol pattern in *Candida albicans*, Sabouraudia 23, 433-442 (1985).
4. A. Polak, and M. Dixon, The antifungal activity of amorolfine (Ro 14-4767/002) in vitro and in vivo, (R. A. Fromtling, ed.) Recent Trends in the Discovery, Development and Evaluation of Antifungal Agents, J.R. Prous Science Publishers, S.A. p 555-573 (1987).
5. A. Polak, Mode of action of morpholine derivates, Antifungal Drugs, Vol. 544, Ann. New York Acad. Scienc. p. 221-228 (1988).
6. A. Polak, Mode of Action Studies, Handbook of Experimental Pharmacology, Vol. 96, Chemotherapy of fungal diseases, (J. F. Ryley, ed.) Springer-Verlag Berlin Heidelberg, p. 153-182 (1990).
7. J. Müller, A. Polak, and R. Jaeger, The effect of the morpholine derivate amorolfine (Roche 14-4767/002) on the ultrastructure of *Candida albicans*, mykosen 30, 528-540 (1987).
8. J. Müller, Electronmicroscopy of fungi and fungous diseases, Electronmicroscopy in Human Medicine, (Johannessen, J.V., ed.) McGraw-Hill Book Company, New York p. 334-390 (1980).
9. W. Melchinger, A. Polak, and J. Müller, The effect of amorolfine and oxiconazole on the ultrastructure of *Trichophyton mentagrophytes*. A comparison, mycoses 33 (1990), in press.

A3

Effect of Amorolfine, a New Antifungal Agent, on the Ultrastructure of *Trichophyton mentagrophytes*

Y.Nishiyama, Y.Asagi, T.Hiratani, H.Yamaguchi, N.Yamada[1], M.Osumi[2]

Teikyo University School of Medicine, Hachioji, Tokyo 192-03
Research Center for Medical Mycology
Japan Women's University, Bunkyo-ku, Mejirodai, Tokyo 112
[1]Laboratory of Electron Microscopy
[2]Department of Biology

Amorolfine(AMOR), a new class of morpholine derivative, is an antifungal agent with high activity against dermatophytes, pathogenic yeasts and filamentous fungi(1). In this study, the effect of AMOR on the ultrastructure of *Trichophyton mentagrophytes* grown in a liquid medium was revealed by scanning (SEM) and transmission(TEM) electron microscopy.

MATERIALS AND METHODS

T.mentagrophytes strain TIMM 1189 was used. Cultures were grown in Sabouraud dextrose broth with or without AMOR (0.8-80

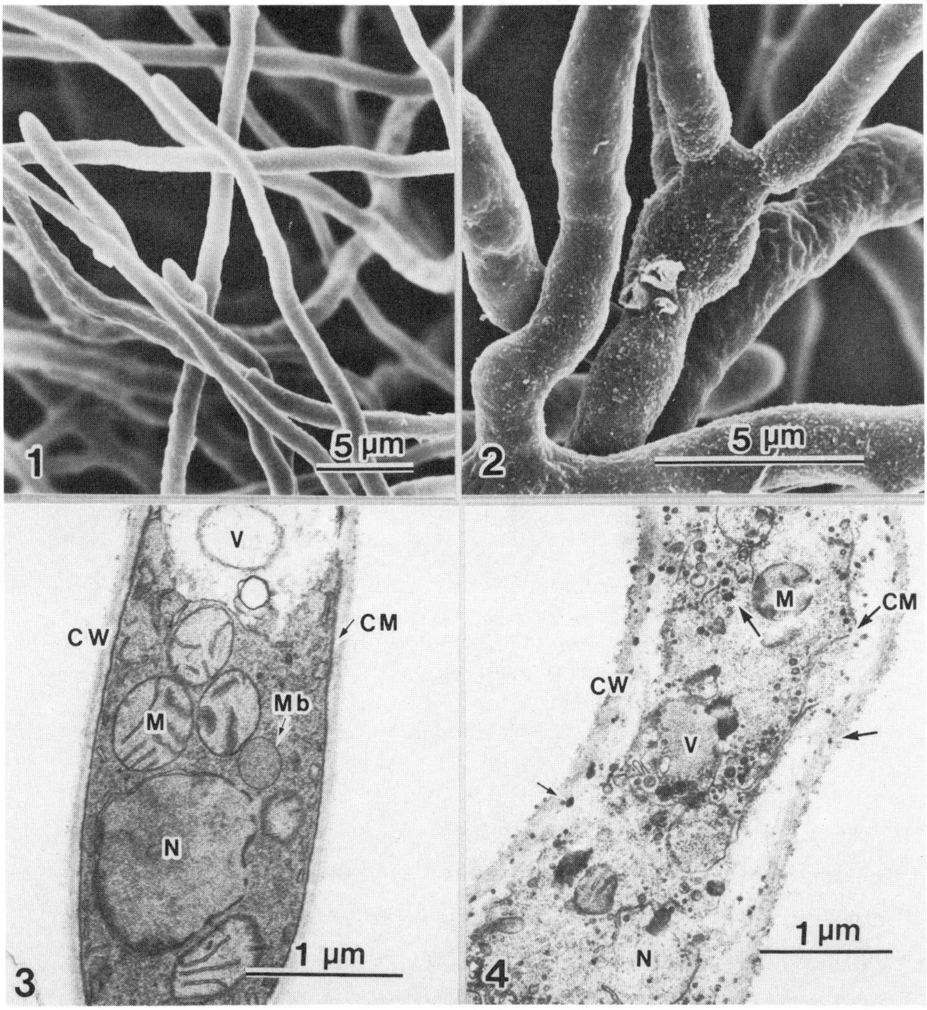

FIG.1. SEM image of untreated control culture of *T. mentagrophytes* grown for 24 hr showing straight elongated hyphae with smooth surface.
FIG.2. SEM image of 24 hr-culture grown with 80 ng/ml of AMOR showing deformed hyphae.
FIG.3. Thin section of untreated control culture of *T.mentagrophytes* grown for 24 hr. CW:cell wall, CM:cytoplasmic membrane, N:nucleus, M:mitochondria, V:vacuole, Mb:microbody
FIG.4. Thin section of a hypha grown with 80 ng/ml of AMOR for 24 hr. Numerous electron dense granules(arrows) are localized in the cell wall and the region between the wall and cytoplasmic membrane. Degeneration of membrane structures of organelles is visible.

ng/ml) at 27 C on a shaker. After various periods of incubation, the hyphal flocs were harvested by centrifugation, prefixed with 2% glutaraldehyde in 0.1 M cacodylate buffer (pH 7.2) for 2 hr and washed with the same buffer. Then the specimens were postfixed with 1% OsO_4 and 1.5% $KMnO_4$ for SEM and TEM, respectively. After dehydration, the specimens were prepared and observed by the methods described previously(2).

RESULTS AND DISCUSSION

Hyphal growth was inhibited at the drug concentration of 0.8 ng/ml, and several morphological changes such as waving of the surface structure and contour deformation were observed by SEM. In thin sections, accumulation of electron dense granular structures formed within both the wall and the cytoplasm was visible. Eighty ng/ml of AMOR caused the collapse and distortion of hyphae and exfoliation of surface structures. Moreover, degeneration of the cytoplasmic membrane and alteration of organelles were clearly seen at this concentration of the drug. From the results obtained, it is concluded that ultrastructural changes produced by AMOR lead to the death of fungal hyphae.

REFERENCES

1. A. Polak, Antifungal activity *in vitro* of Ro 14-4767/002, a phenylpropyl-morpholine. Sabouraudia, 21:205 (1983)
2. Y. Nishiyama, K. Maebashi, Y. Asagi, T. Hiratani, H. Yamaguchi, N. Yamada, A. Taki, J.X. Rong, M. Osumi, Effect of SS717 on the ultrastructure of *Trichophyton mentagrophytes* as observed by scanning and transmission electron microscopy. Jpn.J.Med.Mycol., in press

A4

Bifonazole-Urea Ointment: A New Approach in Topical Treatment of Onychomycosis

S. Stettendorf

Department of Clinical Research BAYER AG, Aprather Weg ,5600 Wuppertal 1, Germany

INTRODUCTION

Fungal infections of the nails still pose difficult problems for physicians and patients as existing therapeutic possibilities are not always satisfactory. Any treatment of onychomycosis will inevitably be a lengthy process and a high degree of patient compliance as well as guidance by the attending physician is required. The oral treatment of onychomycosis with Griseofulvin or other antifungals yields some problems, e.g. the length of treatment, the poor overall response rate, and the possibility of side effects. Surgical removal of mycotic nail is a rapid therapeutic method, but it is accompanied by several risk (pain, bleeding, trauma) and not very well accepted by patients.

One of the therapeutic approaches is keratolysis of the infected nail, e.g. using urea. A new combination of 1% Bifonazole and 40% urea, available as an ointment, is suited for this purpose. We know that urea not only effects hydration,but also facilitates the penetration of active substances. This effect can be intensified by applying the ointment under an occlusive dressing . This poster presents an overview of clinical studies carried out in onychomycoses using such a treatment regimen.

CONCEPT OF TREATMENT

The treatment consisted of two phases:

a)Initial therapy,i.e. atraumatic detachment of the fungus-infected nail with Bifonazole-urea ointment under occlusive dressing.
The Bifonazole-urea ointment was spread on the affected nails and left for 24 h under an occlusive dressing, as a rule a waterproof plaster.
Each time the dressing was changed the nails were bathed in warm water and easily detachable fungus-infected nail material was removed. The application of Bifonazole-urea ointment was continued until the nail or parts of the nail infected by the fungus had been completely detached.

b)Continuing therapy,i.e. subsequent treatment of the nail bed with Mycospor® Bayer AG, Leverkusen, Germany, cream 1%, solution 1%, or gel 1% for a period of 4 weeks or longer without occlusion.

The appropriate formulation was applied every 24h, i.e. once a day.

PATIENTS AND METHOD

Patients with evidence of onychomycosis were included in the studies. Diagnosis was confirmed by mycological (KOH and culture) and clinical findings prior to treatment in all cases.

Mycological examinations (KOH and culture) and clinical assessment
-after complete nail detachment
-at the end of the treatment
-1,3,6 and 12 months after end of treatment.

Final assessment for efficacy was based on mycological (KOH and culture) and clinical findings (nail regrowth).

RESULTS

A. Clinical Studies (Phase III) : [1] - [16]

Design:	non-randomized, mycologically controlled
Countries:	Germany, Yugoslavia, Guatemala, Argentina, Great Britain, Spain, Indonesia, Italy
Total no. of studies:	n = 18
Total no. of patients:	n = 555
Time unitl nail removal:	on average 13 days (7-28 days)
Success rate (mean value)	76% (range 47-90%)

B. Post-marketing Surveillance Study

Patients enrolled:	n = 1453
Patients valid for inclusion (mycological positive):	n = 1036
No. patients toenails infected:	n = 793
No. patients fingernails infected:	n = 136
No. patients toe-and fingernails:	n = 71
Time until nail removal (mean value):	18 days
Patients valid for efficacy:	n = 974
All-over success rate (end of follow-up)	87.2%

ADVANTAGES

Bifonazole-urea ointment combines
-keratolytic and hydrating properties of urea
with
-antimycotic effect of Bifonazole
-intensified by occulsive dressing
from the very bebinning of treatment

TOLERABILITY

- Local tolerance of bifonazole-urea ointment is good
- Fungus-intfected nails can be removed without pain
- No necessity to cover the nail surrounding area

IMPORTANT FACTORS FOR SUCCESSFUL TREATMENT

- Good patient compliance
- Detailed instruction and guidance of patients by the attending physician
- Elimination of sources of reinfection (e.g. tinea pedis, socks /shoes)
- Few number of nails (3-4) to be treated simultaneously during a treatment course

CONCLUSIONS

The described treatment scheme is
- non evasive
- Free from risks, i.e. it is not nealy as stressful as systemic or surgical therapeutic measures
- can be repeated at any time
- good suitable also for outpatient treatment

REFERENCES

[1]Döring, H.F.; Ärztl. Kosmetologie 16:441-443(1986) [2]Nolting, S.et al.; "Fortschritte in der lokalen antimykotischen Therapie", Springer Verlag Berlin: 113(1988) [3]Felten, G.et al.; Dt derm. 35,7:743(1987) [4] Kulenkamp,D.; Dt. Derm.36, 8:846(1988) [5]worret W.-I.; "Onychomykosen-Topische Anti-mykotica-Therapie" Springer Verlag Berlin:63(1989) [6]Ernst Th.-M. et al.; "Onychomykosen-Topische Antimykotika-Therapie" Springer Verlag Berlin: 68 (1989) [7]Pierchalla P. et al.; "2. Dermatologisches Forum-Neues in der Therapie" Verlag medical concept München: 126-135(1987) [8]Effendy I.et al.; hautnah 2-April:92 (1990) [9]Lalosevic,J. et al.:"Fortschritte in der lokalen antimykotischen Therapie", Springer Verlag Berlin: 107(1988) [10]Stettendorf,S. et al.; Internal Report(1986) [11]Galimberti,R. L. et al.; In: Proceedings of the Congress of ISHAM, Barcelona:252(1988) [12]Hay,R.J. et al.; Clinical Experimental Dermatology 13:164(1988) [13]Torres-Rodriquez,J.M.et al.; In:Proceedings of the Congress of ISHAM,Barcelona:248(1988) [14]Lecha, v.et al.; Med. cut. I.L.A. XV, 1:53(1987) [15]Hardjoko, F. S. et al.; Mycoses 33(4) 167-171 (1990) [16]Lasagni, A.; Internal Report(1990)

A5

Modulation of Leukotriene Metabolism by Bifonazole

Klaus D. Bremm and Manfred Plempel

Institute for Chemotherapy, Bayer-Research Center
5600 Wuppertal, Aprather Weg 16, Germany

INTRODUCTION

There is increasing evidence from clinical trials that bifonazole shows an antiphlogistic activity which resembles 1% hydrocortisone (Bauer & Vennemann, 1988). The clinical importance of bifonazole's antiinflammatory action is demonstrated by good therapeutical effects during therapy of acne rosacea and seborrhoic dermatitis (Faergamann, 1989). It was the purpose of the study to investigate the influence of bifonazole and other azoles on the leukotriene metabolism of human neutrophil granulocytes (PMN). The accumulation of neutrophils in the infected skin is an early event during dermatomycosis. These cells express receptors for LTB_4 and are also able to synthesize considerable amounts of chemotactic active LTB_4. The omega-oxidation influences the amounts of biologically active LTB_4 that appear in the medium surrounding stimulated PMN. The resulting inactivation of LTB_4 to its metabolites 20-OH-LTB_4 and 20-COOH-LTB_4 is an important mechanism of regulation during an ongoing infection.

RESULTS

Incubation of human PMN (1×10^7/ml) with A23187 (7.3μM) for 15 minutes resulted in the release of 232±18 ng LTB_4 and 137±12 ng 20-OH-LTB_4 and 20-COOH-LTB_4 (omega-LTB_4).

FIGURE 1: Inhibition of leukotriene metabolism by Bifonazole

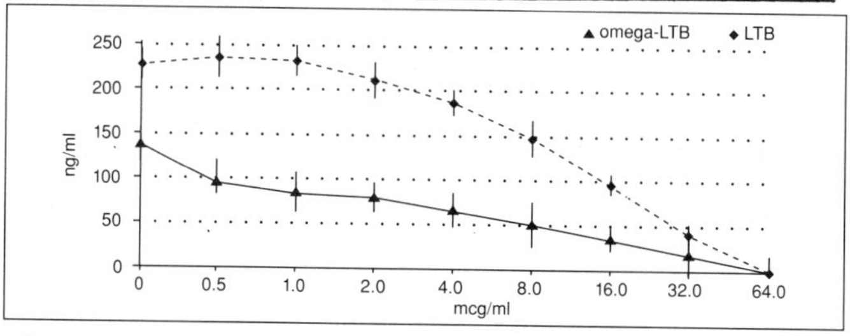

Simultaneous addition of bifonazole modulated LTB_4 generation as well as omega-oxidation. Figure 1 shows that bifonazole already induced decreased omega-oxidation with 0.5 and 1 μg/ml. This inhibition resulted in slightly elevated LTB_4-levels. Starting with 2 μg/ml a dose-dependent inhibition of release and metabolism can be seen. The addition of 64 μg/ml bifonazole resulted in a total inhibition of leukotriene release from human PMN.

Table 1 compares Bifonazole with other topical antifungals and antiphlogistics concerning the leukotriene generation from human PMN It is evident that Bifonazole had a more pronounced effect on the leukotriene formation in human PMN than the other topical antifungals like Clotrimazole, Naftifin and Griseofulvin. During this in vitro studies Cortisol was a more potent inhibitor of the lipoxygenase pathway than Bifonazole, while Betamethason was as potent as Bifonazole.

TABLE 1: Inhibition of leukotriene metabolism by dermatologicals

% inhibition of LTB4-generation				
	0.125 mcg/ml	1 mcg/ml	8 mcg/ml	64 mcg/ml
Bifonazole	2.5	33.8	100	100
Clotrimazole	0	12.8	93.6	100
R3783	0	0	0	54.5
Fluconazole	0	0	0	0
Itraconazole	0	100	100	100
Ketoconazole	0	0	0	100
Naftifine	0	0	0	100
Griseofulvin	0	0	25	50
Betamethasone	0	50	100	100
Cortisol	100	100	100	100

Table 2 shows that Bifonazole induced a significant inhibition of omega-oxidation in dose-dependent manner. The lowest concentration with significant activity was 1 µg/ml which inhibited omega-oxidation by 74%, while 0.125 µg/ml had no detectable effect. Only Itraconazole showed comparable inhibition while all other studied azoles were more than 10 times less active than Bifonazole.

TABLE 2: Inhibition of omega-oxidation by various azoles

% inhibition of omega-oxidation				
	0.125 mcg/ml	1 mcg/ml	8 mcg/ml	64 mcg/ml
Bifonazole	0	74	100	100
Clotrimazole	0	0	24	91
R3783	0	22	50	100
Fluconazole	0	0	10	12
Itraconazole	0	50	100	100
Ketoconazole	0	0	40	100

DISCUSSION

Our data clearly demonstrate that Bifonazole shows a strong potency to inhibit leukotriene generation from human PMN beside its excellent antimycotic activity. The interaction with the lipoxygenase-pathway is one explanation for the observed antiphlogistic effect of Bifonazole (Shoji, 1988). Independent from the molecular mechanism, it is obvious how Bifonazole acts during dermatomycosis and other forms of dermatitis:invading granulocytes face at first low concentrations of Bifonazole and release LTB_4 into the surrounding to attract further PMN. Due to the inhibition of omega-oxidation by low Bifonazole concentration there is additional chemotactic LTB_4 available during the first period. Since Bifonazole shows good penetration into the skin the latter invaded PMN are confronted with higher concentrations of the substance and their LTB_4 synthesis becomes inhibited. Bifonazole cures the symptoms of dermatomycosis very fast, because it regulates inflammation and it eliminates the fungi rapidly.

REFERENCES

Bauer, R & Vennemann, 1988. Steroide in der antimykotischen Therapie. Therapeutische Wirksamkeit des Kombinationspräparates Lotricomb im Vergleich zu einem Monopräparat. Z. Alligemeinmedizin, 64, 996.

Faergemann, J. 1989. Treatment of seborrhoic dermatitis with bifonazole. Mycoses, 32, 309

Shoji,A, 1988. Skin irritation with topical antifungal agents and the anti-inflammatory effects of bifonazole. Int.J.Clin.Pract., Suppl.,55

A6

Treatment of Vulvo-Vaginal Candidiasis with Oxiconazole Vaginal Tablet: Multicenter Double-Blind Trial of Oxiconazole in Comparison with Isoconazole

N.Cho, K.Fukunaga[1] M.Takada[2] S.Matsuda[3] S.Mizuno[1] H.Yamaguchi[4]

Dept. of Obstetrics and Gynecology, Fujigaoka Hospital, Showa Univ. Sch. of Med., Kanagawa, [1]Dept. of Obstetrics and Gynecology, International Goodwill Hospital, Kanagawa, [2]Dept. of Obstetrics and Gynecology, Juntendo Univ. Sch. of Med., Tokyo, [3]Dept. of Obstetrics and Gynecology, Koto Hospital, Tokyo, [4]Research Center for Medical Mycology, Teikyo Univ., Tokyo, Japan

I.PURPOSE

The purpose of this study was to investigate the therapeutic efficacy of Oxiconazole and the tolerance to the drug in patients with vulvo-vaginal candidiasis. As control Isoconazole was used.

II.METHODS

A.TEST DRUGS

a.Oxiconazole(Oxi) 600mg vaginal tablets:containing 600mg of oxiconazole nitrate
b.Oxiconazole placebo tablets
c.Isoconazole(Iso) 300mg vaginal tablets:containing 300mg of isoconazole nitrate
d.Isoconazole placebo tablets

The drugs [a(1 tab.)+d(2 tab.) or c(2 tab.)+b(1 tab.)] for each patient were supplied in one package.

B.PATIENTS
Patients with vaginal candidiasis or vulvo-vaginal candidiasis diagnosed by clinical examination, microscopic examination and fungal identification in culture were entered in the study.

C.ADMINISTRATION
Three vaginal tablets were inserted into the posterior part of the fornix vaginae (a single dose).

D.OBSERVED ITEMS AND SCHEDULE

Items	Before	1st follow-up (after 1 week)	2nd follow-up (after 3 weeks)
Application of drug	↑		
Clinical assessment	↑	↑	↑
Mycological examination	↑	↑	↑

III.RESULTS

In 24 hospitals, 285 patients were subjected to the 1-day treatment with Oxi or Iso vaginal tablets.

A.RATING OF CLINICAL SYMPTOMS GLOBAL IMPROVEMENT
Clinical symptoms global improvement rate at 1st follow-up was 95.4% for Oxi and 90.5% for Iso. At 2nd follow-up, this was 92.3% for Oxi and 90.8% for Iso. No significant differences were found between the two groups at both 1st and 2nd follow-ups(Table 1).

Table 1 Rating of clinical symptoms global improvement

( ):cumulative %

Follow-up	Group	Rating of clinical symptoms global improvement				No. of cases	U-test
		Disappeared	Improved	Unchanged	Aggravated		
1st	Oxi	53(48.6)	51(95.4)	5	0	109	N.S.
	Iso	40(38.1)	55(90.5)	9	1	105	
2nd	Oxi	64(61.5)	32(92.3)	8	0	104	N.S.
	Iso	62(63.3)	27(90.8)	8	1	98	

B.MYCOLOGICAL EFFECT
Mycological cure rate at 1st follow-up was 89.7% in the Oxi group and 86.7% in the Iso group. At 2nd follow-up, this was 83.7% for Oxi, and 78.4% for Iso. No significant differences were found between the two groups at both 1st and 2nd follow-ups(Table 2).

From the results of a separate examination on the different pathogens, Oxi was as effective as Iso(Table 3).

Table 2 Mycological effect

( ):cumulative %

Follow -up	Group	Mycological effect*				No. of cases	U-test
		Negative	Remarkable decrease	Slight decrease	Unchanged or increased		
1st	Oxi	85(79.4)	11(89.7)	2	9	107	N.S.
	Iso	86(81.9)	5(86.7)	2	12	105	
2nd	Oxi	79(76.0)	8(83.7)	1	16	104	N.S.
	Iso	72(74.2)	4(78.4)	0	21	97	

*The results were compared with the pretreatment status and classified as follows.

Culture result	Change in the number of colonies
Negative	:innumerable ~ ≧30 → 0
Remarkable decrease	:innumerable ~ ≧30 → 10 ~ 1
Slight decrease	:innumerable ~ ≧30 → 29 ~ 11
Unchanged or increased	:innumerable ~ ≧30 → innumerable ~ ≧30

Table 3 Mycological effect in each fungus at 1st follow-up

( ):cumulative %

Spec -ies	Group	Mycological effect				No. of cases	U-test
		Negative	Remarkable decrease	Slight decrease	Unchanged or increased		
C.A.*	Oxi	76(82.6)	9(92.4)	1	6	92	N.S.
	Iso	78(89.7)	4(94.3)	2	3	87	
C.G.**	Oxi	6(50.0)	2(66.7)	1	3	12	N.S.
	Iso	7(43.8)	0	0	9	16	

*C.A.: C. albicans **C.G.: C. glabrata

C. RATING OF GLOBAL IMPROVEMENT

Global improvement rate at 1st follow-up was 89.7% for Oxi and 83.8% for Iso. At 2nd follow-up, this was 83.7% for Oxi and 77.3% for Iso. No significant differences were found between the two groups at both 1st and 2nd follow-ups(Table 4).

Table 4 Rating of global improvement

( ):cumulative %

Follow -up	Group	Rating of global improvement: Remarkably effective	Effective	Slightly effective	Failure	Aggra-vated	No. of cases	U-test
1st	Oxi	87(81.3)	9(89.7)	1	10	0	107	N.S.
	Iso	84(80.0)	4(83.8)	2	15	0	105	
2nd	Oxi	83(79.8)	4(83.7)	0	17	0	104	N.S.
	Iso	72(74.2)	3(77.3)	0	21	1	97	

D. SAFETY RATING

There were no remarkable findings regarding side effects and laboratory tests in either group.

IV. CONCLUSIONS

We conclude that Oxi is effective in vulvo-vaginal candidiasis; its efficacy is similar to that of Iso. Oxi may be a good alternative drug in vulvo-vaginal candidiasis.

A7

Treatment of Vulvo-Vaginal Candidiasis with Oxiconazole Vaginal Tablet: Multicenter Double-Blind Trial of Oxiconazole Compared to Clotrimazole

N.Cho, K.Fukunaga[1] M.Takada[2] S.Matsuda[3] S.Mizuno[1] H.Yamaguchi[4]

Dept. of Obstetrics and Gynecology, Fujigaoka Hospital, Showa Univ. Sch. of Med., Kanagawa, [1]*Dept. of Obstetrics and Gynecology, International Goodwill Hospital, Kanagawa,* [2]*Dept. of Obstetrics and Gynecology, Juntendo Univ. Sch. of Med., Tokyo,* [3]*Dept of Obstetrics and Gynecology, Koto Hospital, Tokyo,* [4]*Research Center for Medical Mycology, Teikyo Univ., Tokyo, Japan*

I. PURPOSE

The purpose of this study was to investigate the therapeutic efficacy of Oxiconazole and the tolerance to the drug in patients with vulvo-vaginal candidiasis. As control Clotrimazole was used.

II. METHODS

A. TEST DRUGS

a. Oxiconazole(Oxi) 100mg vaginal tablets: containing 100mg of oxiconazole nitrate
b. Oxiconazole placebo tablets
c. Clotrimazole(Clo) 100mg vaginal tablets: containing 100mg of clotrimazole
d. Clotrimazole placebo tablets

The drugs (a+d or c+b) for each patient (6 days dosage) were supplied in one package.

B. PATIENTS
Patients with vaginal candidiasis or vulvo-vaginal candidiasis diagnosed by clinical examination, microscopic examination and fungal identification in culture were entered in the study.

C.ADMINISTRATION
Two vaginal tablets were inserted into the posterior part of the fornix vaginae once per day for 6 consecutive days.

D.OBSERVED ITEMS AND SCHEDULE

Items	Before	1st follow-up (after 1 week)	2nd follow-up (after 3 weeks)
Application of drug	↑ ↑ ↑ ↑ ↑ ↑		
Clinical assessment	↑	↑	↑
Mycological examination	↑	↑	↑

III.RESULTS

In 24 hospitals, 265 patients were subjected to the 6-day treatment with Oxi or Clo vaginal tablets.

A.RATING OF CLINICAL SYMPTOMS GLOBAL IMPROVEMENT
Clinical symptoms global improvement rate was 96.8% for both Oxi and Clo at 1st follow-up and 95.7% at 2nd follow-up(Table 1).

Table 1 Rating of clinical symptoms global improvement
( ):cumulative %

Follow -up	Group	Rating of clinical symptoms global improvement				No. of cases	U-test
		Disappeared	Improved	Unchanged	Aggravated		
1st	Oxi	54(57.4)	37(96.8)	3	0	94	N.S.
	Clo	45(47.9)	46(96.8)	3	0	94	
2nd	Oxi	67(72.8)	21(95.7)	4	0	92	N.S.
	Clo	68(73.9)	20(95.7)	4	0	92	

B.MYCOLOGICAL EFFECT
Mycological cure rate at 1st follow-up was 96.8% for Oxi and 89.4% for Clo. At 2nd follow-up, this was 90.2% for Oxi and 83.7% for Clo. No significant differences were found between the two groups at both 1st and 2nd follow-ups(Table 2).
From the results of a separate examination on the different pathogens, Oxi was more effective than Clo in the mycological cure rating against <u>Candida glabrata</u>(Table 3).

Table 2 Mycological effect

( ):cumulative %

Follow -up	Group	Mycological effect*				No. of cases	U-test
		Negative	Remarkable decrease	Slight decrease	Unchanged or increased		
1st	Oxi	89(94.7)	2(96.8)	1	2	94	N.S.
	Clo	83(88.3)	1(89.4)	2	8	94	
2nd	Oxi	81(88.0)	2(90.2)	0	9	92	N.S.
	Clo	75(81.5)	2(83.7)	1	14	92	

*The results were compared with the pretreatment status and classified as follows.

Culture result	Change in the number of colonies
Negative	:innumerable~≧30⟶ 0
Remarkable decrease	:innumerable~≧30⟶ 10 ~ 1
Slight decrease	:innumerable~≧30⟶ 29 ~ 11
Unchanged or increased	:innumerable~≧30⟶ innumerable~≧30

Table 3 Mycological effect in each fungus at 1st follow-up

( ):cumulative %

Spec -ies	Group	Mycological effect				No. of cases	U-test
		Negative	Remarkable decrease	Slight decrease	Unchanged or increased		
C.A.*	Oxi	74(97.4)	1(98.7)	0	1	76	N.S.
	Clo	75(97.4)	1(98.7)	0	1	77	
C.G.**	Oxi	12(85.7)	0	1	1	14	$p<0.05$
	Clo	5(38.5)	0	2	6	13	

*C.A.:C. albicans **C.G.:C. glabrata

C.RATING OF GLOBAL IMPROVEMENT

Global improvement rate at 1st follow-up was 95.7% for Oxi and 89.4% for Clo. At 2nd follow-up, this was 90.2% for Oxi and 83.7% for Clo. No significant differences were found between the two groups at both 1st and 2nd follow-ups(Table 4).

Table 4 Rating of global improvement

( ):cumulative %

Follow -up	Group	Rating of global improvement					No. of cases	U-test
		Remarkably effective	Effective	Slightly effective	Failure	Aggra-vated		
1st	Oxi	89(94.7)	1(95.7)	1	3	0	94	N.S.
	Clo	83(88.3)	1(89.4)	2	8	0	94	
2nd	Oxi	82(89.1)	1(90.2)	0	9	0	92	N.S.
	Clo	75(81.5)	2(83.7)	0	15	0	92	

D.SAFETY RATING

There were no remarkable findings regarding side effects and laboratory tests in either group.

IV. CONCLUSIONS

We conclude that Oxi is effective in vulvo-vaginal candidiasis; its efficacy is similar to that of Clo. Oxi may be a good alternative drug in vulvo-vaginal candidiasis.

A8

NND-318, a New Antifungal Imidazole: Its *in Vitro* and *in Vivo* Activity Against Pathogenic Fungi of Dermatomycosis

Tetsuto Ohmi, Shigeo Konaka, Matazaemon Uchida and Hideyo Yamaguchi*

Institute of Life Science Research, Nihon Nohyaku Co., Ltd., Osaka and **Research Center for Medical Mycology, Teikyo University, Tokyo, Japan*

I . INTRODUCTION

NND-318 is a new antifungal agent with an unique structure, 1,3-dithiolanylidenemethylimidazole (Fig. 1), and the clinical phase II trials on superficial mycoses have been initiated in Japan (under the name of TJN-318). This paper presents a brief summary of preclinical studies on this material conducted so far.

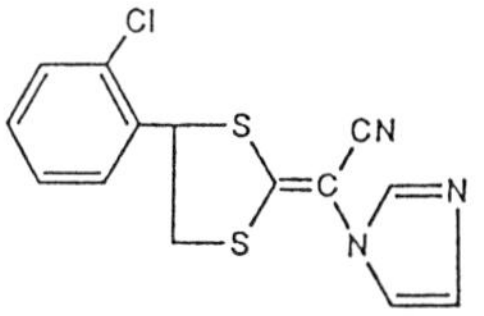

Fig. 1. Chemical structure of NND-318 〔 (±)-(*E*)-[4-(2-chlorophenyl)-1,3-dithiolan-2-ylidene]-1-imidazolylacetonitrile 〕

Table 1. Minimum inhibitory concentration (MIC) against *Trichophyton* spp.

Strain	MIC (μg/ml)				Strain	MIC (μg/ml)			
	NND-318	CTZ[a]	BFZ[b]	TOL[c]		NND-318	CTZ	BFZ	TOL
T. mentagrophytes					*T. rubrum*				
IFO 5466	0.004	0.25	2.0	0.125	IFO 5467	0.016	0.5	2.0	0.031
IFO 5809	0.031	1.0	2.0	0.5	IFO 5807	0.016	0.5	2.0	0.031
IFO 5810	0.008	0.5	2.0	0.031	IFO 5808	0.008	0.5	2.0	0.063
IFO 5811	0.016	0.25	2.0	0.125	IFO 6203	0.016	0.5	2.0	0.016
IFO 5812	0.016	0.25	4.0	0.125	IFO 6204	0.008	0.5	2.0	0.031
IFO 5929	0.031	0.25	0.25	0.125	IFO 9185	0.008	0.25	1.0	0.125
IFO 6124	0.016	1.0	2.0	0.031					

a: Clotrimazole b: Bifonazole c: Tolnaftate

II. *IN VITRO* ANTIFUNGAL ACTIVITY OF NND-318

The *in vitro* antifungal activity was evaluated using conventional broth dilution and agar dilution techniques. MICs of NND-318 and reference drugs against *Trichophyton* spp. are summarized in Table 1. The *in vitro* activities of NND-318 against *Trichophyton* spp. (MIC: 0.004-0.031 μg/ml) were 1-500 times higher than those of clotrimazole (MIC: 0.25-1.0 μg/ml), bifonazole (MIC: 0.25-4.0 μg/ml) and tolnaftate (MIC: 0.016-0.5 μg/ml).

III. THERAPEUTIC EFFICACY OF NND-318 AND TJN-318 IN *IN VIVO* TINEA MODELS

A. TINEA PEDIS MODEL

Tinea pedis was produced on the sole of male Hartley guinea pigs by inoculating *Trichophyton mentagrophytes* IFO 5466 [1]. Therapeutic efficacy of NND-318 and TJN-318 in this model is shown in Tables 2 and 3, respectively.

B. TINEA CORPORIS MODEL

Tinea corporis was produced on the back of male Hartley guinea pigs by inoculating *T. mentagrophytes* IFO 5466 [2,3]. Therapeutic efficacy of NND-318 in this model is shown in Table 4.

Topical application of NND-318 or TJN-318 to these two *in vivo* models offered higher therapeutic efficacy than that of clotrimazole, bifonazole and/or tolnaftate.

Table 2. Therapeutic efficacy of NND-318, bifonazole and tolnaftate in the tinea pedis model

Treatment [a]		Fungus-positive loci (%) from infected loci
None		100
Placebo (solvent)[b]		100
NND-318	0.25% solution	60
	0.5% solution	20
	1.0% solution	0
BFZ	0.5% solution	100
	1.0% solution	100
TOL	0.5% solution	100
	1.0% solution	100

a: From day-10 after the inoculation, testing compounds (0.1 ml/locus) were topically applied once a day for 10 consecutive days. Five days after the last application, skin blocks from the sole were cultured to detect fungi. b: PEG-300 was used as a solvent for every solution.

Table 3. Therapeutic efficacy of TJN-318, and bifonazole in the tinea pedis model

Treatment [a]		Fungus-positive loci (%) from infected loci
None		100
TJN-318	1.0% cream [b]	10
BFZ	1.0% cream [c]	100

a: From day-10 after the inoculation, testing agents (0.1 g/locus) were topically applied once a day for 5 consecutive days. Five days after the last application, skin blocks from the sole were cultured to detect fungi.
b: TJN-318 is a cream preparation used for clinical trials and contains 1.0% NND-318.
c: Mycospor®

Table 4. Therapeutic efficacy of NND-318, clotrimazole, bifonazole and tolnaftate in the tinea corporis model

Treatment [a]		Fungus-positive loci (%) from infected loci	Treatment		Fungus-positive loci (%) from infected loci
None		100	None		100
Placebo (solvent)[b]		100	Placebo (solvent)		100
NND-318	0.3% solution	88	NND-318	0.3% solution	70
	1.0% solution	13		1.0% solution	0
CTZ	0.3% solution	100	CTZ	0.3% solution	100
	1.0% solution	75		1.0% solution	60
TOl	0.3% solution	75	BFZ	0.3% solution	100
	1.0% solution	50		1.0% solution	90

a: From day-3 after the inoculation, testing compounds (0.2 ml/locus) were topically applied once a day for 11 consecutive days. Five days after the last application, skin blocks from the back were cultured to detect fungi. b: PEG-300 was used as a solvent for every solution.

These preclinical studies demonstrate that NND-318 is promising for a topical antifungal agent potentially useful for most kinds and types of superficial mycoses.

REFERENCES

1. Fujita, S. and T. Matsuyama, Experimental tinea pedis induced by non-abrasive inoculation of *Trichophyton mentagrophytes* arthrosporea on the plantar part of a guinea pig foot, J. Med. Vet. Mycol., 25: 203-213 (1987).

2. Sakai, S., T. Kada, G. Saito, N. Muraoka and Y. Takahashi, Studies on chemotherapy of *Trichophyton* infections. 1. Antifungal properties of halogen phenol esters, J. Sci. Res. Inst., 46: 113-117 (1952).
3. Noguchi, T., A. Kaji, Y. Igarashi, A. Shigematsu and K. Taniguchi, Antitrichophyton activity of naphthiomates. Antimicrob. Agents Chemother., 1962: 259-267 (1963).

A9

Clinical Studies of 5-Fluorocytosine for Fungal Urinary Infection

T. Matsumoto, N. Ogata and J. Kumazawa

Department of Urology, Faculty of Medicine
Kyushu University
3-1-1, Maidashi, Higashi-ku, Fukuoka, 812, Japan

I. INTRODUCTION

Fungal urinary infection is common in patients with catheter, urinary tract cancer, obstructive uropathy, etc.[1] Clinical usefulness of 5-fluorocytosine (5-FC) was examined for such patients and susceptibility of 5-FC, amphotericin-B (AMPH) or miconazole (MCZ) for urinary fungal isolates was studied. Furthermore, serum and urinary ß-glucan and D-arabinitol were measured to estimate the significance of such indicators in fungal urinary infections.

II. PATIENTS AND METHODS

A. Patient specifications: 16-years or older patients of both sexes suffering from significant fungiuria ($\geqq 10^4$ cfu/ml) including mixed infection with bacteria were subjects of this study.

B. Treatment: Patients were divided randomly into four treatment groups as described below. Each treatment was continued for at least 2 weeks.

1) Mixed infection with bacteria

Group A: 5-FC was administered at a dose of 3 to 4.5g per day and Ofloxacin (OFLX) or Ciprofloxacin (CPFX) was also administered at a dose of 400 or 600mg per day.

Group B: OFLX or CPFX was administered at a dose of 400 or 600mg per day.

2) Single infection of fungus

Group C: 5-FC was administered at a dose of 3 to 4.5g per day.

Group D: No treatment.

C. Isolation of fungus and/or bacteria was performed by dip slide (BCB slide ®) before treatment and 1 or 2 weeks after initiation of treatment. Concentration of ß-D-glucan was measured in serum and urine by Toxicolor and Endospecy methods. Serum concentration of D-arabinitol was also measured.

III. RESULTS

A. Clinical and mycological response to 5-FC: The elimination rate of fungus of groups A, B, C and D was 66.7, 55.6, 71.4 and 60.0%, respectively. Mycological response in the 5-FC treatment group (Group A+C) was thus 70.7% in elimination rate and spontaneous elimination occurred in 57.1% of the group not treated for fungus (Group B+D) (Table 1).

B. Minimum inhibition concentration (MIC) distribution of fungus against 5-FC, AMPH and MCZ: MIC distribution of *C. albicans*, *C. glabrata* and other Candida species were more susceptible to 5-FC than against AMPH and MCZ.

C. ß-D-glucan and D-arabinitol concentration: Serum and urine concentrations of Toxicolor and Endospecy were measured and ß-D-glucan concentration was estimated by the value of the former minus the latter. Serum concentration of ß-D-glucan was not correlated with

Table 1. Mycological response in treatment and non-treatment groups

Group	Mycological response *				Elimination rate (%)
	E	D	U	O	
A + C	7	2	1	2	70.0
B + D	8	1	5	2	57.1

* E: Eliminated D: Decreased U: Unchanged O: Others

urinary fungal count. Urine concentration of ß-D-glucan was, however, correlated with urinary fungal count in single fungal infection. Serum D-arabinitol concentration was not related with urinary fungal count.

IV. CONCLUSION

These results suggest that 5-FC is useful in *Candida* urinary infection and that ß-D-glucan concentration is one of the useful indicators of fungiuria.

V. REFERENCE

1) Koginm, P. J. et al. Advances in the diagnosis of renal candidiasis. J. Urol. 119: 184 (1978).

A10

Differential Therapeutic Efficacy of Fluconazole in the Murine Model of Systemic Cryptococcosis Produced with Two Different Types of *Cryptococcus neoformans*: Histopathological and Biochemical Analyses

K. Shibuya, M. Wakayama, S. Naoe, K. Uchida* and H. Yamaguchi*

Department of Pathology, Ohashi Hospital *(2-17-6, Ohashi, Meguro)*
Toho University School of Medicine
Tokyo, Japan 153

*Research Center for Medical Mycology *(359, Otsuka, Hachioji)*
Teikyo University
Tokyo, Japan 192-03

Fluconazole(FCZ) demonstrated different efficacies in two strains of *Cryptococcus neoformans* , and was virulent to mice infected with F37 but less efficacious to mice infected with F13. Histopathological study on whole organs and biochemical examination of peripheral blood were carried out to determine the difference in therapeutic effect by strain.

1. MATERIALS AND METHODS

Animals: ICR SPF mice, 4-weeks-old, male

Strains: *Cryptococcus neoformans* F13 & F37

Method: To produce a saline suspension of the above two strains, $1X10^6$ cell/mouse was inoculated into a vein. On the ninth day after inoculation, mice were sacrificed immediately after obtaining blood from the heart, and paraffin sections were prepared in the routine manner for histological study.

2. RESULTS

1) *BIOCHEMICAL EXAMINATION OF PERIPHERAL BLOOD*

The examination revealed increase of gross protein, alpha-1 globulin, GOT and LDH, and decrease of albumin.

2) *HISTOPATHOLOGICAL STUDIES*

Group inoculated with Cr. neoformans F13(Group F13): Focal proliferation of yeast was recognized in all of lung, liver, kidney, spleen and brain. However, the response of inflammatory cells was weak and found only in liver and spleen. In other organs, a cystic lesion had developed by the proliferation of yeast, and in brain the volume increased especially prominently.

Group inoculated with Cr. neoformans F37(Group F37): In liver and spleen, numerous aggregations of histiocytes were observed surrounding the yeast. The infiltration of chronic inflammatory cells such as lymphocytes in this area brought about a corresponding change in granuloma. In liver and kidney, the response of histiocytes was minimal, and in brain, although cystic lesions similar to that of the Group F13 developed, they were fewer in number and smaller.

3. DISCUSSION

Biochemical examination suggests the existence of a systemic inflammatory disease, especially a chronic infectious disease. In Group F37, as the decrease of albumin and alpha-1 globulin was prominent, and with the slight increase of gamma globulin, a more severe chronic infectious disease or liver cell damage is suspected. The higher increase of GOT and LDH in Group F37, and the fact that no increase of enzyme originating from the bile tract was seen in either group, indicates that chronic inflammatory disease existed and that liver cell damage was more severe in this group.

Histologically, in Group F37, numerous granulomas were developed in the reticuloendothelial system such as liver and spleen. The above results of biochemical examination seemed to derive not from the organic involvement by yeast, but from the necrosis of liver cells by the inflammatory cell response induced by the invading yeast. In kidney, the main change was proliferation of yeast in the interstitium, and little functional disorder was seen. Therefore, the possibility that this directly affects the death of animals is very slight.

In summary, the fundamental difference between Groups F13 and F37 is whether or not granulomatous inflammation exists in the living body. With *Cr. neoformans* F13, which does not cause granulomatous inflammation, it is considered difficult to restrain the proliferation by a usual dose of antibiotic injection. Infected animals are fatally affected by a great proliferation of yeast in the central nervous system. On the other hand, *Cr. neoformans*F37 stimulates the defense mechnisms of the body, i.e. morphologically recognized granulomas. Therefore, infected animals were probably able to exist owing to the combined effects of suppressing yeast proliferation through the injection of antibiotics to infected animals and the natural defense mechanisms of the body.

A11

SM-9164, an Active Enantiomer of SM-8668 (Sch39304): Oral and Parenteral Activity in Systemic Fungal Infection Models

T. Tanio, N. Ohashi, I. Saji and M. Fukasawa

Research Laboratories, Sumitomo Pharmaceuticals Co., Ltd., Osaka, Japan

I. INTRODUCTION

SM-8668 has excellent activities by oral administration in various deep and superficial infection models (1-8). We confirmed that the antifungal activity of SM-8668 depended mostly on its RR-enantiomer (SM-9164) and found that SM-9164 was superior to SM-8668 in water-solubility and chemotherapeutic index. In this study, we have evaluated the efficacy of SM-9164 against murine systemic candidiasis, cryptococcosis and aspergillosis by oral and intravenous treatment.

II. EXPERIMENTAL METHODS

Male albino ddY mice, five weeks old, were inoculated via the tail vein with the following numbers per mouse of saline-washed organisms: 2.0 x 10^6 for *Candida albicans* KB-8, 2.0 x 10^7 for *Cryptococcus neoformans* TIMM0418, and 2.0 x 10^7 for *Aspergillus fumigatus* MTU6001. Appropriate doses of each drug were orally or intravenously administered to groups of 10 mice at 0, 24 and 48 h after infection. For the therapeutic regimen, drug treatment was started on day 1 after infection and continued once daily for 3 days. The survival rates of mice were recorded for 10 days (candidiasis and aspergillosis) or 20 days (cryptococcosis). The 50% effective dose (ED_{50}) values were calculated from the survival rates of each group on the final day using probit analysis.

III. RESULTS

The prophylactic and therapeutic efficacies of SM-9164 and other drugs are shown in Table 1. In this study, all mice of the solvent-treated control group died within 9 days after infection with candidiasis, within 15 days after infection with cryptococcosis or within 4 days after infection with aspergillosis. SM-9164 showed excellent efficacy in each infection model by both oral and intravenous treatment, while the efficacy of fluconazole was high against candidiasis, low against cryptococcosis and poor against aspergillosis. In aspergillosis, SM-9164 was less efficient than amphotericin B when treatment was begun on day 0. However, when treatment was started on day 1, amphotericin B was inactive even at the maximum non-lethal dose of 2.5 mg/kg, although SM-9164 still showed efficacy.

IV. DISCUSSION

Fluconazole became available in several countries including Japan recently and was rapidly adapted for clinical use. In this study, we showed the superiority of SM-9164 to fluconazole against systemic fungal infection models. SM-9164 showed good oral absorption (the bioavailability was approximately 100%, similar to that of fluconazole), and the elimination half-life in serum was longer than that of fluconazole. SM-9164 was therefore more efficient than fluconazole not only against aspergillosis (MICs were

Table 1. Efficacy of SM-9164 against murine systemic fungal infection

Inoculated organism	Drug	Route	ED_{50} (µg/ml)	95% confidence limit
I. Prophylactic regimen (treatment was started on day 0)				
C. albicans	SM-9164	p.o.	0.27	0.12 - 0.63
KB-8	SM-8668		0.38	0.15 - 1.0
	Fluconazole		1.4	0.23 - 9.0
	SM-9164	i.v.	0.10	0.031 - 0.35
	Fluconazole		1.3	0.37 - 4.3
	Miconazole		>25	
	Amphotericin B		0.10	0.045 - 0.22
C. neoformans	SM-9164	p.o.	0.71	0.32 - 1.6
TIMM0418	SM-8668		1.9	1.0 - 3.5
	Fluconazole		29	10 - 85
	SM-9164	i.v.	1.1	0.67 - 1.7
	Fluconazole		>25	
	Miconazole		>25	
	Amphotericin B		0.62	
A. fumigatus	SM-9164	p.o.	4.1	1.4 - 12
MTU6001	SM-8668		18	12 - 25
	Fluconazole		>125	
	SM-9164	i.v.	8.2	3.9 - 17
	Fluconazole		>25	
	Miconazole		>25	
	Amphotericin B		0.27	0.10 - 0.71
II. Therapeutic regimen (treatment was started on day 1)				
A. fumigatus	SM-9164	p.o.	5.5	1.6 - 19
MTU6001	SM-9164	i.v.	8.5	3.8 - 19
	SM-8668	p.o.	12	5.6 - 25
	Fluconazole	p.o.	>125	
	Miconazole	i.v.	>25	
	Amphotericin B	i.v.	>2.5	

6.25 and 200 μg/ml, respectively) but also against candidiasis and cryptococcosis (in vitro activities were similar). The superiority of SM-9164 to amphotericin B against aspergillosis in the therapeutic regimen was probably due to its good penetration of into the cerebrospinal fluid, since colonies of *A. fumigatus* were detected in mouse brain on day 1 after infection.

These results confirm that SM-9164 is useful in deep fungal infection.

V. REFERENCES

1. K. A. Mcintyre, and J. N. Galgiani, *In vitro* susceptibilities of yeasts to a new antifungal triazole, Sch 39304: Effects of test conditions and relation to *in vivo* efficacy, Antimicrob. Agents Chemother., 33: 1095. (1989).

2. B. I. Restrepo, J. Ahrens, and J. R. Graybill, Efficacy of Sch 39304 in murine cryptococcosis, Antimicrob. Agents Chemother., 33: 1242. (1989).

3. J. R. Perfect, K. A. Wright, M. M. Hobbs, and D. T. Durack, Treatment of experimental cryptococcal meningitis and disseminated candidiasis with Sch 39304, Antimicrob. Agents Chemother., 33: 1735. (1989).

4. G. S. Kobayashi, S. J. Travis, M. G. Rinaldi, and G. Medoff, *In vitro* and *in vivo* activities of Sch 39304, fluconazole, and amphotericin B against *Histoplasma capsulatum*, Antimicrob. Agents Chemother., 34: 524. (1990).

5. J. Defaveri, S. H. Sun, and J. R. Graybill, Treatment of murine coccidioidal meningitis with Sch 39304, Antimicrob. Agents Chemother., 34: 663. (1990).

6. A. M. Sugar, M. Picard, and L. Noble, Treatment of murine pulmonary blastomycosis with Sch 39304, a new triazole antifungal agent, Antimicrob. Agents Chemother., 34: 896. (1990).

7. K. V. Clemons, L. H. Hanson, A. M. Perlman, and D. A. Stevens, Efficacy of Sch 39304 and fluconazole in a murine model of disseminated coccidioidomycosis, Antimicrob. Agents Chemother., 34: 928. (1990).

8. T. Tanio, K. Ichise, T. Nakajima, and T. Okuda, *In vivo* Efficacy of SM-8668 (Sch 39304), a new triazole antifungal agent, Antimicrob. Agents Chemother., 34: 980. (1990).

A12

Chronotoxicity of Amphotericin B in Mice

Y. YOSHIYAMA, S. NAKANO*, T. KOBAYASHI and F. TOMONAGA

School of Pharmaceutical Sciences, Kitasato University, Tokyo, Japan

*Department of Clinical Pharmacology and Therapeutics, Medical College of Oita, Oita, Japan

Amphotericin B (AMPH) is still the most useful agent for treating various deep-seated fungal infections. It is difficult for general physicians to use AMPH in certain clinical situations, because the drug has serious side effects. Recent research indicates that biosusceptibility to a variety of drugs follows circadian rhythms (1). Circadian rhythmicity has been reported in the toxic effects of many drugs (2-5). If the circadian biosusceptibility rhythm exists in AMPH toxicity, the time of AMPH administration should be strictly regulated. We studied the circadian variation of mortality rate induced by AMPH in mice.

Materials and Methods

One hundred and twenty male ICR mice weighing between 26 and 38 g were used. The animals were housed from 4 weeks old at ten per cage in a standardized light-dark (LD) cycle of lights on from 7:00 to 19:00 (LD 12:12) at a temperature of 24+1 C and humidity of 60+10 % with food and water ad libitum for three weeks. Groups of ten animals each were injected at one of six times :9:00, 13:00, 17:00, 21:00, 1:00 and 5:00. Each animal was injected 1.25 mg/kg, 2.5 mg/kg and 5.0 mg/kg AMPH intravenously. After injection, animals were returned to their home cages (10 mice per cage) and observed at 4 hour intervals for 24 hours after injection. Dead animals were removed at each observation.

Results and Discussion

There was a significant variation in mortality depending on the time of injection. The highest mortality was found in animals injected with the drug at 17:00, toward the latter half of the light-on phase. The lowest mortality was found in animals injected with the drug at 1:00, toward the middle of the light-off phase (Fig. 1.).

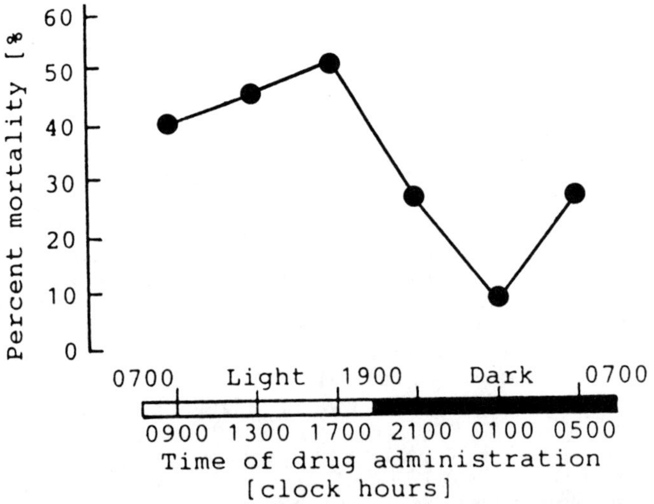

Fig.1. Circadian rhythm of mortality after an i.v. injection of amphotericin B (2.5 mg/kg). Each point represents the data from 10 mice.

In the present study, the AMPH-induced death occurred within 10 to 30 minutes after the end of the infusion and was preceded by tremors and convulsions. Thus, the AMPH-induced death was clearly attributable to respiratory insufficiency resulting from neuromuscular blockade. LD_{50} values for cholinergic drugs, such as acetylcholine Cl, carbachol Cl, pilocarpine HCl and oxotremorine, have been reported to be minimum in mice injected during the light-off phase (6). On the other hand, LD_{50} values for anticholinergic drugs, such as atropine SO_4, scopolamine HCl and atropine HCl, have been reported to be minimum in mice injected during the light-on phase (6). The finding in the present study nicely corresponds to this cholinergic drug data.

The choice of the most appropriate time of day for drug administration may help to achieve rational chronotherapeutics of some drugs including AMPH under certain experimental and clinical situations.

Conclusion

Time-of-day of drug administration is an important determinant in toxicological studies with AMPH.

References

1. Y. Yoshiyama, S. Nakano and N. Ogawa, Chronopharmacokinetic study of valproic acid in man: Comparison of oral and rectal administration, J. Clin. Pharmacol. 29: 1048. (1989)
2. S. Nakano, K. Nagai and N. Ogawa, Role of feeding schedule and pharmacokinetics in chronopharmacology of drugs acting on the central nervous system, Annu. Rev. Chronopharmacol. 1:263. (1984)
3. S. Nakano, S. Ohdo and N. Ogawa, Manipulation of feeding schedule can modify the circadian rhythms of toxicity and kinetics of theophylline in mice, Annu. Rev. Chronopharmacol. 5: 317. (1988)
4. S. Nakano and N. Ogawa, Chronotoxicity of gentamicin in mice, IRCS Med. Sci. 10: 592. (1982)
5. S. Nakano, C. Hara and N. Ogawa, Circadian rhythm of apomorphine-induced stereotypy in rats, Pharmacol. Biochem. Behav. 12: 459. (1980)
6. A. H. Friedman, Chronobiology, Igaku Shoin Ltd., Tokyo, p.163. (1974)

A13

Enactins, a Family of Hydroxamic Acid Antimycotic Antibiotics: Isolation, Characterization, and Structure Elucidation

Katsumi Yamamoto, Yoshikazu Shiinoki, Hiromasa Okada, Yoshio Inouye, Shoshiro Nakamura

Institute of Pharmaceutical Sciences
Hiroshima University School of Medicine
Hiroshima 734, Japan

Enactins (ENs) and neo-enactins (NEs) are antimycotic antibiotics showing similar antimicrobial spectra and potentiating polyene antifungal antibiotics [1, 2]. Both ENs and NEs are composed of several congeners, though EN congeners are far more hydrophilic and far less active against fungi and yeasts than NE congeners. All EN and NE congeners contain L-serine to form the hydroxamic acid structure. The structures of NE congeners were previously reported [3, 4, 5, 6]. A crude EN mixture was recovered from the cultured broth of *Streptomyces roseoviridis* by adsorption on Diaion HP-20 and following elution with aqueous acetone. EN congeners were further isolated by repeated reverse-phase HPLC and named EN-Ia, -Ib, -IIa, -IIb, -IIc, -III, -IVa, -IVb, -Va, -Vb, -VIa and -VIb in an elution order. Among them, EN-IVa, -IVb, -Vb, -VIa and -VIb were proved to be identical with NE-M_1, -A, -M_2, -B_1 and -B_2, respectively [7]. In contrast, the others were found to be new and the structures of

Table 1. ^{1}H NMR Data (400MHz, $CDCl_3$) of DNP Derivatives of Novel Enactin Congeners

Assignment (Position)	Chemical shift(δ, ppm)		
	DNP-EN-Ia (27℃)	DNP-EN-Ib_1 (27℃)	DNP-EN-Va (50℃)
$CHCH_3$ (20,21)		0.88 (3H,d,J=6.9,H-21), 1.13 (3H,d,J=6.5,H-20)	
$C(CH_3)_2$ (20,21)	1.12 (6H,s)		
$CH(CH_3)_2$ (19,20)			0.89 (6H,d,J=6.8)
CH_2 and CH (10,11,12,13,15,16,17,18)	1.26 (8H;m;H-10,11,17,18)	1.26 (7H;m;H-10,11,17,18)	1.20∿1.43 (15H,m)
CH_2CH_2CO (9,12,16)	1.54 (6H,m)	1.56 (6H,m)	1.55 (2H,m,H-9)
CH_2CO (8,13,15)	2.42 (6H,m,)	2.41 (6H,m)	2.43 (2H,t,J=7.4,H-8)
NCH_2CH_2CO (6)	2.84 (2H,t,J=5.2)	2.84 (2H,t,J=5.0)	2.84 (2H,t,J=5.9)
CHOH (14,19)		3.75 (1H;dq;J=4.2,6.5;H-19)	3.59 (1H,br,H-14)
NCH_2CH_2CO (5)	4.01 (1H;dt;J=5.2,14.5), 4.28 (1H;dt;J=5.2,14.5)	4.02 (1H;dt;J=5.0,14.5), 4.27 (1H;dt;J=5.0,14.5)	4.04 (1H;dt;J=5.9,14.5), 4.26 (1H;dt;J=5.9,14.5)
$HOCH_2$ (1)	4.09 (1H;ddd;J=4.5,4.5,11.0), 4.17 (1H;ddd;J=4.5,4.5,11.0)	4.10 (1H;ddd;J=5.2,5.2,11.5), 4.17 (1H;ddd;J=5.2,5.2,11.5)	4.09 (1H;ddd;J=5.2,5.2,11.5), 4.13 (1H;ddd;J=5.2,5.2,11.5)
NHCHCO (2)	4.86 (1H,br m)	4.85 (1H,br m)	4.87 (1H,br m)
H-Ar (6')	6.88 (1H,d,J=9.0)	6.88 (1H,d,J=9.2)	6.90 (1H,d,J=9.1)
H-Ar (6")	7.60 (1H,d,J=9.0)	7.60 (1H,d,J=9.2)	7.58 (1H,d,J=9.1)
H-Ar (5')	8.27 (1H;dd;J=2.7,9.0)	8.27 (1H;dd;J=2.6,9.2)	8.26 (1H;dd;J=2.8,9.1)
H-Ar (5")	8.52 (1H;dd;J=2.7,9.0)	8.52 (1H;dd;J=2.7,9.2)	8.50 (1H;dd;J=2.8,9.1)
H-Ar (3')	9.12 (1H,d,J=2.7)	9.12 (1H,d,J=2.6)	9.09 (1H,d,J=2.8)
H-Ar (3")	8.93 (1H,d,J=2.7)	8.94 (1H,d,J=2.7)	8.92 (1H,d,J=2.8)
CHNHAr	9.17^{b} (1H,d,J=8.0)	9.17^{b} (1H,d,J=8.0)	9.08^{b} (1H,d,J=8.0)

Tetramethylsilane (0 ppm) was used as an internal standard. Number of protons, multiplicity, coupling constants in Hz and position of protons where necessary are indicated in parenthesis. b) Temperature dependent.

Table 2. ^{13}C NMR Data[a] ($CDCl_3$) of DNP Derivatives of Novel Enactin Congeners

Position	Chemical shift (δ, ppm)						
	DNP-EN-Ia		DNP-EN-Ib_1	DNP-EN-Ib_2		DNP-EN-Va	
	Exptl	Calcd	Exptl	Exptl	Calcd	Exptl	Calcd
C-1	62.11		62.10	62.11		62.31	
C-2	56.26		56.25	56.25		56.28	
C-3	172.50		172.50	172.50		172.50	
C-5	43.50		43.50	43.50		43.76	
C-6	38.82		38.82	38.83		38.80	
C-7	208.33		208.32	208.35		208.15	
C-8	42.86[b]		42.84[b]	42.84[b]		43.01	
C-9	23.39[c]		23.36[c]	23.37[c]		23.47	
C-10	28.69[d]		28.67[d]	28.67[d]		28.97[b]	
C-11	28.67[d]		28.66[d]	28.65[d]		29.25[b]	
C-12	23.21[c]		23.19[c]	23.20[c]		25.34	
C-13	42.57[b]		42.60[b]	42.60[b]		37.93[c]	
C-14	211.73		211.84	211.93		72.09	
C-15	42.76		42.99	42.92		37.35[c]	
C-16	24.30		21.52	21.01		23.47	23.3
C-17	23.94	22.0	32.18	32.00	31.1	39.10	39.4
C-18	43.57	46.7	39.54	40.03	42.3	27.98	27.8
C-19	70.98	68.3	70.88	71.63	70.3	22.59	21.6
C-20	29.29	30.6	20.10	19.86	19.3	22.59	21.6
C-21	29.29	30.6	14.06	14.87	14.1		
C-1'	146.67[e]		146.66[e]	146.67[e]		146.66[d]	
C-2'	131.62[e]		131.61[e]	131.62[e]		131.84[d]	
C-3'	124.25		124.25	124.25		124.16	
C-4'	137.19[e]		137.17[e]	137.18[e]		137.44[d]	
C-5'	130.50		130.49	130.50		130.46	
C-6'	113.99		114.27	114.00		113.96	
C-1"	154.87		154.87	154.88		154.84	
C-2"	137.34[e]		137.17[e]	137.34[e]		137.44[d]	
C-3"	122.84		122.83	122.84		122.74	
C-4"	143.06[e]		143.05[e]	143.06[e]		143.22[d]	
C-5"	129.90		129.90	129.90		129.77	
C-6"	115.43		115.42	115.43		115.41	

a) ^{13}C NMR spectra were recorded on a Jeol GX 400. Tetramethylsilane (0 ppm) was used as an internal standard. b∿e) Values with identical superscript within a column may be interchanged.

Fig. 1. Structures of EN and NE Congeners and Their DNP Derivatives

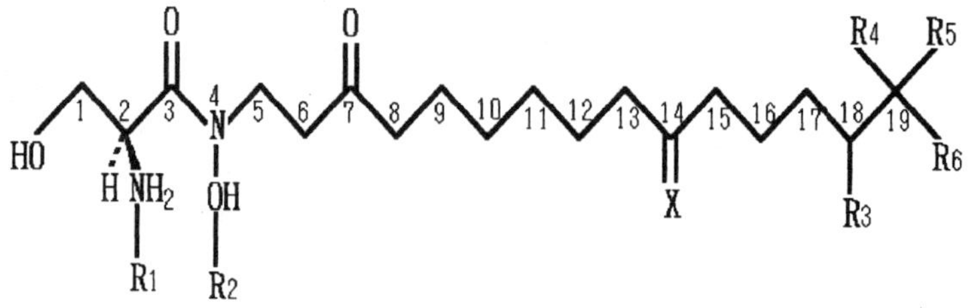

Compound	R_1	R_2	X	R_3	R_4	R_5	R_6
EN-Ia	H	H	=O	H	OH	CH_3	CH_3
EN-Ib$_1$	H	H	=O	CH_3	H	OH	CH_3
EN-Ib$_2$	H	H	=O	CH_3	OH	H	CH_3
EN-IVa (=NE-M$_1$)	H	H	=O	CH_3	H	H	H
EN-IVb (=NE-A)	H	H	=O	H	H	H	CH_3
EN-Va	H	H	$<^{OH}_{H}$	CH_3	H	H	H
EN-Vb (=NE-M$_2$)	H	H	$<^{OH}_{H}$	H	H	H	CH_3
EN-VIa (=NE-B$_1$)	H	H	=O	CH_3	H	H	CH_3
EN-VIb (=NE-B$_2$)	H	H	=O	H	H	CH_3	CH_3
NE-NL$_1$	H	H	=O	H	H	H	H
NE-NL$_2$	H	H	=O	H	H	H	C_2H_5

DNP derivatives, R_1: R_2:

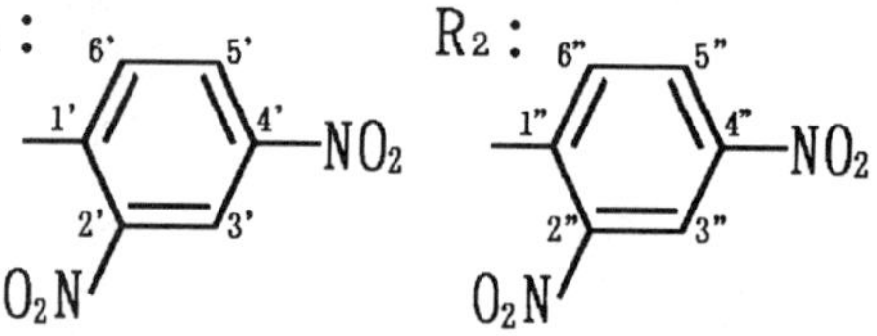

EN-Ia, -Ib and -Va were elucidated by studying ^{1}H and ^{13}C NMR spectra and MS of their DNP derivatives.

In the ^{1}H NMR spectrum of DNP-Ib, however, the unexplainable proton signals were observed at δ 3.63 (*ca.* 0.5H, dq) and δ 3.75 (*ca.* 0.5H, dq); these two protons were not coupled with each other Based on these observations, EN-Ib was considered to consist of an almost equal amount of two closely related isomers which were separated by normal-phase HPLC and named EN-Ib_1 and -Ib_2.

As in the case of NE congeners, the unstable free bases of EN congeners were converted to the corresponding stable bis-DNP derivatives. Structural elucidation of EN-Ia, -Ib_1, -Ib_2 and -Va was aided by comparing their NMR data (Tables 1, 2) with those for NE-B_2, -B_1 and -M_1 (data not shown). The structures of EN-Ia and -Ib_1 were disclosed to be 19-hydroxy-NE-B_2 and -B_1, respectively, whereas the 14-carbonyl group in NE-M_1 was reduced to the hydroxyl group in EN-Va (Fig. 1). The ^{1}H NMR data of DNP-EN-Ib_1 and -Ib_2 were essentially the same except the double quartet (1H; J=6.2,6.2) at δ 3.75 in the former shifted to δ 3.63 (1H; J=4.2, 6.5) in the latter. Therefore, EN-Ib_2 is postulated to be the epimer of EN-Ib_1 at 19 position, though the steric configuration still remains to be solved.

REFERENCES

1. T. Otani, S. Arai, K. Sakano, Y. Kawakami, K. Ishimaru, H. Kondo, and S. Nakamura, H 646-SY3 substance, a potentiator for polyene antifungal antibiotics, J. Antibiotics, 30: 182. (1977).
2. H. Kondo, H. Sumomogi, T. Otani, and S. Nakamura, Neo-enactin, a new antifungal antibiotic potentiating polyene antifungal antibiotics, J. Antibiotics, 32: 13. (1979).
3. S.K. Roy, S. Nakamura, J. Furukawa, and S. Okuda, The structure of neo-enactin A, a new antifungal antibiotic potentiating polyene antifungal antibiotics, J. Antibiotics, 39: 717. (1986).
4. S.K. Roy, Y. Inouye, S. Nakamura, J. Furukawa, and S. Okuda, Isolation, structural elucidation and biological properties of neoenactins B_1, B_2, M_1 and M_2, neoenactin congeners, J. Antibiotics, 40: 266. (1987).
5. H. Okada, K. Yamamoto, S. Tsutano, and S. Nakamura, A new group of antibiotics, hydroxamic acid antimycotic antibiotics. I. Precursor-initiated changes in productivity and biosynthesis of neoenactins NL_1 and NL_2, J. Antibiotics, 41: 869. (1988).
6. H. Okada, K. Yamamoto, S. Tsutano, Y. Inouye, S. Nakamura, and J. Furukawa, A new group of antibiotics, hydroxamic acid antimycotic antibiotics. II. The structure of neoenactins NL_1 and NL_2 and structure-activity relationship, J. Antibiotics, 42: 276. (1989).
7. K. Yamamoto, Y. Shiinoki, M. Nishi, Y. Matsuda, Y. Inouye, and S. Nakamura, A new group of antibiotics, hydroxamic acid antimycotic antibiotics. III. Isolation and characterization of enactin congeners, J. Antibiotics, 43: 1012. (1990).

A14

BMY-28864, a Water-Soluble Pradimicin Derivative

T. Oki, M. Kakushima, M. Nishio, H. Kamei, M. Hirano, Y. Sawada and M. Konishi

Bristol-Myers Squibb Research Institute, Bristol-Myers Squibb K.K. 2-9-3 Shimo-meguro, Meguro-ku, Tokyo 153, Japan

I. INTRODUCTION

The pradimicins are a group of antibiotics produced by *Actinomadura hibisca* P157-2 with potent antifungal activities (1,2) apparently resulting from Ca^{2+}-dependent binding to the fungal cell surface that induces an alteration in plasma membrane permeability (3). Although the pradimicins are relatively nontoxic, their limited solubilities in aqueous media at physiological pHs posed difficulties in further development. In order to improve the water solubility, we embarked on microbial and chemical modifications primarily focused on the D-alanine moiety of pradimicin A and have developed a water soluble derivative, BMY-28864 (4,5).

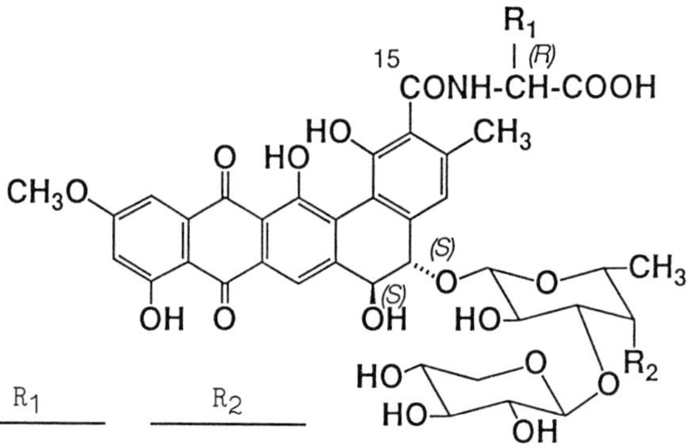

	R_1	R_2
Pradimicin A	CH_3	$NHCH_3$
BMY-28864	CH_2OH	$N(CH_3)_2$

II. WATER SOLUBILITY AND ACUTE TOXICITY IN MICE

BMY-28864 was highly soluble in aqueous media (e.g., >20 mg/ml in Dulbecco's phosphate buffered saline containing 0.9 mM Ca^{2+} and 0.5 mM Mg^{2+}, pH 7.2, 25°C) and appeared to be well tolerated in mice following intravenous administration at doses up to 600 mg/kg.

III. ANTIFUNGAL ACTIVITY

BMY-28864 was active against a wide range of pathogenic fungi including *Candida albicans*, *Candida tropicalis*, *Cryptococcus neoformans*, and *Aspergillus fumigatus*. As shown in Tables 1-3, the MIC results remained within 2-fold of each other with inoculum between 10^4 and 10^6 cells/ml, medium pH from 5.0 to 8.5, and serum concentration up to 50%. Figure 1 shows the effect of BMY-28864 on growing cells of *C. albicans* A9540; the antibiotic, at MIC or higher concentrations, yielded a 3-log (99.9%) reduction of the initial inoculum in 8 hours or less.

BMY-28864 was effective in protecting mice from lethal systemic infections with *C. albicans* A9540 (PD_{50} 12 mg/kg), *C. neoformans* IAM 4514 (11 mg/kg), and *A. fumigatus* IAM 2034 (36 mg/kg) by a single intravenous administration.

TABLE 1

Effect of inoculum size on antifungal activities

Organism	Inoculum size	MIC (μg/ml) BMY-28864	AMPH-B	KCZ
C. albicans A9540	1.5×10^4	12.5	0.4	6.3
	1.5×10^5	12.5	0.4	6.3
	1.5×10^6	25	0.4	50
C. albicans ATCC 32354	1.1×10^4	6.3	0.4	6.3
	1.1×10^5	6.3	0.4	12.5
	1.1×10^6	12.5	0.4	50

MICs were determined by the broth dilution method in Sabouraud dextrose broth containing 4% glucose, pH 7.0. Incubation: 37°C, 24h.

TABLE 2

Effect of medium pH on antifungal activities

		MIC (μg/ml)					
		BMY-28864			KCZ		
Organism	pH	5.0	7.0	8.5	5.0	7.0	8.5
C. albicans A9540		3.1	3.1	3.1	100	25	3.1
C. albicans ATCC 32354		3.1	3.1	3.1	100	25	3.1

MICs were determined by the agar dilution method on Difco yeast morphology agar containing 0.1M KH_2PO_4 that had been adjusted to appropriate pH values with 5N NaOH. Inoculum size: 10^4 cells/spot. Incubation: 28°C, 40h.

TABLE 3

Effect of serum on antifungal activities

		MIC (μg/ml)					
		BMY-28864			KCZ		
Organism	Serum(%)	0	20	50	0	20	50
C. albicans A9540		6.3	6.3	6.3	25 (0.05)	50 (12.5)	100 (50)
C. albicans ATCC 32354		3.1	3.1	6.3	50 (0.05)	100 (50)	100

MICs were determined by the broth dilution method in Difco yeast nitrogen broth containing 1% glucose that had been supplemented with 0, 20 or 50% fetal bovine serum. Figures in parentheses denote 90% inhibitory concentrations (IC_{90}). Inoculum size: 10^5 cells/ml. Incubation: 37°C, 24h.

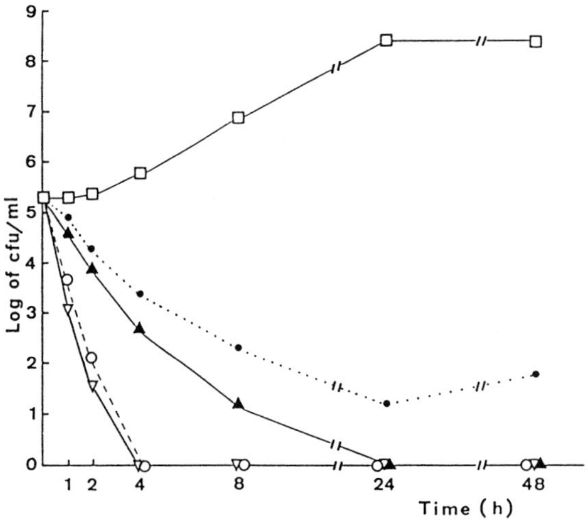

FIGURE 1. Time course of the cell viability of *C. albicans* A9540 exposed to MIC (6.3 μg/ml, ●), 4MIC (▲) and 16MIC (O) units of BMY-28864 in yeast nitrogen broth containing 1% glucose, pH 7, with shaking (100 rpm) at 28°C. ∇, amphotericin B (1.6 μg/ml). □ , control. Initial inoculum: 2 x 10^5 cfu/ml

REFERENCES

1. T. Oki, O. Tenmyo, M. Hirano, K. Tomatsu, and H. Kamei. Pradimicins A, B, and C, new antifungal antibiotics. II. *In vitro* and *in vivo* biological activities. J. Antibiotics 43: 763 (1990).

2. Y. Sawada, M. Nishio, H. Yamamoto, M. Hatori, T. Miyaki, M. Konishi, and T. Oki. New antifungal antibiotics, pradimicins D and E: glycine analogs of pradimicins A and C. J. Antibiotics 43: 771 (1990).

3. Y. Sawada, K. Numata, T. Murakami, H. Tanimichi, S. Yamamoto, and T. Oki. Calcium-dependent anticandidal action of pradimicin A. J. Antibiotics 43: 715 (1990).

4. Y. Sawada, M. Hatori, H. Yamamoto, M. Nishio, T. Miyaki, and T. Oki. New antifungal antibiotics pradimicins FA-1 and FA-2: D-Serine analogs of pradimicins A and C. J. Antibiotics 43(10): in press.

5. T. Oki, M. Kakushima, M. Nishio, H. Kamei, M. Hirano, Y. Sawada, and M. Konishi. Water-soluble pradimicin derivatives, synthesis and antifungal evaluation of *N,N*-dimethyl pradimicins. J. Antibiotics 43(10): in press.

A15

Selective Fungicidal Activity of *N,N*-Dimethyl-pradimicin FA-2 (BMY-28864): Ca^{++}-Dependent Plasma Membrane Perturbation in *Candida albicans*

Y. Sawada, T. Murakami, T. Ueki, Y. Fukagawa, M. Konishi, T. Oki and Y. Nozawa*

Bristol-Myers Squibb Research Institute, Bristol-Myers Squibb K.K., 2-9-3 Shimo-meguro, Meguro-ku, Tokyo 153, Japan

**Department of Biochemistry, Gifu University School of Medicine, 40 Tsukasamachi, Gifu 500, Japan*

I. INTRODUCTION

BMY-28864, *N,N*-dimethyl-pradimicin FA-2, is a water-soluble antifungal compound of therapeutic interest (1). In this report, we describe the characteristics of its binding to the cell surface mannan of *Candida albicans* that induce perturbation of the plasma membrane and ultimately cell death.

II. FORMATION AND CHARACTERIZATION OF A TERNARY COMPLEX

Yeast mannan (M7504, Sigma, 2 ml of 0.25 mg/ml, 10 nmoles), Ca^{++} (2 ml of 1 mM $CaCl_2$, 2 μmoles) and BMY-28864 (6 ml of 100 μg/ml, 0.69 μmole) were mixed and left to stand overnight at 25°C. The resulting precipitate was collected by centrifugation, washed twice with water and dissolved in 1 ml of DMSO. Concentration of BMY-28864 in the solution was estimated spectrophotometrically at 498 nm, and the concentration of Ca^{++} was measured with a flame photometer. Molar ratio of mannan, Ca^{++} and BMY-28864 in the precipitate was calculated based on the following MWs; mannan: 5×10^4 (mean MW), Ca^{++}: 40, BMY-28864: 870. As a result, the approximate molar ratio of mannan: Ca^{++}: BMY-28864 in the precipitate was 1 : 18 : 45.

III. BINDING KINETICS

In the presence of 200 μM Ca^{++} in 50 mM Na^+-phosphate, pH 7.0, 60 μg/ml BMY-28864 showed 83% (50 μg) binding to the resting cells (1×10^7 cells/ml) of *C. albicans* A9540 in 30 minutes at 25°C, while insignificant binding of BMY-28864 was observed in the absence of Ca^{++}. The Bmax value of this binding was estimated to be 82 μg (94 nmoles)/1×10^7 cells as determined by the Scatchard analysis. The binding of BMY-28864 to both *C. albicans* cells and yeast mannan was irreversible upon washing with water, and was uncompetitive with 500 μg/ml concanavalin A.

IV. ALTERATION OF MEMBRANE PERMEABILITY

FIG. 1 demonstrates effect of BMY-28864 on the membrane permeability of *C. albicans* A9540, as determined by K^+ leakage. Induction of K^+ leakage from BMY-28864-treated cells occurred only when 200 μM Ca^{++} existed. EGTA (2 mM) totally reversed the BMY-28864-dependent K^+ leakage. These results are consistent with those of pradimicin A in the Ca^{++}-dependent perturbation of the candidal plasma membrane (2). In contrast, 60 μg/ml BMY-28864 neither induced K^+ leakage from, nor showed binding to erythrocytes (1×10^8 cells/ml saline) in the presence of 200 μM Ca^{++} at 37°C.

EFFECT OF BMY-28864 ON THE MEMBRANE PERMEABILITY OF *C. albicans*

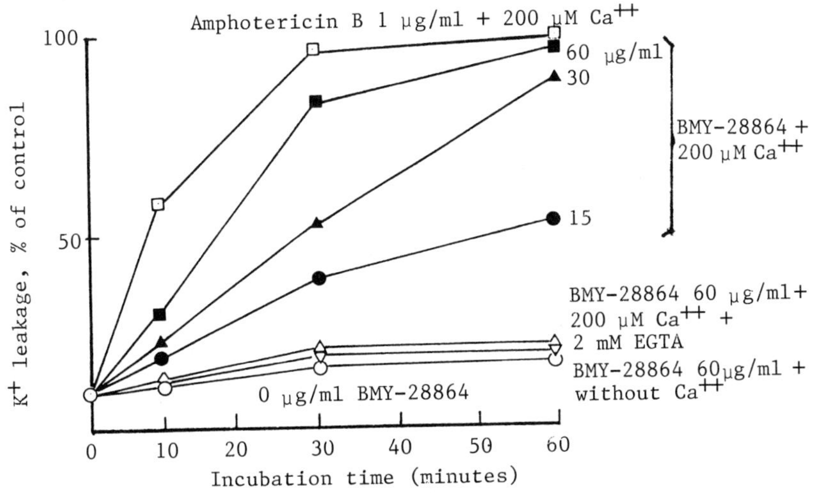

FIG. 1. *C. albicans* (2×10^7 cells/2 ml) was incubated at 37°C with and without BMY-28864 or amphotericin B in the presence and absence of 200 μM $CaCl_2$ in 50 mM Na^+-phosphate, pH 7.0. Concentration of K^+ was determined with a flame photometer. 100% = 4.2 ppm.

V. CONCLUSION

Pradimicins including BMY-28864 were active against a wide variety of yeasts, fungi and certain mannan-containing bacteria such as *M. luteus* (3). The *in vitro* candidacidal action of BMY-28864 against *C. albicans* A9540 cells is described in this Proceedings (T. Oki, N. Kakushima, N. Nishio, H. Kamei, M. Hirano, Y. Sawada and M. Konishi, "BMY-28864, a water soluble pradimicin derivative"). The candidacidal action of BMY-28864 begins with its avid and irreversible binding to the cell surface mannan in the presence of Ca^{++}, which induces an alteration of plasma membrane integrity leading to cell death. Mannan and mannoprotein on the cell surface of pathogens are the primary target for pradimicin action.

REFERENCES

1. T. Oki, M. Kakushima, M. Nishio, H. Kamei, M. Hirano, Y. Sawada and M. Konishi. Water-soluble pradimicin derivatives, synthesis and antifungal evaluation of *N,N*-dimethyl pradimicins, J. Antibiotics 43(10): in press.

2. Y. Sawada, K. Numata, T. Murakami, H. Tanimichi, S. Yamamoto and T. Oki. Calcium-dependent anticandidal action of pradimicin A. J. Antibiotics 43: 715-721(1990).

3. S. J. Tonn and J. E. Gander. Biosynthesis of polysaccharides by prokaryotes. Ann. Rev. Microbiol. 33: 169-199(1979).

A16

Electron Microscopic Studies on the Antifungal Action on BMY-28864, a Highly Water-Soluble Analog, Against *Candida albicans*

K. Numata*, N. Naito, N. Yamada, H. Kobori, H. Yaguchi, M. Osumi and T. Oki*

Department of Biology and Laboratory of Electron Microscope, Japan Women's University
2-8-1 Mejirodai, Bunkyo-ku, Tokyo 112, Japan

**Bristol-Myers Squibb Research Institute, Bristol-Myers Squibb K.K. 2-9-3 Shimo-meguro, Meguro-ku, Tokyo 153, Japan*

I. INTRODUCTION

BMY-28864 is a highly water-soluble pradimicin analog with broad antifungal activity *in vitro* and demonstrable efficacy *in vivo* (1). The anticandidal action of pradimicin A includes binding to the mannan components on the yeast cell surface and the subsequent perturbation in the cell membrane, causing potassium leakage and cell death, in calcium-dependent manner (2). As part of mechanism study of pradimicins, we have examined the morphological effects of BMY-28864 on *C. albicans* A9540 cells by electron and light microscopy.

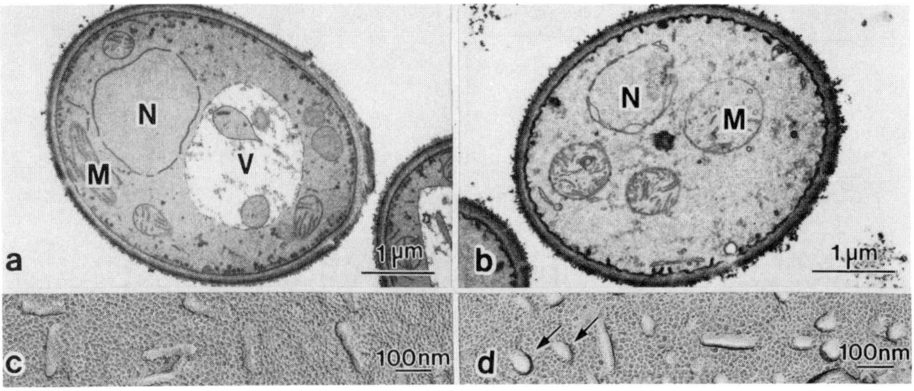

FIG. 1. TEM images of the cellular components and cell membrane surfaces in thin-sectioned (a & b) and freeze-fractured (c & d) *C. albicans* A9540 cells: (a & c) drug-free control, (b & d) treated with 100 µg/ml BMY-28864 in PBS(+) at 30°C for 4 hrs.

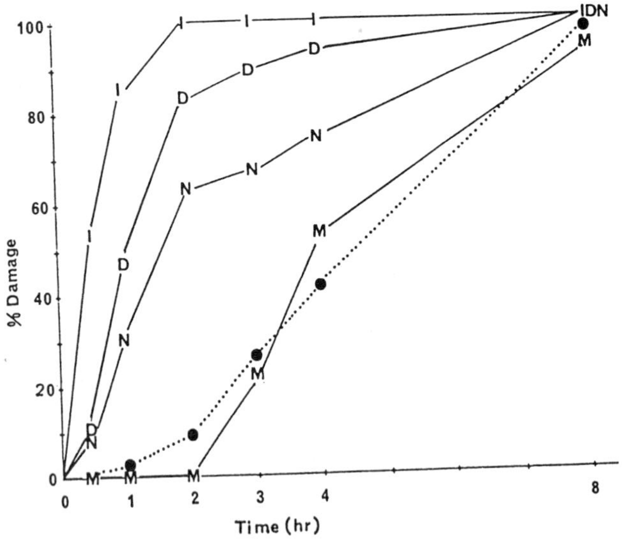

FIG. 2. Effects of BMY-28864 on ultrastructures and cell viability of *C. albicans* A9540.
The cells (10^7/ml) were incubated in PBS(+) in the presence of 100 µg/ml BMY-28864 with gyratory shaking at 30°C. The morphological changes and cell death were monitored by TEM and methylene blue staining. I, cell membrane invagination; D, cell membrane detachment; N, nuclear membrane damage; M, mitochondrion aberration; ●, cell death.

II. RESULTS AND DISCUSSION

BMY-28864 exhibited fungicidal action against *C. albicans* A9540 in Dulbecco's buffered saline containing calcium and magnesium ions [PBS(+)]. Scanning electron microscopy revealed that the cell surface alterations induced by 100 µg/ml BMY-28864 for 4 hours at 30°C, such as abnormal swelling and bulging, occurred often around budding sites and bud scars. The major detrimental effects of BMY-28864 on the cells are classified as cell membrane invagination, cell membrane detachment, nuclear membrane fragmentation and mitochondrion aberration by transmission electron microscopy (TEM) with thin-sectioned specimens (FIGs. 1a & 1b). The invagination of the cell membrane was visualized as deep pits (indicated by arrows in FIG. 1d) more clearly by the freeze-fracturing technique. Together with nuclear membrane damage, abnormal transposition of the nuclei ($P<0.1$) was observed only among BMY-28864 (50 and 100 µg/ml)-treated cells, compared with the drug-free control and amphotericin B (1 µg/ml)-treated cells by the 2 x 2 contingency method. The immunofluorescence microscopy with YOL 1/34 antitubulin demonstrated clear damage of microtubules only in the cells treated with BMY-28864. The transposition of nuclei might be associated with the antimicrotubular effect of BMY-28864. The above results and the time course study (FIG. 2) by TEM allow us to draw a conclusion that BMY-28864 first attacks the cell membrane and then damages the nuclei, resulting in expression of the candidacidal effect.

REFERENCES

1. T. Oki, M. Kakushima, M. Nishio, H. Kamei, M. Hirano. Y. Sawada and M. Konishi. Water soluble pradimicin derivatives, synthesis and antifungal evaluation of *N,N*-dimethyl pradimicins., J. Antibiotics 43(10) in press.

2. Y. Sawada, K. Numata, T. Murakami, H. Tanimichi, S. Yamamoto and T. Oki. Calcium-dependent anticandidal action of pradimicin A. J. Antibiotics 43, 715-721 (1990).

A17

Aureobasidins, a New Family of Antifungal Antibiotics: Isolation, Structure, and Biological Properties

K. Takesako, K. Ikai, H. Kuroda, I. Kato, *T. Hiratani, *K. Uchida and *H. Yamaguchi

Takara Shuzo Co., Ltd., Seta, Otsu, Shiga 520-21, Japan.

**Research Center for Medical Mycology, Teikyo University, Otsuka, Hachioji, Tokyo 192-03, Japan.*

I. ISOLATION AND STRUCTURE OF AUREOBASIDINS A~R.

Aureobasidins A~R (Fig. 1) were produced by fermentation of *Aureobasidium pullulans* R106 and were isolated by several procedures, including C18-HPLC and SiO2-HPLC.

The structure of aureobasidin A (Ab A) was determined by NMR, MS, and amino acid analysis of Ab A and its derivatives. The structures of Abs B~R were determined by their physicochemical properties and FAB-MS fragmentation analysis.

II. *IN VITRO* ANTIFUNGAL ACTIVITY OF AUREOBASIDINS.

Ab A was highly active *in vitro* against pathogenic fungi, including *Candida, Cryptococcus, Histoplasma, Blastomyces,* and some species of *Aspergillus* (Table 1). Except against some fungi such as *Aspergillus* and *Trichophyton,* Ab A showed higher activity than amphotericin B (AMPH). Ab A was not active against bacteria. Ab A showed fungicidal effects on growing cells of *C. albicans,* but showed little cytotoxic effect on not-growing cells.

The hydroxyl group of βHOMeVal at X4 was important for their high activity. Abs A, E, and I had much higher activity than the others.

Fig. 1. Structures of Aureobasidins A~R.

```
   CH3
   |
R- CH- CHCO——→MeVal———→Phe——→X1———→Pro———→X2——→X3———→Leu———→X4—┐
       |                                                         |
       O ————————————————————————————————————————————————————————┘
```

Aureobasidin	R	X1	X2	X3	X4
A	Et	MePhe	aIle	MeVal	βHOMeVal
B	Me	MePhe	aIle	MeVal	βHOMeVal
C	Et	MePhe	Val	MeVal	βHOMeVal
D	Et	MePhe	aIle	MeVal	γHOMeVal
E	Et	βHOMePhe	aIle	MeVal	βHOMeVal
F	Et	MePhe	aIle	Val	βHOMeVal
G	Et	MePhe	aIle	MeVal	MeVal
H	Et	MePhe	aIle	MeVal	Val
I	Et	MePhe	Leu	MeVal	βHOMeVal
J	Et	MePhe	aIle	MeVal	N,βMeAsp
K	Me	MePhe	aIle	MeVal	MeVal
L	Et	MePhe	Val	MeVal	MeVal
M	Et	Phe	aIle	MeVal	MeVal
N	Et	MePhe	aIle	MeVal	$MeDH_{3,4}Val$
O	Et	MePhe	aIle	MeVal	βHOMePhe
P	Et	MePhe	aIle	Val	MeVal
Q	Et	MePhe	aIle	MeVal	MePhe
R	Et	βHOMePhe	aIle	MeVal	MeVal

Et: ethyl, Me: methyl, MeVal: N-methylvalyl, βHOMeVal: β-hydroxy-N-methylvalyl, $MeDH_{3,4}Val$: N-methyl-3,4-didehydrovalyl, γHOMeVal: γ-hydroxy-N-methylvalyl, N,βMeAsp: N,β-dimethylasparaginyl.

III. *IN VIVO* ANTIFUNGAL ACTIVITY OF AUREOBASIDIN A.

Against murine systemic candidiasis, Ab A was highly effective (Table 2). The activities of AMPH, fluconazole (FCZ), and Ab A were comparable. *C. albicans* cells present in the kidneys of infected mice were removed by Ab A treatment.

The acute toxicity of Ab A was very low; LD50 for mice were 231 mg/kg (iv) and >1000 mg/kg (sc or po).

Table 1. Antifungal Spectrum of Ab A and AMPH.

Strain	TIMM No.	MIC (μg/ml)	
		Ab A	AMPH
Candida albicans	0144	0.04>	2.5
C. tropicalis	0312	0.08	2.5
C. parapsilosis	0287	0.16	5
C. krusei	0270	0.04>	2.5
C. guilliermondii	0257	0.08	1.25
C. glabrata	1062	0.04>	2.5
Cryptococcus neoformans	0354	0.63	2.5
Cr. neoformans	0363	1.25	2.5
Aspergillus fumigatus	0063	20	5
A. fumigatus	0068	>80	5
A. clavatus	0056	0.16	2.5
A. flavus	0058	>80	20
A. nidulans	0112	0.16	10
Trichophyton mentagrophytes	1189	10	5
T. mentagrophytes	1196	>80	5
Sporothrix schenckii	0959	>80	5
Histoplasma capsulatum	0713	0.16	2.5
H. capsulatum	0714	0.08	5
Paracoccidioides brasiliensis	0878	80	20
P. brasiliensis	0880	0.31	2.5
Blastomyces dermatitidis	1690	0.04>	0.31
B. dermatitidis	0126	0.31	2.5

Table 2. Antifungal Activity against Murine Candidiasis.

Drugs	ED_{50} (mg/kg)*					
	single	qdx6 (d0-5)			qdx6 (d5-9)	
	sc	iv	sc	po	sc	po
Ab A	15.1	3.3	6.5	16.8	6.6	26.0
AMPH	nt	nt	0.9	nt	1.9	nt
FCZ	nt	nt	4.1	20.0	>40	24.7

Infection: *C. albicans* TIMM 1768, $1x10^6$ cells/mouse, iv.
Treatment: single; once at 4 hours after infection. qdx6 (d0-5); once daily from day 0 to day 5.
*ED_{50} was calculated by fitting of survival data at day 20 to a logistic dose-response model. Untreated mice died 5 to 16 days post-infection. nt, not tested.

A18

Chemical and Biological Studies of Maniwamycin A and Its Stable Analogues

M.Nakayama, H.Itoh, I.Watanabe, T.Deushi and M.Shiratuchi

Tokyo Research Laboratories
Kowa Co., Ltd.
Higashimurayama, Tokyo 189, Japan

Novel antifungal antibiotic maniwamycin A (MMA) was isolated from the culture broth of a strain of actinomycetes which was classified as Stretomyces prasinopilosus KC-7367. This strain was isolated from a soil sample collected in Maniwa-gun, Okayama prefecture, Japan. MMA was isolated by resin adsorption and extraction with EtOAc and purified by column chromatography [1].

MMA is colorless oil. The antibiotic is soluble in MeOH, acetone, EtOAc and benzene but insoluble in water. Through the high-resolution electron impact (HREI)-MS, the molecular formula of MMA was established as $C_{10}H_{18}N_2O_2$. The UV absorption maximum at 235 nm (ϵ 12,400) and the characteristic band near 1500 cm^{-1} in the IR spectrum implied the presence of an azoxy group. The structure of MMA was determined to be Z-(3S)-2-oxobutane-NNO-azoxy-1'-(E-1'-hexene) as shown in Fig.1 by means of spectral analyses and chemical studies [2].

Only four antibiotics: elaiomycin [3], LL-BH872 [4], valanimycin [5] and jietacins [6] have been reported to contain an azoxy moiety. MMA is a new compound of this class and the first natural compound possessing a trans- α,β -unsaturated azoxy chromophore.

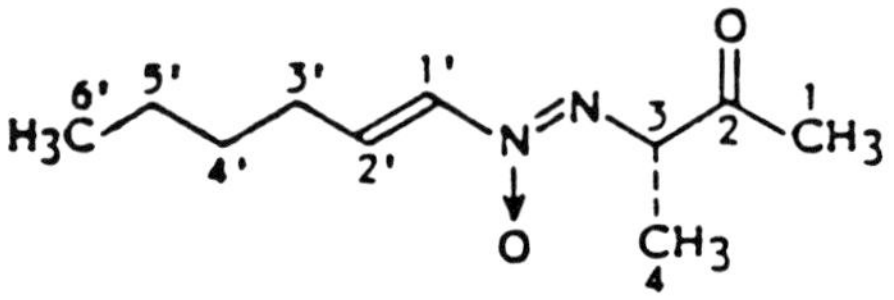

Fig. 1. The structure of maniwamycin A.

MMA is stable in acidic conditions but undergoes decomposition at pH above 7.0. Therefore, we have studied chemical transformation of MMA to give its stable analogues. In these studies we found that the oxime analogues of MMA were stable compounds. The oximes were synthesized as shown in Fig. 2 in high yield. The oxime analogues had less <u>in vitro</u> activities than MMA (Table 1).

The toxicity (LD_{50}, iv) of MMA, analogue **2** and **7** in rats were 6.25~ 12.5 mg/kg, 50~ 100 mg/kg and >200 mg/kg, respectively.

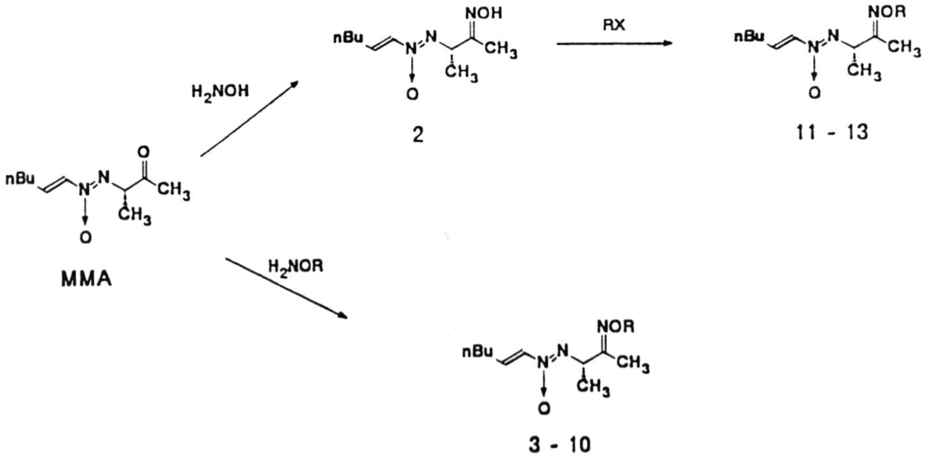

Fig. 2. Syntheses of stable analogues.

Table 1. Activities of the Oximes of MMA

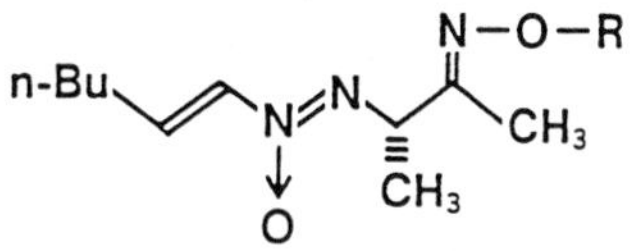

Compound	R	Minimum Inhibitory Concentration (μg/ml) *C.a.*	*C.n.*	*T.m.*	*T.r.*
1	MMA	1.6	3.1	3.1	3.1
2	H	12.5	12.5	6.2	6.2
3	CH_3	25	25	25	12.5
4	$(CH_2)_2OCH_2CH_3$	25	25	25	12.5
5	$(CH_2)_4N(CH_3)_2$	>100	50	50	50
6	$CH_2C_6H_3Cl_2$-2,4	>100	>100	100	100
7	CH_2COOH	25	12.5	6.2	6.2
8	$C(CH_3)_2COOH$	12.5	12.5	6.2	6.2
9	$CH_2C_6H_4COOH$-4	50	50	100	100
10	$CH(COOH)C_6H_3Cl_2$-2,4	50	50	>100	>100
11	$COCH_3$	50	25	25	25
12	$CO(CH_2)_7CH{=}CH(CH_2)_7CH_3$	100	100	>100	>100
13	COC_6H_5	50	12.5	6.2	6.2

NOTE : *C.a.* : *Candida albicans* ; *C.n.* : *Cryptococcus neoformans* ; *T.m.* : *Trichophyton mentagrophytes* ; *T.r.* : *Trichophyton rubrum.*

REFERENCES

1. M. Nakayama, Y. Takahashi, H. Itoh, K. Kamiya, M. Shiratuchi, and G. Otani, Novel antifungal antibiotics maniwamycin A and B. I. Taxonomy of the producing organism, fermentation, isolation, physico-chemical properties and biological properties, J. Antibiotics, 42: 1535 (1989).
2. Y. Takahashi, M. Nakayama, I. Watanabe, T. Deushi, M. Shiratuchi, and G. Otani, Novel antifungal antibiotics maniwamycin A and B. II. Structure determination, J. Antibiotics, 42: 1541 (1989).
3. C. L. Stevens, B. T. Gillis, J. C. French, and T. H. Haskell, Elaiomycin. An aliphatic α, β - unsaturated azoxy compound, J. Am. Chem. Soc., 80: 6088 (1958).
4. W. J. McGahren, and M. P. Kunstmann, A novel α, β-unsaturated azoxy-containing antibiotic, J. Am. Chem. Soc., 91: 2808 (1969)
5. M. Yamamoto, H. Iinuma, H. Naganawa, Y. Yamagishi, M. Hamada, T. Masuda, H. Umezawa, Y. Abe, and M. Mori, Isolation and properties of valanimycin, a new azoxy antibiotic, J. Antibiotic, 39: 184 (1986).
6. S. Omura, K. Otoguro, N. Imamura, H. Kuga, Y. Takahashi, R. Masuma, Y. Tanaka, H. Tanaka, S. Xue-hui, and Y. En-tai, Jietacins A and B, new nematocidal antibiotics from a Streptomyces sp. Taxonomy, isolation, and physico-chemical and biological properties, J. Antibiotic, 40: 623 (1987).

A19

Antifungal Activity of *Odontella sinensis*

A. Subramanian, R. Selvaraj and S. Manivasaham

Centre of Advanced Study in Marine Biology
Annamalai University
Parangipettai, Tamil Nadu, India, 608502

Marine microalgae are rich sources of natural products showing a wide range of bioactivity[1]. The marine diatom Odontella sinensis was cultured under laboratory conditions and the solvent extracts of the diatom were tested against the fungus Candida albicans.

Odontella sinensis was cultured in the laboratory following the method of Selvaraj et al.[2] in F/2 medium[3]. Dry algal powder was steeped in hexane and the residue was steeped in methanol. The methanol extract was run through a silica cartridge and eluted with 20ml of the following solvents in sequence: dichloromethane, 5 and 50% acetone in dichloromethane, 100% acetone and absolute methanol. These fractions (known weight) were transferred to 5 mm dia filter paper discs and tested against Candida albicans on Sabouraud dextrose

Table 1.

Antifungal Activity of Odontella sinensis

Solvents	*A*	*B*	*C*	*D*	*E*
Dry wt. (mg)	*0.04*	*0.25*	*0.20*	*0.11*	*0.45*
Zone of inhibition in mm (mean)	*-*	*12.5*	*18.03*	*8.96*	*8.43*
Specific activity	*-*	*50.0*	*90.1*	*81.5*	*21.0*

A = Dichloromethane

B = 5% Acetone in Dichloromethane

C = 50% Acetone in Dichloromethane

D = 100% Acetone

E = Methanol

agar medium. The mean values of triplicate measurements of the inhibition zone are shown in Table 1.

Maximum activity was seen in 50% acetone in dichloromethane followed by 100% acetone fraction, as shown in the table. However, 5% acetone in dichloromethane and absolute methanol fractions also showed activity. This indicates that both non-polar and polar constituents are active in Odontella sinensis. Identification of these compounds is in progress.

REFERENCES

1. B. Metting and J. W. Pyne. Biologically active compounds from microalgae, Enzyme Microb. Technol., 8: 386 (1986)

2. R. Selvaraj. S. Manivasaham, A. Purushothaman and A. Subramanian. Preliminary investigation on antibacterial activity of some marine diatoms, Indian J. Med. Res., 89: 198 (1989)

3. R. R. L. Guillard. Culture of phytoplankton for feeding marine invertebrate. In "Culture of Marine Animals" (W. L. Smith and M. H. Chanley, ed.), Plenum Publishing Corp., New York, p. 29 (1975).

A20

Ajoene, a Component of Garlic (*Allium sativum*), Affects Growth and Dimorphism in *Paracoccidiodes brasiliensis*

Gioconda San-Blas, Felipe San-Blas, and Leonardo Mariño

Instituto Venezolano de Investigaciones Científicas (IVIC), Centro de Microbiología y Biología Celular, Apartado 21827, Caracas 1020A, Venezuela.

I. INTRODUCTION

Garlic (Allium sativum) has been used for centuries as a folk medicine (1). A novel compound derived from garlic, ajoene (Fig. 1), which is a potent inhibitor of platelet aggregation (2), also possesses in

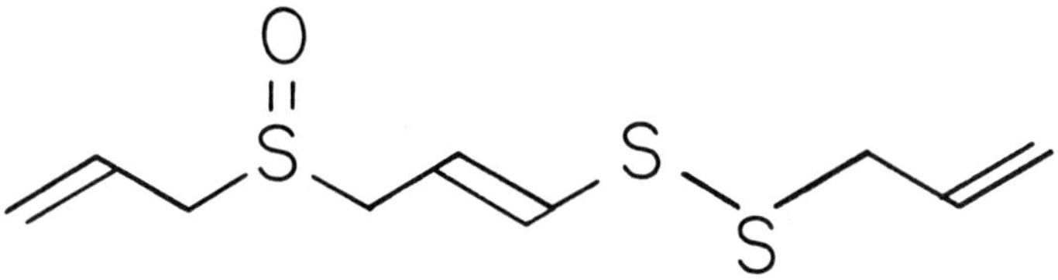

FIG. 1. Chemical structure of ajoene.

vitro antifungal activity against several pathogenic species (3). Recently, the inhibition of growth of *Paracoccidioides brasiliensis*, a dimorphic pathogenic fungus, by ajoene, was reported (4). In this paper we explore the effect of ajoene on the dimorphism of *P. brasiliensis*, and initiate studies on its mode of action.

II. MATERIALS AND METHODS

P. brasiliensis strain IVIC Pb73 was grown under conditions described before (4), and light and electron microscopic observations followed in the same way. The effect of ajoene on the synthesis *in vitro* of glucans was traced as described elsewhere (5), adding ajoene (0-100 uM) to the assay mixtures.

III. RESULTS AND DISCUSSION

The yeast (Y) phase of *P. brasiliensis* was more sensitive to the presence of ajoene than the mycelial (M) one, through perturbations in the cytoplasmic membrane (4). While Y → M transformation proceeded normally in the presence of ajoene, the reverse M → Y process was blocked. The synthesis *in vitro* of glucan was not inhibited by ajoene, though the activity of glucan synthetase was sensitive to temperature, being less active at 37°C (Fig. 2).

Ajoene has been proposed to act at the level of lipid composition of the membrane (6). However, the presence of a disulfide bridge in its molecule, and the fact that it blocks M → Y transformation

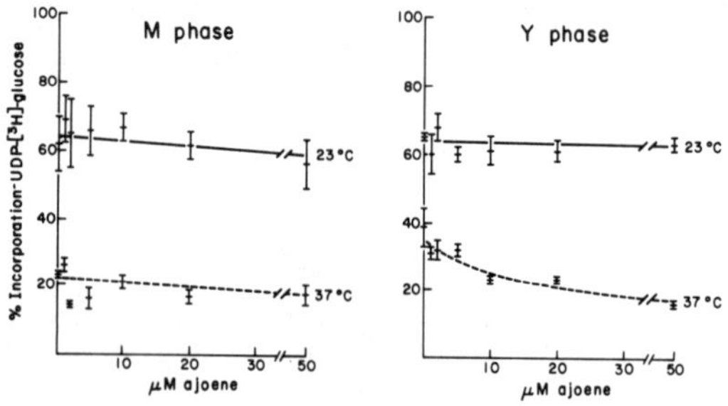

FIG. 2. Effect of ajoene on glucan synthetase activity of M and Y phases of *P. brasiliensis*.

but not the reverse, tend to suggest that its mechanism of action might be related to the activity of protein disulfide reductase, enzyme that has been postulated as one of the enzymes involved in P. brasiliensis transformation (7). Therefore, the possibility that ajoene interferes with protein disulfide reductase is under consideration.

REFERENCES

1. M. K. Jain, C. Scanzello, and R. Apitz-Castro, Wirkung des knoblausch. Wahrheit und Dichtung. Chem. Unserer Zeit. 22: 193-200 (1988).

2. R. Apitz-Castro, E. Ledezma, J. Escalante, A. Jorquera, F. Piñate, J. Moreno-Rea, G. Carrillo, O. Leal, and M. K. Jain, Ajoene {(E,Z)-4,5,9-trithiadodeca-1,6,11-triene 9-oxide}, reversibly prevents platelet activation in dogs under extracorporeal circulation. Arzneim. Foprsch. 38: 901-904 (1988).

3. S. Yoshida, S. Kasuga, N. Hayashi, T. Ushiroguchi, H. Matsuura, and S. Nakagawa, Antifungal activity of ajoene derived from garlic. Appl. Environm. Microbiol. 53: 615-617 (1987).

4. G. San-Blas, F. San-Blas, F. Gil, L. Mariño, and R. Apitz-Castro, Inhibition of growth of the dimorphic fungus Paracoccidioides brasiliensis by ajoene. Antimicrob. Ag. Chemother. 33: 1641-1644 (1989).

5. G. San-Blas, Biosynthesis of glucans by subcellular fractions of Paracoccidioides brasiliensis. Exp. Mycol. 3: 249-258 (1979).

6. M. A. Ghannoum, Studies on the anticandidal mode of action of Allium sativum (garlic). J. Gen. Microbiol. 134: 2917-2924 (1988).

7. F. Kanetsuna, L. M. Carbonell, I. Azuma, and Y. Yamamura, Biochemical studies on thermal dimorphism of Paracoccidioides brasiliensis. J. Bacteriol. 110: 208-218 (1972).

A21

Effect of Protein Inhibitors on Extracellular Proteinase Activity and Cell Growth of *Sporothrix schenckii*

R. Tsuboi, T. Sanada and H. Ogawa

Department of Dermatology, Juntendo University School of Medicine 2-1-1 Hongo, Bunkyo-ku, Japan 112

I INTRODUCTION

Sporotrichosis is a widely distributed fungal infection caused by *Sporothrix schenckii*. However, the parasitic invasive factors which lead to the instigation of these lesions have not yet been clarified. Proteolysis of insoluble skin constituents is speculated to be an important biochemical factor.

Recently, we purified two extracellular proteinases from the yeast form of *S. schenckii* grown in albumin- or collagen-supplemented liquid medium (1). Proteinase I, a serine proteinase, had an optimal pH of 6.0, and its activity was strongly inhibited by chymostatin. Proteinase II, a carboxyl proteinase, had an optimal pH of 3.5, and its activity was strongly inhibited by pepstatin. Our previous investigations with *Candida albicans* (2) suggested that these two proteinases may be expressed to allow fungal growth. We investigated the inhibitory effect of either or both of the proteinase inhibitors pepstatin and chymostatin on the cell growth of *S. schenckii* to clarify the role of proteinases in fungal infection.

II MATERIALS AND METHODS

Organism and cultivation method (1). The liquid culture medium was prepared with the following contents in 1 liter of distilled water: 10 g of yeast carbon base (Difco), 50 mg of inositol, 10 mg of thiamine, 10 mg of pyridoxine, and 2.5 g of bovine serum albumin. A yeast form of precultivated *S. schenckii* was prepared to give 10^4 cells per ml in culture medium. Liquid medium (70 ml) in 200-ml Erlenmeyer flasks was incubated in a shaking bath (80 cycles/min) at 27°C for 10 days. Cell counts were done with a hemacytometer. Proteinase activity was assayed with azocoll (Sigma) as a substrate (1).

Influence of proteinase inhibitors on extracellular proteinase production and cell growth of *S. schenckii*. To examine the inhibitory effect of proteinase inhibitors, chymostatin (an inhibitor of proteinase I, Peptide Institute) or pepstatin (an inhibitor of proteinase II, Peptide Institute) or both were added to the culture medium at the commencement of cultivation. Proteinase activities were measured in culture filtrates after 48h of dialysis against distilled water to remove the effect of inhibitors in the medium.

III RESULTS AND COMMENTS

Fig. 1 shows the effect of proteinase inhibitors on extracellular proteinase production and cell growth of *S. schenckii*. Proteinase I activity (Fig. 1A) was detected in control (no inhibitor) and pepstatin-containing media but was barely detected in medium containing either chymostatin or both pepstatin and chymostatin. Proteinase II (Fig. 1B) was detected in control (no inhibitor) and chymostatin-containing media but was barely detected in medium containing either pepstatin or both pepstatin and chymostatin. Cell growth

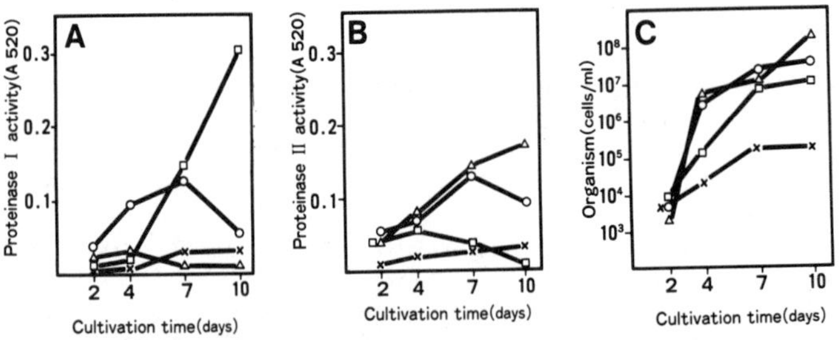

Fig.1. Effect of proteinase inhibitors on extracellular proteinase production and cell growth of *S. schenckii*. A:Proteinase I activity; B:Proteinase II activity; C:culture density. Symbols:○,no inhibitor (control);△,chymostatin (10μg/ml);□,pepstatin (10μg/ml);×,pepstatin (10μg/ml plus chymostatin (10μg/ml).

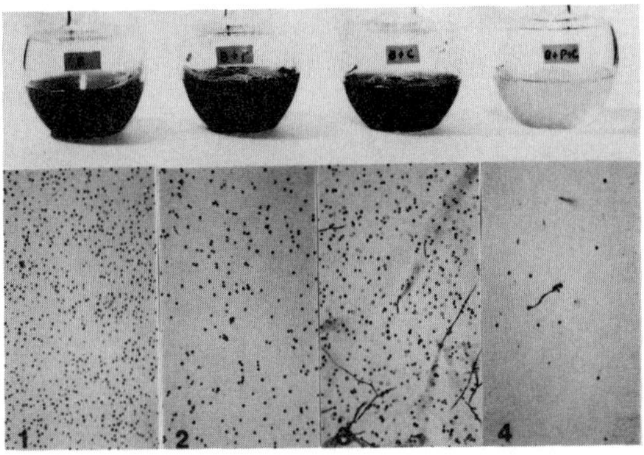

Fig.2. Macro- and micro-scopic appearance of cell growth on the 10th cultivation day. 1:no inhibitor (control); 2:pepstatin (10ug/ml); 3: chymostatin (10ug/ml); 4:pepstatin (10 ug/ml) plus chymostatin (10ug/ml).

of *S. schenckii* (Fig. 1C) was inhibited to fewer than 10^5 cells per ml only in the medium containing both pepstatin and chymostatin. Fig. 2 shows macro and micro-scopic appearance of cell growth on the 10th cultivation day. Only pepstatin/chymostatin containing medium could strongly inhibit the cell growth.

These results suggested that at least one of the two proteinases was expressed to allow fungal growth in albumin-supplemented media. To inhibit fungal growth, the addition of both pepstatin and chymostatin was required. In the case of *C. albicans*, the addition of pepstatin was sufficient to inhibit cell growth, because *C. albicans* produces only one major extracellular proteinase (2). These inhibitory profiles suggest that extracellular proteinases are essential for fungal growth in nitrogen-restricted media and that the number of extracellular proteinases related to cell growth differs according to the fungus species. Although the antifungal effect of pepstatin and chymostatin was an indirect fungistatic action caused by inhibition of the activities of proteinases, their nontoxic and selective action may lead to their use as new topical therapeutic agents.

IV REFERENCES

1. R.Tsuboi, T.Sanada, K.Takamori and H.Ogawa. Isolation and properties of extracellular proteinases from *Sporothrix schenckii*, J.Bacteriol., 169: 4104 (1987).

2. R.Tsuboi, Y.Kurita, M.Negi and H. Ogawa. A specific inhibitor of keratinolytic proteinase from *Candida albicans* could inhibit the cell growth of *C. albicans*. J.Invest.Dermatol. 85: 438 (1985).

A22

Electrophoretic Enzyme Patterns of *Aspergillus fumigatus* Isolated from Clinical Specimens

H. Matsuda, S. Maesaki, H. Yamada, H. Koga, S. Kohno, K. Hara, E. S. Rahayu* and J. Sugiyama*

2nd. Department of Internal Medicine, Nagasaki University School of Medicine, Nagasaki, Japan
*Institute of Applied Microbiology, Tokyo University, Tokyo, Japan

INTRODUCTION

Aspergillus species have been increasingly recognized as opportunistic pathogens, and their identification is still based on morphological characteristics. Recently enzyme electrophoresis has been developed as a chemotaxonomic tool for the classification of *Aspergillus* species (1). We evaluated the usefulness of electrophoretic enzyme patterns of *Aspergillus fumigatus* isolated from clinical specimens for identification.

MATERIALS AND METHODS

Isolates were 17 strains of *A. fumigatus*, 3 of *A. flavus*, 1 of *A. nidulans* and 3 of *A. nigar* from clinical specimens, and 3 strains of *A. fumigatus*, 1 of A. flavus, 2 of A. terreus, 1 of A. nidulans, 2 of A. nigar, 1 of A. oryzae and 2 of N. fischeri from soil.

Isolates from slant agar were inoculated into 5 ml Yeast-Malt (YM) broth (0.3 % yeast extract, 0.3 % malt extract, 0.3 % polypeptone, 2 % glucose, pH 7.0) as preculture medium, and incubated on a reciprocal shaker at 26℃ for 24 hours. Precultures were transferred into 100 ml YM broth, and incubated on a reciprocal shaker at 26℃ for 24 hours. The mycelial cells were harvested by filtration, washed with 0.05 M Tris-HCl buffer (pH 7.8), and then added 2× volume of 0.05 M Tris-HCl buffer (pH 7.8). Sonication was done on ice. The disrupted cells were centrifuged at 9,000 rpm at 4℃ for 30 minutes and at 40,000 rpm at 4℃ for 2 hours, and the supernatant was collected. Electrophoresis was performed in horizontal slab gels of 3.75 % polyacrylamide (2). Extracts were mixed with 40 % sucrose, and enzymes were separated using Tris-HCl buffer (pH 8.9) in gel and Tris-glycine buffer (pH 8.3) in electrode vessels with 15 to 25 mA current at 5℃ for about 5 hours. Bromophenol blue was used as the tracking dye. After electrophoresis, the gel was removed from the mould and stained to visualize the enzymes. The relative mobility (Rm) of the enzyme bands was calculated as the ratio of the distance that the enzyme moved from the origin to the distance that the tracking dye moved. The following five enzymes were examined: glucose-6-

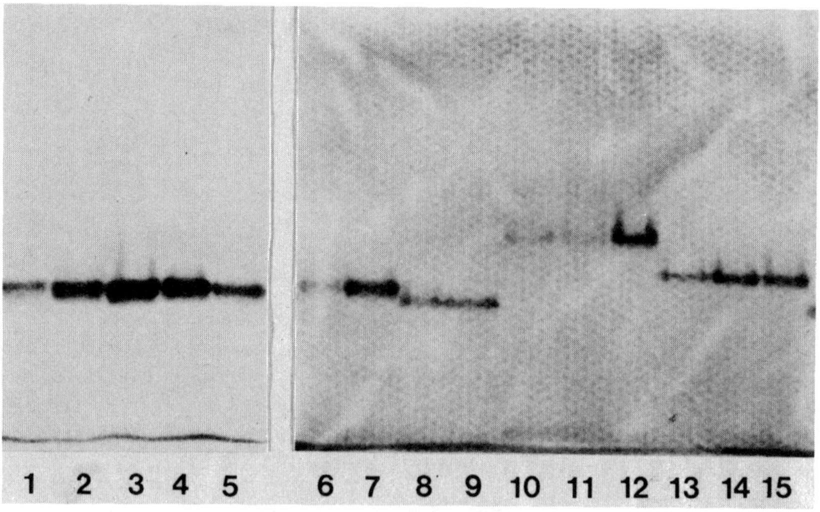

Figure 1. GDH electrophoretic patterns of 15 Aspergillus strains. 1 - 7 are the bands of A. fumigatus. 8 and 9 are A. flavus. 10 is A. terreus. 11 and 12 are A. nidulans. 13 - 15 are A. nigar. The patterns are characteristic for each species.

phosphate dehydrogenase (G6PDH, NADP-dependent), lactate dehydrogenase (LDH, NAD -dependent), glutamate dehydrogenase (GDH, NADP-dependent), fumarase (Fmase, NAD-dependent) and malate dehydrogenase (MDH, NAD-dependent).

RESULTS AND DISCUSSION

The isolates within the same species showed identical or similar enzyme patterns regardless of whether they were from clinical specimens or soil, and differences were detected between species. Figure 1 shows GDH pattern of 15 Aspergillus strains. This enzyme produced a single band in all strains. The Rm value of A. fumigatus was 65, and different from other species. The Rm value of G6PDH of A. fumigatus was 47, and was identical in this species. However, the strains of A. fumigatus were divided into two groups by the enzyme patterns of Fmase, one band or two bands. They were divided into five groups by LDH, and seven by MDH. Electrophoretic enzyme patterns are considered to be useful as an aid to the identification of A. fumigatus isolated from clinical specimens. Especially, GDH and G6PDH patterns could be better indexes for identification than other enzymes. For the purpose of clinical application, more strains should be investigated.

REFERENCES

1. K. H. Nealson and E. D. Garber, An electrophoretic survey of esterases, phosphatases, and leucine amino-peptidases in mycelial extracts of species of Aspergillus, Mycologia 59 p.330-336 (1967)

   S. Nasuno, Differentiation of Aspergillus sojae from Aspergillus oryzae by polyacrylamide gel disk electrophoresis, Journal of General Microbiology 71 p.29-33 (1972)

2. J. Sugiyama and K. Yamatoya, Electrophoretic comparison of enzymes as a chemotaxonomic aid among Aspergillus taxa : (1) Aspergillus sects. Ornati and Cremei, Modern Concepts in Penicillium and Aspergillus Classification, Plenum Press, New York and London p.385-393

   K. Yamatoya, J. Sugiyama and H. Kuraishi, Electrophoretic comparison of enzymes as a chemotaxonomic aid among Aspergillus taxa : (2) Aspergillus sect. Flavi, Modern Concepts in Penicillium and Aspergillus Classification, Plenum Press, New York and London p.395-405 (1990)

A23

Candida psychrofermentans, a New Yeast Species Isolated from a Water Sample of Lake Vanda in South Victoria Land, Antarctica

Jiro Nishikawa, Hideyuki Nagashima, Genki I. Matsumoto, and Hiroshi Iizuka

Department of Applied Biological Science, Faculty of Science and Technology, Science University of Tokyo
2641 Yamazaki, Noda, Chiba 278

Department of Biology, Faculty of Industrial Science and Technology, Science University of Tokyo (address as above)

Department of Chemistry, College of Arts and Science the University of Tokyo
8-1 Komaba, 3-chome, Meguro, Tokyo 153

INTRODUCTION

Lake Vanda in the Dry Valleys of South Victoria Land, Antarctica is an interesting meromictic lake. It is covered with thick ice all the year round. In the upper layer down to a depth of 50 m the temperature is always about 7°C and chlorinity is low, while in the deeper layer below 50 m the temperature rises markedly with depth up to 24°C near the bottom (69 m) and the chlorinity greatly increases up to four times that in usual sea water. Dissolved oxygen in the upper layer is saturated, but the bottom layers are anoxic[1,2].

Some reports have appeared on the distribution of bacteria and fungi, and twelve species of yeasts were found[3-6]. We also reported the characterization and habitats of yeast as well as bacteria isolated from Lake Vanda[7]. We report here the isolation, characterization and nomenclature of a new species of yeast from water samples from the lake.

RESULTS AND DISCUSSION

Eight strains of yeast were isolated from a single water sample taken at a depth of 5 m. The isolation was carried out on seven kinds of agar plates. Seven yeast strains were isolated at 7°C, one strain at 22°C, but no strains at 30°C. Taxonomical studies revealed that all eight strains were the same species in the genus *Candida*. The strains were able to grow in the temperature range of -1°C to 25°C, and the optimum temperature was 15°C, which shows that these strains are obligate psychrophilic. The above results are well consistent with the environment of the lake where the sample was collected. Our strains are fermentable, CoQ 8 type, with 53% of G+C content, and their isolation origin is water from Lake Antarctica. The closest species to our strains are: *C. curiosa*, *C. frigida* (*Leuco. frigidum*), *C. gelida* (*Leuco. gelidum*), *C. nivalis* (*Leuco. nivalis*) and *Leuco. stokesii*. *C. curiosa* with 53% of G+C content has been isolated from frozen foods in Japan. From a chemotaxonomic viewpoint, good coincidence was observed among our strains and *C. curiosa*. However, clear differences were found among our strains and *C. curiosa* in other physiological properties such as assimilation of carbon compounds, splitting of arbutin, vitamin requirement and DBB reaction. On the other hand, four species other than *C. curiosa* are yeasts of *Basidiomycetes* and have been isolated from soils in Antarctica. In taxonomy of microorganisms, the original place isolated is a very important ecological factor. Moreover, it must be pointed out that neither sporidium not taliospore were found in our strains. In *C. frigida* physiological characteristics such as assimilation of carbon compounds, growth on 50% glucose medium, splitting of arbutin and vitamin requirements were different from our strains. In the cases of C. gelida, C. nivalis and Leuco. stokesii, many similarities in physiological characteristics were observed, but important differences were also not neglected in our studies. Overall, from the above results, it was concluded that our isolated strains must be a new species, and we called it: Candida psychrofermentans Nishikawa et Iizuka sp. nov.

This new species is an obligate psychropilic and fermentable yeast, and may be useful in many fields of fermentation technology.

REFERENCES

1) Torii, T., Yamagata, N., Nakaya, S., Murata, S, Hashimoto, T., Matsubaya, O. and Sakai, H. Inst. Polar Ros., Issue 4, 5-29 (1975)

2) Matsumoto, G. I., Torii, T. and Hayama, T. Hydrobiologia, 111, 119-126 (1984)

3) Meyer, G. H., Morrow, M. B., Wyss, C., Borg, T. E. and Littlepage, J. J. Science 138, 1103-1104 (1962)

4) Kriss, A. E., Mitskevich, I. N., Rozanova, E. P. and Osnitskaya, L. K. Microbiology 45, 917-922 (1976)

5) Takii, S., Honda, T., Hiraishi, A., Matsumoto, G. J., Kawana, T. and Torii, T. Hydrobiologia 135, 15-21 (1986)

6) Sugiyama, J., Sugiyama, Y., Iizuka, H. and Torii, T. Nankyoku shiryo (Antarctic Record), 28, 213-232 (1967)

7) Nagashima, H., Nishikawa, J., Matsumoto, G. I. and Iizuka, H. Proc. NIPR. Symp. Polar Biol. 3, 190-200 (1990)

Author Index

Subject Index

A

B

C

D

E

F

G

H

I

K

L

M

N

O

P

Q

R

S

T

W

Z

About the Editors

HIDEYO YAMAGUCHI is a Professor and Director of the Research Center for Medical Mycology at Teikyo University School of Medicine, Tokyo, Japan. The author or coauthor of over 200 monographs, book chapters, and journal articles, and editor of the book Catalogue of Medically Important Fungal Strains Collected in Japan, he is a member of the American Society for Microbiology, International Society for Human and Animal Mycology, and Japan Antibiotics Research Association. Professor Yamaguchi received the M.D. (1958) and Doctor of Medical Sciences (1963) degrees from the University of Tokyo, Japan.

GEORGE S. KOBAYASHI is a Professor in the Departments of Internal Medicine and Molecular Microbiology, Washington University School of Medicine, and Associate Director of the Microbiology Laboratories, Barnes Hospital, St. Louis, Missouri. The author or coauthor of over 260 abstracts, book chapters, and journal articles, he is a Fellow of the American Academy of Microbiology and Infectious Diseases Society and a member of the New York Academy of Sciences, American Society for Microbiology, and Medical Mycological Society of the Americas, among others. Professor Kobayashi received the B.S. degree (1952) from the University of California, Berkeley, and Ph.D. degree (1963) from Tulane University, New Orleans, Louisiana.

HISASHI TAKAHASHI is a Professor and Chairman of the Department of Dermatology, Teikyo University School of Medicine, Tokyo, Japan. The Author of several journal articles and book chapters, he is a member of the International Society of Human and Animal Mycology and American Society for Microbiology, as well as treasurer of the Japanese Society for Medical Mycology and councilor of the Japanese Dermatological Association. Professor Takahashi received the M.D. (1955) and Ph.D. (1972) degrees from the University of Tokyo, Tokyo, Japan.